Stabilization in Trauma Treatment

Regina Lackner

Stabilization in Trauma Treatment

A Holistic Cross-method Practical Guide

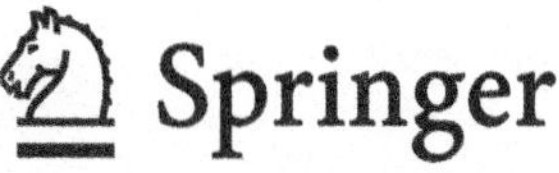

Springer

Regina Lackner
Vienna, Austria

ISBN 978-3-662-67479-6 ISBN 978-3-662-67480-2 (eBook)
https://doi.org/10.1007/978-3-662-67480-2

Translation from the German language edition: "Stabilisierung in der Traumabehandlung" by Regina Lackner, © Springer-Verlag GmbH Deutschland, ein Teil von Springer Nature 2021. Published by Springer Berlin Heidelberg. All Rights Reserved.

This book is a translation of the original German edition „Stabilisierung in der Traumabehandlung" by Lackner, Regina, published by Springer-Verlag GmbH, DE in 2021. Marianne Thatcher and Regina Lackner translated the book based on the first draft of translation that was done by an artificial intelligence machine translation tool. Springer Nature works continuously to further the development of tools for the production of books and on the related technologies to support the authors.

This Springer imprint is published by the registered company Springer-Verlag GmbH, DE, part of Springer Nature.
The registered company address is: Heidelberger Platz 3, 14197 Berlin, Germany

Love and gratitude
to my parents
Gerda and Hans Lackner

Preface to the English edition

Dear Readers,
After the book was first published in 2021 (in German) I was repeatedly asked if it was also available in English or whether it would be published In English. So, I talked to Renate Eichhorn from Springer Vienna, who was committed to implementing this idea as were Nathalie Huilleret, Sylvana Freyberg and Claus-Dieter Bachem from Springer Heidelberg who made it possible.

Based on the first draft translated by AI, Marianne Thatcher and I have tried very hard to translate the book accurately and to make it as readable as possible. Christopher Thatcher supported us with his precise suggestions and advice.

I hope that the book will support you in accompanying your clients even more effectively and comprehensively, thus, contributing to their healing from trauma and to their being able to live their lives more freely and self-empowered.

In doing so, I wish you all the best.

Vienna
February 2024

Warmly
Regina Lackner

Preface of the original German edition

Dear readers,

As a teenager, I was moved by the life stories of people who had experienced trauma. It always touched and amazed me that many of them could continue to live, go their own way and master their lives despite their experiences.

On the one hand, my mother´s life story has deeply influenced me; as a young girl she experienced destruction and violence in South Moravia in 1945 and had to flee to Austria with her family. On the other hand, the life stories and narratives of Holocaust survivors have moved and interested me since my school days. Finally, my own early traumatizations, especially the early death of my father, let me feel the scope of traumatic experiences.

From the beginning of my Psychology studies, especially through my research on intimate and family violence, the topics of trauma and coping with trauma have taken hold of me. I also dealt with this in the context of my dissertation on women coping with sexual violence. My great interest from that developed into possible tools that can strengthen and stabilize traumatized people. Through my work as a lecturer on the stabilization module of the Trauma Curriculum of the Austrian Academy of Psychology, I finally decided to publish these tools as a compendium. Hence this book.

There is now a wealth of research on the effects of traumatic experiences and some well-documented, sound and efficient methods to process them. However, stabilization, the foundation and heart of trauma treatment, has so far been little explored. It is my heartfelt desire to show the importance and far-reaching effectiveness of stabilization with this book, thus contributing to the treatment of trauma being even more effective and supporting our clients more comprehensively on their way to healing.

Warmly
Regina Lackner

Contents

Stabilization—Necessity, Effect, Benefit

1

Contents

Stabilization is the foundation and the heart of every trauma treatment. It establishes the beginning and should determine the entire treatment process; like a continuous ribbon that runs through it and embeds it at the same time.

If the trauma treatment resembles a path, then it is stabilization that enables and facilitates us to follow it; to overcome all the hurdles and difficulties, to find our way through the terrain, to cope with the weather and to get closer to our goal step by step. The stabilizing exercises and interventions are then our equipment, our provisions, our first aid kit as well as all the impressions and experiences that we collect on our way, which strengthen and enrich us.

The necessity of stabilization is often emphasized and highlighted in the literature and in further education in trauma treatment; however, to this day there has been no in-depth discussion on this. What does stabilization actually mean? How comprehensively effective is it? How significantly can it contribute to the healing of our clients, and how much does it support and facilitate the processing of traumatic experiences? These questions have so far remained mostly unconsidered.

By default, stabilization is described as the first of 3 treatment stages:

- Stage 1: Stabilization—applies to the establishment of safety, stabilization and symptom-related treatment
- Stage 2: Processing—applies to processing and solving traumatic memories

R. Lackner, *Stabilization in Trauma Treatment*,
https://doi.org/10.1007/978-3-662-67480-2_1

- Stage 3: Integration—applies to the integration of what could be gained in stages 1 and 2 and the reintegration of the personality (e.g. Herman 1992; Rothschild 2017; van der Kolk et al. 2000)

This stage-oriented model goes back to Pierre Janet, a French psychiatrist, who first presented it at the end of the 19th century. For a long time it had been forgotten. It was not until the late 1980s that it was taken up again by the two trauma experts Bessel van der Kolk and Onno van der Hart and since then described in several articles and books (e.g. van der Hart et al. 1989). Judith Herman, another trauma expert, made it known to a larger readership with her book *Trauma and Recovery* published in 1992. Today, Janet's model is considered the "gold standard" of every trauma treatment (Rothschild 2017, p. 12). It gives us a structure and shows that a successful trauma treatment is based on all 3 stages. Thereby, stabilization has a special significance. The more stable our clients are, the sooner and better they can cope with the effects of their traumatization, master their everyday life and living as well as the challenges of processing their traumatic memories.

However, we must not see Pierre Janet's model exclusively as linear as if one stage were to follow the other and then the process were completed. In the case of a single event (like an accident) that does not have any further consequences such as serious injuries, operations, or permanent physical impairments, the treatment may indeed correspond to these 3 stages. In the case of multiple, repeated, chronic, and complex traumatization this model only reflects the rough course of treatment. Within this, stabilization, processing and integration are not just repeated several times; rather, they interlock. So there is processing and integration after stabilization, then further processing and again stabilization and integration. Even during the processing of the traumatic memories, stabilization plays a key role; stabilization and trauma processing go hand in hand.

Thus, stabilization is far more than just the 1st stage of trauma treatment; it runs through the entire treatment process and at the same time embeds it, like a riverbed.

Stabilization essentially focuses on the empowerment of our clients and the improvement of their quality of life. In this sense and from a comprehensive and holistic perspective, it aims to support our clients in:

- relieving their symptoms
- developing (again) a feeling of safety and support
- gaining a feeling of control over their body, emotions, thoughts and life
- acquiring strength and vitality
- (re)connecting with themselves, their inner self and body
- achieving confidence and
- experiencing an increase in self-efficacy and autonomy through all of this

Hence, stabilization counteracts the burden of trauma and works against its force. Its relationship to traumatization can be imagined as a balance beam with two plates; one plate carries the burden of trauma, the other the balancing force of stability and stabilization. The greater the burden of traumatization, the greater the force of stability and stabilization must be in order to counteract it.

On the one hand, with the help of stabilizing techniques the symptoms of our clients can be alleviated, transformed and even resolved. On the other hand, these techniques enable them to influence their well-being and to regulate and stabilize themselves by reinforcing their strengths and resources and counteracting stressful emotions, memories, physical states and thoughts. Therefore, in the sense of empowerment, stabilization is also an aid for self-help. Furthermore, our clients can re-experience a feeling of safety, support, strength and vitality. These experiences correct those of loss of control, helplessness and powerlessness that they had during and through their traumatic experiences and thus strengthen their self-efficacy, autonomy and self-esteem. In this way with increasing stabilization, our clients´ "window of tolerance" gradually widens, so that they can better deal with their traumatic memories and no longer react so intensely to them (Siegel 2012).

So far, the focus of trauma treatment is often primarily on processing traumatic memories. Stabilization only plays a preparatory role in this; it is almost exclusively seen as a prerequisite for trauma processing. Usually only a few, mainly the same stabilizing interventions, are recommended and applied. For example, in Germany and Austria these always include the imagining of an inner safe place, and often that of a safe or inner helpers (e.g. Peichl 2018; Reddemann 2001). The inner safe place is assumed to be essential for stabilization. Accordingly, it is prescribed to clients as standard and presented to them as a necessary prerequisite without which processing their traumatic memories would not be possible. The various other stabilizing approaches, ways and techniques are often overlooked. In order to enable our clients an effective and efficient stabilization, we should offer them a number of different stabilizing interventions and exercises, so that they can discover and select those that are suitable, easy to use and most effective for them.

The more stable our clients are, the better they can cope with the force of their traumatic memories during trauma processing and stay in the here and now (Rothschild 2017), and the better they can deal with any after-effects that may occur. Furthermore, an in-depth stabilization seems to reduce the risk of severe after-effects. If our clients are (still) not sufficiently stable and processing their traumatic memories takes place too early, there is a risk their condition deteriorates, causing further destabilization or even retraumatization. Therefore, neither time and financial resources nor our clients' desire to process their memories as quickly as possible should lead us to neglect or shorten stabilization.

Comprehensive stabilization facilitates the process of trauma processing and significantly improves the symptoms of our clients, their general well-being and their quality of life. Some feel so strengthened by their stabilization that they are no longer (so) burdened by their traumatic experiences and consequently no longer find it necessary to process them. Some of our clients only want to work on stabilization and do not want to deal with their traumatic memories in more detail (Rothschild 2017).

On the one hand stabilization is based on our presence, our attitude and the way we accompany our clients, on the other hand on the variety of stabilizing techniques that we use. These should be easy for our clients to learn and implement; we should not demand too much effort from them to acquire and apply them. Trauma treatment itself is burdensome and challenging enough so that stabilization should be as effortless and gentle as possible and, ideally, should always bring some joy.

Example from practice

Bettina, 29, is severely traumatized due to her multiple, partly life-threatening experiences of violence and the massive neglect by her parents. It is very difficult for her to deal with her intrusive thoughts and memories, and uncontrollable bodily reactions and emotions; she feels helplessly exposed to them. Most of the time Bettina's body is in a highly aroused and tense state. One of the first stabilization exercises I suggest to Bettina is to become aware of the backrest touching her back. Bettina finds this easy. While doing so she notices how her body gradually relaxes. Amazed that this is possible, and so easy and relatively fast, she then applies this small exercise again and again in her everyday life. Another stabilizing exercise also amazes Bettina: perceiving an area in her body that feels good.[1] She is surprised that her body and her inner self can calm down simply by becoming aware of a body part—namely her feet—which feel pleasant and observing that. Both experiences make Bettina feel happy; through them she can experience an immediate improvement in her well-being and learn that she can influence it. ◄

This example shows how simple and fast stabilizing exercises can work. However, this presupposes that we have a broad range of different stabilizing options we can offer our clients, depending on the goal—for example to strengthen their feeling of safety or to reduce tension. Together we can explore and find out which techniques appeal to them, are easy to implement and effective.

This is the reason I wrote this book. It should serve as a compendium for your practice, in which you find a variety of interventions and exercises in addition to numerous suggestions. In Part IV I have collected and sorted these according to symptoms or needs. In Part III we discuss the fundamental conditions for successful trauma treatment. Part II gives an extensive overview of the multitude of possible ways and means of stabilization. Before that, in Part I, I invite you on a tour of the most practical relevant points about trauma and traumatization.

To adress all genders I use the female and male forms alternately throughout the book.

The practice examples are intended to illustrate a particular aspect in a condensed form. To maintain the anonymity of my clients, I have changed their names and ages and omitted or altered details. At the end of Part II and in Part IV you

[1] The significance of perceiving pleasant body sensations and using them as a resource is described in detail by Peter Levine (1998, 2011).

will find some reconstructed, shortened dialogues from my practice. Here too I have changed the names of my clients and completely omitted their age and other information.

References

van der Hart O, Brown P, van der Kolk BA (1989) Pierre Janet's treatment of post-traumatic stress. J Trauma Stress 2(4):379–395

Herman JL (1992) Trauma and recovery. The aftermath of violence – from domestic abuse to political terror. Basic Books, New York.

van der Kolk BA, van der Hart O, Marmar CR (2000) Dissoziation und Informationsverarbeitung beim posttraumatischen Belastungssyndrom. In: van der Kolk BA, McFarlane AC, Weisaeth L (Hrsg) Traumatic Stress. Grundlagen und Behandlungsansätze, Theorie, Praxis und Forschung zu posttraumatischem Streß sowie Traumatherapie. Junfermann, Paderborn, pp 241–261 (Dissociation and Information Processing in Posttraumatic Stress Disorder. In: van der Kolk BA, MacFarlane AC, Weisaeth L (Eds) Traumatic Stress. The Effects of Overwhelming Experiences on Mind, Body, and Society. 1996, Guildford Press, New York)

Levine PA, Frederick A (1998) Trauma-Heilung. Das Erwachen des Tigers. Unsere Fähigkeit, traumatische Erfahrungen zu transformieren. Synthesis, Essen (Waking the Tiger: Healing Trauma: The Innate Capacity to Transform Overwhelming Experiences. 1997, North Atlantic Books, Berkeley)

Levine PA (2011) Sprache ohne Worte. Wie unser Körper Trauma verarbeitet und uns in die innere Balance zurückführt. Kösel, München (In an Unspoken Voice. How the Body Releases Trauma and Restores Goodness. 2011, North Atlantic Books, Berkeley)

Peichl J (2018) Integration in der Traumatherapie. Vom Opfer zum Überlebenden. Klett-Cotta, Stuttgart

Reddemann L (2001) Imagination als heilsame Kraft. Zur Behandlung von Traumafolgen mit ressourcenorientierten Verfahren. Klett-Cotta, Stuttgart (Who You Were Before Trauma: The Healing Power of Imagination for Trauma Survivors. 2020, The Experiment, New York)

Rothschild B (2017) The body remembers. Volume 2. Revolutionizing trauma treatment. W.W. Norton, New York

Siegel D (2012) Mindsight. Die neue Wissenschaft der persönlichen Transformation. Goldmann, München (Mindsight. The New Science of Personal Transformation. 2010, Bantam Books, New York)

Part I
Basics Relevant to Practice

To be able to accompany traumatized people in the best possible way, basic knowledge about the variety of traumas, their dynamics and biological foundations as well as the range of their possible effects is necessary. This knowledge enables us to not only understand and assess our clients in their experience and their burden, but also to inform them sufficiently in the context of psychoeducation. This is an important component of stabilization; the more our clients know about trauma and its possible consequences, the better they can understand their symptoms and reactions and so themselves. This gives them clarity, reduces their feeling of helplessness and strengthens their experience of normality.

Furthermore, this knowledge enables us to explain the significance and necessity of stabilization to our clients and to impart the effect and benefit of the individual stabilizing exercises and interventions.

Varieties of Traumatization 2

Contents

Traumatization can be triggered by a variety of different events and circumstances that threaten our life or integrity and in which we have little or no option for action, cannot carry out or complete our defense impulses, and feel powerless and helpless. They can have a variety of effects, like a continuum, ranging from individual symptoms to complex symptom pictures. Just as they vary in their complexity, they can be experienced differently in terms of intensity and scope.

2.1 The Variety of Traumatizing Events and Circumstances

Classically, a distinction is made between Trauma type I and Trauma type II (Terr 1994); that is, between single traumatic events, such as accidents, and ongoing or recurring traumatic incidents, like sexual abuse in childhood. However, this differentiation is not exact, as many traumatic experiences of type I, such as accidents, often involve further traumatizing circumstances, such as hospital stays, operations, medical treatments and drastic personal, family and/or professional changes.

R. Lackner, *Stabilization in Trauma Treatment*,
https://doi.org/10.1007/978-3-662-67480-2_2

The events and circumstances that can be traumatizing are infinitely varied and multifaceted. Many people think of trauma as torture and war, severe physical violence, sexual abuse and rape, serious accidents or natural disaster. However, traumatization can also be caused by quite different, often more "silent", inconspicuous, less obviously dramatic events. This is particularly true for children and adults who have experienced this in their childhood. A fall while riding, getting lost in a shopping center, capsizing in an inflatable boat and being rescued at the last moment, or choking while eating are just a few examples of events that can traumatize children. In addition to accidents, medical examinations, interventions and treatments have a high potential to be traumatizing; after violence, the latter are the most common cause of trauma in children (Levine & Frederick 1998). However, many of these events can also be traumatizing for us adults.

In our practice, clinic or facility, we see clients with different traumatizations and at different times after they have occurred; whether it is acute from a recent event, or after an incident that happened a long time ago, which is now expressed through symptoms. Often people come to us after experiencing chronic traumatizations such as neglect, physical, sexual and/or psychological violence in their childhood and youth. Many people seek our help for symptoms whose cause is unclear, but which on closer questioning can frequently be discovered in early or previous traumatic events or circumstances. Even if they have already received a diagnosis, which does not initially suggest a trauma, such as depression or obsessive-compulsive disorder, traumatic experiences are often found in the life stories of our clients. For exemple, a large proportion of people diagnosed with borderline personality disorder have experienced chronic sexual, physical and psychological violence as well as neglect in their childhood and youth (e.g. Herman et al. 1989). These experiences or other traumas, such as medical interventions, examinations and treatments, e.g. tonsillectomies, often hide underneath depression, anxiety disorders or obsessive-compulsive disorders. In particular, painful treatments and examinations, such as lumbar punctures or dressing changes after burns, as well as operations in which the anaesthetic was insufficient, can be traumatic. This can also be pre-birth events, like violence experienced by the expectant mother or intrauterine medical interventions, birth complications or an immediate separation after birth or early loss of the mother. Frequently various forms of repeated subtle psychological violence can be found in the life stories of our clients; for example, when their parents demanded obedience from them and restricted and suppressed their needs and development through strict rules, norms, prohibitions and punishments. It is often the continuous non-recognition of the child and her needs or her "use" by her parents to fulfil their own needs that can be traumatic. Long-term, progressive or psychiatric illness of a parent, his care and/or a long or repeated separation, for instance, due to his hospital stays, can also traumatize children as can the death of a parent or sibling and witnessing violence within her family. Furthermore, children can be burdened or even traumatized by their parents' trauma. This phenomenon, the transgenerational traumatization, was first observed in the 1960s in children of Holocaust survivors, Vietnam veterans and, more recently, World War II survivors. It is even seen in their grandchildren (e.g. Yehuda et al. 1998). This transgenerational effect can be caused by other events, too, such as intra-family sexual or physical violence, or early loss experiences, like the suicide of a close family member. In addition, witnessing the death or serious injury of another person can lead to trauma. Finally, as already mentioned, it is often the seemingly insignificant or less dramatic appearing, "subtle" (Levine 2008, p. 20) events through which our clients were traumatized in their childhood.

In adulthood, too, incidents can have a traumatic effect, which we think should not burden us, or we should be able to endure; these often include medical examinations, interventions, or operations.

Example from practice

Mathilde, 65, has been suffering from severe anxiety, uncertainty and strong emotional instability for some time; she feels very clingy, tearful and hopeless. Until a few months ago, Mathilde was a self-confident, independent and energetic woman. Now she has changed so much. Mathilde had knee operation half a year ago and has been suffering from severe pain since then. She wonders if her change could be related to the intervention and its consequences. In our initial meeting, Mathilde vaguely remembers her surgery and snippets of the doctors´ conversation during it. She also remembers a conversation with a nurse on her hospital discharge, who told her confidentially that not everything had gone smoothly during the operation and that the anaesthetic had not been strong enough. In the course of processing Mathilde's anxiety and memories of the operation, she gradually becomes aware that she was not fully anaesthetised; she was partly conscious, and aware of what was happening and had incredible pain. Due to the effect of the anaesthesia she could neither communicate by means of gestures nor verbally. Through the processing, both Mathilde's anxiety and uncertainty as well as her pain gradually subside and she regains her original strength and autonomy. ◀

Parents or other adults often do not recognise that certain events are threatening, dramatic and burdensome for the affected children; over the years they fall into oblivion or are no longer given any importance. Consequently, no connection is made between the former experiences and the current symptoms nor is it even considered. Through careful questioning about possible traumatic, burdensome events and experiences in childhood and adolescence as part of the anamnesis and at other points in the course of treatment, our clients often recall these events. Frequently they become aware of the effect and significance of these experiences at that time. Sometimes they feel that these still have an effect on them, so that a connection between the former experience and the current symptomatology becomes clearly perceptible and recognisable.

Example from practice

Bernhard, 42, a successful and popular manager, has been suffering from a deep sadness for a long time, which overwhelms him repeatedly, sometimes completely unexpectedly and with strong crying spells. He is at a loss and can find no explanation for his state. On my routine questions about bad, threatening, decisive events, Bernhard tells that he lost his best friend at the age of 5; immediately after they had seen each other for the last time, Bruno drowned in the pond in which they had been swimming together before. While telling me this, Bernhard notices how much the death of his best friend shocked him and left him feeling completely lost and helpless at the time. He was alone with his pain; nobody comforted him, explained to him what had happened or talked to him about Bruno's death. Through recounting this event, Bernhard recognises the connection between his current sadness and depression and the sudden and so painful loss at that time. ◄

Previous traumatic experiences form the basis for current or recent events; if these more recent traumatizations are processed, they may not be completely resolved and still have an effect. If we ask again about earlier experiences or already know about them, we often discover events that lie behind the current ones or are intertwined with them. Frequently these resemble each other or have the same theme, for example, the experience of loss. In this case, the symptoms of both events usually mix; those of the former are overlaid by the current ones or reappear stronger.

Example from practice

Agnes, 24, experienced a terrorist attack in France a few years ago. Afterwards she suffered from a number of post-traumatic symptoms: flashbacks, a high level of arousal with restlessness, sleep disturbances and a strong impairment of concentration and memory as well as fear and panic attacks. These could largely be resolved after some time through stabilization exercises and trauma-specific processing. However, Agnes still had massive fear and panic attacks when she participated in events with many people; especially when she knew that she could not leave the room quickly, such as a concert hall. Then she often had great fear that someone would rush into the room and do something to her. Agnes has the impression that her fear is not related to the terrorist attack. When I ask her again about earlier experiences, which could remind her, Agnes remembers a Perchtenlauf (a traditional Tyrolean procession with scary devilish costumes) that she had visited as a little girl with her aunt. Suddenly the Perchten (the costumed people), which looked terrifying to her, ran into the crowd and also towards Agnes. She was terribly frightened at the time and tried to hide behind her aunt, who was just immersed in a conversation and did not notice Agnes's fear. All this comes back to Agnes now and while it does, she re-experiences the fear and paralysis of that time. We decide to process this situation using EMDR (Eye Movement Desensitization and Reprocessing). Afterwards Agnes feels freer; the thought of an upcoming concert is now less frightening for her. In fact, she experiences the next performances much more relaxed than before. ◀

It is important that we know about the wide range of possible traumatic events in order to be as attentive as possible to seemingly less dramatic incidents that could have traumatized our clients. This trauma-sensitive attitude allows us to investigate and explore in detail the causes of their respective symptomatology. It is less the event itself than our clients reaction to it that plays a decisive role (Porges 2018). Therefore, it is so important that we observe them attentively; when we ask them questions and while they are talking they reveal through their physical and emotional reactions whether a certain event was traumatizing and is still in effect. When our clients are having specific memories and we ask them what happens when they just think or talk about them, they often mention physical sensations such as pressure in the chest or stomach or a lump in the throat. Frequently we can observe that our clients become restless, breathe more heavily or appear frozen. They often tell us that they become afraid or panicked or feel like in a fog, dazed or dizzy when they think of what happened. These all are signs of a traumatization that has not yet been (sufficiently) processed.

2.2 Trauma-focused Anamnesis: A Necessity

Basically, we should routinely ask in every initial consultation and as part of every anamnesis about different dramatic, decisive and threatening events and circumstances, and incorporate these questions into the further course of treatment, for example when we investigate a certain symptomatology in more detail.

Often I meet traumatized people who were not asked about traumatic experiences in their previous examinations, consultations or treatments. Subsequently, these experiences were not reported; partly because they did not think of them or did not consciously remember them, partly because they did not attach any importance to these—sometimes distant—events or circumstances. People who have experienced sexual, psychological or physical violence often keep it to themselves if they are not asked; mostly out of shame or fear of not being taken seriously or being denigrated. Frequently they are concerned about overwhelming or burdening their counterpart with these experiences.

Targeted questioning about possible explicitly named traumatic experiences enables and facilitates our clients to mention what happened; especially if they are or have been affected by sexual, physical or psychological violence. If we omit these questions in the anamnesis or at the beginning of a treatment, we mostly do not find out about important experiences underlying the respective topic. Then we cannot properly assess the respective symptomatology and run the risk of making a wrong diagnosis, and consequently not suggesting an adequate and effective treatment. By asking questions about various traumatic events and circumstances, we enable our clients to report traumatic experiences, that they would otherwise not have mentioned. This is important because these give us an insight into the cause of their symptomatology making an appropriate and effective therapeutic accompaniment possible.

By routine questioning, we signal our openness to all possible traumatic experiences and our willingness and ability to deal with them. Due to this questioning many of our clients entrust themselves to someone for the first time and reveal their experiences. Frequently this is the first opportunity to have their symptoms recognized and to receive an appropriate and effective treatment.

In order to clarify whether the traumatic experiences still affect and burden our clients, it is important to observe closely how they react when they mention them; do they, for example, breathe faster, become restless or immobile, this would indicate that they have not yet been able to process the experience sufficiently. At the same time, it is necessary to ask our clients how they feel when they mention the experiences or even just think about them. If they say, for instance, they feel uncomfortable, have a feeling of constriction, get scared or tremble inside, then this also indicates that the experiences are not yet completely processed. We should make them aware of this, explain that these feelings and emotions are an expression of an increased (or decreased) level of arousal caused by the event, and recommend that they process the experience in a trauma-therapeutic way.

However, in the anamnesis or the initial meeting, we should not go into the experiences in detail or even ask for details; this could lead our clients into reactivation of their traumatic memories and the body sensations and feelings associated with them, triggering a corresponding defensive reaction. That could overwhelm, (further) destabilize and possibly re-traumatize them. After all, "our body listens" and reacts accordingly when we think or talk about traumatic experiences (Heller 2003). With this metaphor, we can explain to our clients why it is not advisable to go into detail about the experience during the anamnesis or initial conversation. At the same time, it is important to assure them that we will deal with the experience later. This, however, requires getting to know each other better as well as sufficient stabilization.

Memories of traumatic experiences frequently only arise in the course of our therapeutic collaboration. When they have gained trust in us, feel safe and/or have become more stable, our clients often have the courage to entrust us with experiences that they have kept to themselves until then. Furthermore, with their increasing stability, contents often enter their consciousness that were not accessible to them for a long time. For instance, it is well known and proven by several studies that memories of sexual violence in childhood are not remembered for years, frequently even for decades (e.g. Lackner 2000). Through the increase in psychological stability and inner and outer safety, but also through the weakening of defense mechanisms in old age, these or other burdensome memories can enter consciousness that were not previously accessible.

When asking about possible traumatic events, it is advisable to avoid the words traumatizing, trauma or traumatization. Many affected people do not see themselves as traumatized nor perceive the traumatic events they have experienced as such. They would therefore not recognize themselves in questions in which the terms traumatization or traumatic experiences occur. It is more sensible to ask about stressful, drastic, threatening events and circumstances and to give a number of possible incidents as examples: accidents, earthquakes, losses, separations from parents, illnesses, hospitalization, medical interventions, etc.

It is also crucial to routinely ask questions in the anamnesis about possible physical, sexual and psychological violence as well as different forms of neglect—emotional, medical, hygienic, educational and social. Most of those affected tell us their experiences if we ask about them sensitively and openly, but specifically. Without our corresponding questions, however, they usually remain unmentioned (Heise 1994). It is important to avoid terms such as sexual abuse or physical violence. Many affected people, for example, do not experience themselves as sexually abused despite violent sexual experiences and accordingly deny questions with this terminology (Finkelhor 1979). It is much more sensible to ask in a descriptive way, for example: *"Many children and adolescents are touched in their intimate area without their consent or are forced to perform sexual acts. Have you ever experienced something similar?"*

2.3 The Variety of Consequences and Possible Diagnoses

Traumatic experiences can lead to a variety of symptoms and symptom pictures. These include, among others, a greatly increased level of arousal, which is expressed by restlessness, irritability, startle reactions, impaired concentration and memory or difficulty falling and staying asleep. Frequently there are fear, panic, depression and exhaustion states as well as numbness and feelings of inner emptiness and hopelessness. Flashbacks, threatening and burdensome intrusive thoughts and inner images or nightmares are often seen. Dissociative states such as absences, depersonalization and derealization or amnesia are common. Frequently physical symptoms such as chronic pain states, migraine, digestive problems, high blood pressure or cardiac arrythmia manifest (Howard et al. 2018; Levine 2019; Porges 2018; Stensland et al. 2018). The variety of possible consequences of traumatization is comprehensive, their extent and complexity are determined by the form, duration and frequency of the traumatic experiences as well as risk and protective factors.

From a neurobiological point of view, our "brain and body are inherently adaptive"; consequently, post-traumatic symptoms are not to be understood as "evidence of pathology", but rather as "an attempt at adaptation" (Fisher 2019, p. 18). They are "a normal reaction to extreme stress" and thus "a normal adaptive process of reaction to an abnormal situation" (Lifton 1993, p. 12). Post-traumatic stress disorder (PTSD) is therefore not a disorder, but rather reflects the struggle of traumatized people to adapt to the traumatic events and circumstances and to cope with them. If we take this point of view and convey it to our clients, we are already contributing to their stabilization. By not pathologizing the consequences of trauma, but rather presenting them as normal adaptive reactions to non-everyday, terrible events, our clients can experience themselves as "normal" and recognize and acknowledge their efforts to cope with and master the traumatic experiences.

Post-traumatic stress disorder is only one of a number of different symptom pictures that are caused by traumatic experiences. Scientific studies on the consequences of traumatization or on the effectiveness of certain trauma-therapeutic methods or interventions usually involve participants who have been diagnosed with post-traumatic stress disorder. This creates or reinforces the impression that traumatization is expressed exclusively or primarily in PTSD. This is not the case. Not all people who have been traumatized show all the signs of PTSD or meet the criteria as described in the ICD-10 or 11 or DSM-V. Frequently they suffer primarily from depression, anxiety and panic attacks and/or obsessive/compulsive symptoms. In the case of people affected by complex traumatization, an emotionally unstable personality disorder is often diagnosed. Many of the consequences of trauma cannot be assigned to diagnostic categories (Fisher 2019). For instance, only a small proportion of traumatized children show the criteria for PTSD (van der Kolk 2016). Many times I have encountered children, for example, who have been diagnosed with an attention deficit disorder and treated accordingly with medication, but who were traumatized. Their life histories often concealed serious trauma, i.e. accidents or violence, which had not been asked about in the previous anamnesis.

In the context of initial meetings, anamneses and diagnostic examinations, questions about possible traumatic experiences are frequently omitted. In most countries it is not yet a standard procedure to ask these questions routinely. As a result, traumatization all too often remains undiscovered. Since the symptoms of traumatized people often do not correspond to the diagnostic criteria of PTSD and other diagnoses are attributed to them, the possibility of trauma is frequently not taken into account. However, traumatization often hides behind depression, anxiety disorders, substance abuse and personality disorders, many times not asked about and therefore not recognized. Sometimes affected people mention their traumatic experiences to doctors, psychologists or psychotherapists, but these are not given any importance; especially if there has been no previous diagnosis of PTSD. Many are treated according to the diagnoses without investigation of the causes of the current symptoms. This leads to treatments that are inadequate and consequently not effective, which usually intensifies and prolongs the suffering of the affected people.

Example from practice

Jonas, 23, had suffered from severe obsessive-compulsive symptoms and self-harming behavior for years. During a hospital stay after an accident, he was referred and admitted to a psychiatric department. Although Jonas repeatedly said he had experienced massive physical and psychological violence from his parents since he was a child, he was not treated for trauma, only for his compulsions. Jonas did not experience any improvement, instead, his condition deteriorated. Once again he experienced that he was not taken seriously. ◀

2.3.1 Trauma first!

As with Jonas, compulsions and, for instance, depression, fear or anxiety disorders, addictive behavior or dissociative states are often expressions and forms of coping with trauma. As already discussed, they are "attempts at adaptation" that enable those affected to cope with traumatic experiences and circumstances, to endure and continue living with them (Fisher 2019, p. 18). For example, hypervigilance enables a child growing up in a threatening environment to be alert and to protect itself as best it can. Dissociations allow those affected to shield themselves from the force of the events or circumstances and thus to endure the unbearable. Therefore, symptoms are forms of self-regulation and thus also of stabilization; "treating" them without taking into account the underlying trauma can deprive our clients of essential self-regulatory strategies and mechanisms, which can lead to a deterioration of their condition, as happened with Jonas. In the spirit of the principle of "trauma first", it is necessary to focus on the trauma and its effects and to treat these first and only then treat other symptom pictures, such as addictive behavior or eating disorder. With the processing of the traumatic experiences, the latter usually improve by themselves.

2.3.2 Diagnoses: Caution!

Example from practice

Siglinde, 52, was admitted to a psychiatric department of a hospital due to severe depression. From an early age she was exposed to extreme physical and psychological violence and neglect by her parents. In her marriage, Siglinde experienced physical as well as sexual and psychological violence. Nevertheless, her treating doctor assumed that she suffered from depression and not from traumatization and treated her mainly with medication. He considered a trauma treatment unnecessary. ◀

Unfortunately, as in the case of Siglinde, it frequently occurs, that diagnoses lead to only seeing a particular condition of the affected people leaving their causes unexplored or unheeded. That carries the risk that the condition and the symptomatology will be treated, but not the underlying cause. However, it is essential to investigate the causes and triggers of the respective symptoms. That is why it is fundamental to routinely inquire about possible traumatic events as part of the anamnesis. It is also important to recognize the significance of trauma and focus on its processing; knowing that the cause of numerous symptoms and symptom pictures is often found in traumatic experiences.

Diagnoses have their importance and necessity; for example, for communication within or between individual professional groups or for billing with health insurance and insurance companies. They are also significant for our clients who have the need to name their symptoms and assign them to a condition in order to gain clarity. Above all, they are necessary with regard to further treatment steps and recommendations. For that reason, we should consider diagnoses critically and with great care; knowing that they are classifications that reflect symptoms, not their causes. They are attempts to grasp, describe and categorize symptoms and symptom pictures. They are subject to intense debates and decision-making processes within the scientific community from which they are described and formulated. In this respect, diagnoses are always a reflection of the respective state of knowledge and scientific discourse as well as the prevailing opinions and attitudes of the scientists and experts participating in this process. Social and political factors as well as interests of the respective professions also play a role. This was shown, for example, in the recent debates in the preparation of the DSM-V. Although numerous studies and statements of renowned experts pointed to the necessity of introducing the symptom picture "developmental trauma disorder", this was not included in the DSM-V by the American Psychiatric Association (van der Kolk 2016). With regard to the diagnoses that are often made as a result of sexual abuse, violence and neglect in childhood, such as borderline personality disorder, ADHD or social behavior disorder, Bessel van der Kolk (2019) emphasizes that "none of them provides a clue about what has really gone wrong, nor do they offer any suggestions about what can be done to help patients who have them" (p. 45).

Due to all these aspects, we must handle diagnoses very carefully. Regardless of this, we should first and foremost explore and understand the symptomatology of our clients in order to be able to determine, recognize and consequently accompany and support them in their suffering in the best possible way.

References

Finkelhor D (1979) Sexually victimized children. Free Press, New York

Fisher J (2019) Die Arbeit mit Selbstanteilen in der Traumatherapie. Junfermann, Paderborn (Healing the Fragmented Selves of Trauma Survivors. Overcoming Internal Self-Alienation. 2017, Routledge, New York) Quoted from original English version (p 1)

Heise LL (1994) Gender-based violence and women's reproductive health. Int J Gynecol Obstet 46:221–229

Heller L (2003) Somatic Experiencing®. Training, Beginner I, September 2003, Penzberg, DE

Herman JL, Perry JC, van der Kolk BA (1989) Childhood trauma in borderline personality disorder. Am J Psychiatr 146(4):490–495

Howard JT, Sosnov JA, Janak JC, Gundlapalli AV, Pettey WB, Walker LE, Stewart IJ (2018) Associations of initial injury severity and posttraumatic stress disorder diagnoses with long-term hypertension risk after combat injury. Hypertension 71:824–832 van der Kolk BA (2016) Verkörperter Schrecken. Traumaspuren in Gehirn, Geist und Körper und wie man sie heilen kann. G. P. Probst, Lichtenau/Westfalen (The Body Keeps the Score. Mind, Brain and Body in the Transformation of Trauma. 2015, Penguin Books, London).

van der Kolk BA (2019) Sicherheit und Reziprozität: Die Polyvagal-Theorie als Rahmen für Verständnis und Behandlung von entwicklungsbezogenen Traumafolgestörungen. In: Porges SW, Dana D (Hrsg) Klinische Anwendungen der Polyvagal-Theorie. Ein neues Verständnis des Autonomen Nervensystems und seiner Anwendung in der therapeutischen Praxis. G. P. Probst, Lichtenau/Westfalen, pp 43–48 (Safety and Reciprocity: Polyvagal Theory as a Framework for Understanding and Treating Developmental Trauma. In: Porges SW, Dana D (Eds) Clinical Applications of the Polyvagal Theory. The Emergence of Polyvagal-Informed Therapies. 2018, W.W. Norton, New York, pp 27–33) Quoted from original English version (p 29)

Lackner R (2000) Sexueller Missbrauch, spezielle Aspekte seiner Bewältigung, deren Beziehung zueinander und die Bedeutung sozialer Unterstützung, Unveröffentlichte Dissertation. Paris Lodron Universität Salzburg, Salzburg (Sexual Abuse, specific aspects of coping with it, their relationship to each other, and the importance of social support. Unpublished dissertation, Paris Lodron University of Salzburg, Salzburg, AT).

Levine PA, Frederick A (1998) Trauma-Heilung. Das Erwachen des Tigers. Unsere Fähigkeit, traumatische Erfahrungen zu transformieren. Synthesis, Essen (Waking the Tiger: Healing Trauma: The Innate Capacity to Transform Overwhelming Experiences. 1997, North Atlantic Books, Berkeley)

Levine PA (2008) Vom Trauma befreien. Wie Sie seelische und körperliche Blockaden lösen. Kösel, München (Healing Trauma. A Pioneering Program for Restoring the Wisdom of Your Body. 2005, Sounds True, Boulder)

Levine PA (2019) Polyvagal-Theorie und Trauma. In: Porges SW, Dana D (Hrsg) Klinische Anwendungen der Polyvagal-Theorie. Ein neues Verständnis des Autonomen Nervensystems und seiner Anwendung in der therapeutischen Praxis. G. P. Probst, Lichtenau/Westfalen, pp 19–42 (Polyvagal Theory and Trauma. In: Porges SW, Dana D (Eds) Clinical Applications of The Polyvagal Theory. The Emergence of Polyvagal-Informed Therapies. 2018, W.W. Norton, New York, pp 3–26)

Lifton RJ (1993) From Hiroshima to the Nazi doctors. The evolution of psychoformative approaches to understanding traumatic stress syndromes. In: Wilson JP, Raphael B (Eds) International handbook of traumatic stress syndromes. Plenum Press, New York, pp 11–23

Porges SW (2018) Die Polyvagal-Theorie und die Suche nach Sicherheit. Traumabehandlung, soziales Engagement und Bindung. G. P. Probst, Lichtenau/Westfalen

Stensland S, Zwart J-A, Wentzel-Larsen T, Dyb G (2018) The headache of terror. A matched cohort study of adolescents from the Utoya and the HUNT Study. Neurology 90(2):e111–e118

Terr L (1994) Unchained memories. True stories of traumatic memories, lost and found. Basic Books, New York

Yehuda R, Schmeidler J, Wainberg M, Binder-Brynes K, Duvdevani T (1998) Vulnerability to posttraumatic stress disorder in adult offspring of holocaust survivors. Am J Psychiatr 155(9):1163–1171. https://doi.org/10.1176/ajp.155.9.1163

3 Neuroscientific Insights

Contents

In order to effectively help traumatized people, it is necessary to delve into the physiological, especially the neurophysiological effects of traumatic experiences. If we know what happens in our body during a threatening event, we can understand how or why typical trauma-specific symptoms can occur. Then we can also recognize what our body and soul need to find stability and why and how the individual stabilization techniques can be supportive and healing.

3.1 The Nervous System: Short and Sweet

The primary task of our nervous system is to ensure our survival (e.g. Porges 2018). Our nervous system consists of the brain, the brainstem and the spinal cord as well as the cranial or brain nerves, the spinal and the peripheral nerves (e.g. Rothschild 2017). It can be divided into two areas:

R. Lackner, *Stabilization in Trauma Treatment*,
https://doi.org/10.1007/978-3-662-67480-2_3

- the central nervous system (CNS), to which the brain and the spinal cord belong, and
- the peripheral nervous system (PNS), to which the rest of the nerve tissue belongs, which runs through our body. This transmits information from our body and our environment to our brain and spinal cord, as well as in the opposite direction from our brain and spinal cord to our body (in order to enable, for example, the performance of a movement).

Functionally, our nervous system is divided into two units:

- the somatic or voluntary and
- the autonomic or vegetative, involuntary nervous system

However, this separation is not exact, since firstly parts of the somatic nervous system, such as reflexes, are not consciously controllable. Secondly, we can indirectly influence the autonomic nervous system through physical movement and other activities such as breathing, mindfulness exercises or inner images (e.g. van der Kolk 2016).

With regard to traumatization, the autonomic nervous system is particularly important. It controls our vital functions, such as breathing, blood pressure, heart rate, body temperature, fluid and electrolyte balance, digestion and metabolism. Generally, two branches of the autonomic nervous system are described:

- The sympathetic nervous system (SNS), that enables us to react quickly to stimuli and mobilize our body to fight or flight in danger. The SNS is performance-enhancing.
- Its so-called counterpart, the parasympathetic nervous system (PNS), that reduces the activity of our body (e.g. slows down our heart rate) and lets us relax and regenerate, and thus is essential for our health. The PNS is recovery-promoting.

The enteric nervous system is also assigned to the autonomic nervous system. It is an independent nervous system consisting of a complex network of nerves that runs along the wall of the entire gastrointestinal tract. Due to its size and complexity, it is also called the gut brain (Enders 2019). It is in constant exchange with the brain, the vagus nerve being the most important connection between the two.

3.1.1 The Vagus Nerve

The most important neural path of the PNS is the vagus nerve. It is one of the ten brain or cranial nerves, more precisely the tenth (X), which exits the brain stem and wanders through our body by branching out multiple times (hence "vagus", lat. for wandering). It is connected to almost all internal organs and involved in the regulation of their activity. Moreover, it is an important part of our immune system. However, the vagus nerve is not just a single nerve, but rather a "whole family of nerve pathways" that have their origin "in several areas of the brain stem" (Porges 2010, p. 51). 80% of the fibers of the vagus nerve are of a sensory nature, i.e. viscerosensitive: they send information from the internal organs or sensations from the organs to our brain. Therefore, we can influence our level of arousal through slow breathing, singing and slow movements and thus have a calming effect on our organism (Dana and Grant 2019; Porges 2018; van der Kolk 2016). The remaining 20% are of a motor nature, i.e. visceromotor: they influence our physiological state by controlling the involuntary movement in our organs (e.g. our intestinal activity). In addition, the vagus nerve is receptive to consciously perceived body sensations, so it is also somato-sensitive.

Functionally, according to the American psychiatrist and neuroscientist Stephen Porges (2018), the vagus nerve is an inhibitory nerve. It has a calming effect on our organism. For example, it causes our heart rate to slow down and to calm us. However, the vagus, which is generally understood as an anti-stress system, can also lead to a drastic slowing of the heart rate up to its complete standstill and thus to death. Hence, so Stephen Porges, it is a nerve that can both protect us and be deadly for us. Stephen Porges has dealt intensively with this phenomenon, the so-called vagus paradox, and discovered in his long-term research, that the vagus nerve has two paths; so the parasympathetic nervous system is divided.

3.1.2 Stephen Porges' Polyvagal Theory

In his Polyvagal Theory, Stephen Porges (2010, 2018) describes how the autonomic nervous system not only consists of the sympathetic and the parasympathetic, but of three branches that maintain the balance in our body through their interaction:

- the sympathetic nervous system (which mobilizes our body and enables us to fight or flight) and
- the two-part parasympathetic nervous system, namely
  - the older non-myelinated vagus branch, also called dorsal vagus, and
  - the new myelinated (i.e. surrounded by an insulating, fatty layer) vagus branch, also called ventral vagus.

The two vagus branches originate from different areas of the brain stem, run through our body on different paths and have different functions. Accordingly, they have different effects on our physiological state, our emotional reactions and our behavior.

The vagus path, whose nerve fibers are not surrounded by myelin sheath, is the phylogenetically older vagus. It can be found in reptiles and enables them to freeze in danger, to reduce their heart rate and inhibit their breathing, thus pretending to be dead in order to ensure their survival. On the other hand, mammals and therefore humans have two vagus circuits: the older one, like in reptiles, and a younger one that has evolved over time.

Older, Dorsal Vagus Branch

The older vagus branch is primarily responsible for the regulation of the organs below our diaphragm, such as our stomach and our intestine. It is also called dorsal (posterior) or vegetative vagus. It is usually activated when we are confronted with a threat or danger in which we have little or no option for action. For instance, if we are driving in a car and suddenly, without being able to notice it in time, a car shoots out of an exit and crashes into us; then we may be able to impulsively step on the brake, but we will probably remain paralyzed or frozen in the car and feel numb, empty or out of it, i.e. we are dissociated. We may feel dizzy or even faint, or we might feel nauseous and have to vomit, or urinate involuntarily. These are signs that our older vagus or our immobilization system is active. This is also the case when women (or men) are raped; they often experience an immobilization reaction, feel paralyzed or frozen, and can neither defend themselves nor call for help. Their body is in a kind of frozen state. At the same time, their pain threshold increases, so that they no longer perceive pain so intensely, and they dissociate, are so to speak drifted or beamed away; this protects them from having to experience the event so intensely or consciously and be able to endure it. All this is an expression of the fact that their nervous system is reacting to the dangerous situation and adapting to it, ensuring their survival.

It is important to explain this mechanism to our clients so that they can understand why their body was paralyzed and why they could not defend themselves or call for help. The information that the immobilization is a volitionally uncontrollable, instinctive survival reaction of our body that ensures our survival is enormously relieving and stabilizing for our clients. Usually they suffer from massive feelings of guilt and shame that they did not defend themselves. Questions or even accusations from others as to why they did not defend themselves and fight back only increase these feelings. If our clients recognize that their immobilization was a protective reaction controlled by their nervous system, without which they might not have survived and which protected them from experiencing something even worse, they can more easily accept their freezing. This reduces their feelings of guilt and shame, as well as their fear, that their body could do something that they don't understand. We can support this by inviting them to "take a little time" to "appreciate what your body has done for you" (Porges 2018, p. 149), helping our clients to regain a positive, reconciling approach to their body. This is particularly helpful if they feel betrayed, cheated and abandoned by their body due to their freezing and the inability to defend themselves.

New, Ventral Vagus Branch

Besides to the older one, we also have a phylogenetically younger vagus branch. Its nerve fibers are surrounded by a myelin layer, an insulating fat layer, which allows for rapid conduction of stimuli. This new vagus is also referred to as the ventral (front), smarter or wiser vagus. It is primarily connected to the organs above the diaphragm, specifically to our heart and our lungs, where it exerts a regulatory effect. Hence, it acts as vagus brake and inhibits the activity of the sinoatrial node, the pacemaker of our heart, so that our original (intrinsic) heart rate slows down (Porges 2019). If the tone of the ventral vagus and its inhibitory function decreases, the heart rate corresponding to the sinoatrial node is expressed; then our heart beats unrestrained and therefore much faster. However, the vagus brake can not only be switched on and off, but also inhibits the activity of the sinoatrial node in stages. By increasing or decreasing the tone of the ventral vagus, it can change the heart performance so that it is possible for us to calm down and allow closeness to other people, or to distance ourselves from others and withdraw (Porges 2010). If the ventral vagus is in an optimal tone, the defense mechanisms of the sympathetic nervous system are inhibited, we are relaxed and can connect with others. If its tone is low, then our heart beats faster, the influence of the sympathetic nervous system increases and the fight or flight mechanism is initiated. The vagus brake is thus "a neurophysiological mechanism that enables rapid transitions between physiological states that either promote social communication or mobilization" (ibid. p. 228–229).

A special characteristic of the ventral vagus is that it interacts in the brainstem with structures that control the striped facial and head muscles, which are responsible for our mimic (facial muscles), our vocal expression (laryngeal and pharyngeal muscles) and our hearing (middle ear muscles). Consequently, there is a connection between heart and face, voice and melody of speech as well as hearing. According to Stephen Porges (2018), we can "read" in the face of a person and hear in his voice what „is going on in his heart" (p. 94). That is why we can have a calming effect on others with a melodious, pleasant voice. Thus, the ventral vagus is involved in our social interactions and bonds. These are enabled and determined by eye contact, mimic, voice and speech melody as well as hearing. Primarily, we get in touch with someone through eye contact and speaking, whereby we can recognize in his or her gaze and in his or her mimic and voice whether we can feel safe with him or her, or whether he or she is threatening to us. "From a face-heart connection, that coordinates the heart with the muscles of the face and head", a complex neurological system "emerges", which Stephen Porges calls the "Social Engagement System" (2019, p. 72). It can only be found in mammals, for whom social relationships and social integration are essential for survival. If the ventral vagus and the associated system for social engagement work optimally, our "health, development and healing" are supported (ibid.).

Commonalities and differences between the two Vagus Branches

The two vagus branches work harmoniously together to ensure "the smooth running of important biological processes, but they also respond to the environment, and we use them for defensive reactions" (Porges 2018, p. 123); namely, to freeze in the face of danger (dorsal vagus) or to seek someone's protection (ventral vagus).

The commonality between the two vagus pathways is their inhibition of mobility. However, this has a very different effect on both. The dorsal vagus causes our body to freeze or collapse in the face of danger. On the other hand, the ventral vagus enables us to relax in a safe environment and to allow social closeness. When we feel safe, the ventral vagus is active and the other two systems are inhibited, namely the dorsal vagus and the sympathetic nervous system, and with it our fight or flight mechanisms. Then there is an "optimal 'autonomic balance'" between the dorsal vagus and the sympathetic nervous system (Porges 2019, p. 79). The mobilization can be maintained, although we do not use it as defense, but "pro-socially" to contact others, to establish closeness and form bonds. For example, we experience this when playing or dancing; we make eye contact with our counterpart to ensure he or she does not mean us any harm and that we can feel safe. Then we can be relaxed and mobile at the same time.

Hierarchy of our defense mechanisms

The three branches of our autonomic nervous system developed at different stages of evolution. From an evolutionary point of view, the older dorsal vagus (in cartilaginous fish) developed first, then the sympathetic nervous system (in bony fish) and finally in mammals the new, ventral vagus (Porges 2018). In danger, these three systems, forming a three-stage hierarchy, are used in reverse order of their emergence:

- First, the phylogenetically youngest circuit, i.e. the newer or ventral vagus or the social engagement system is activated. In danger, we look for eye contact with someone else, talk to him or grab the hand of someone close to us or hug him to make us feel safe.
- If this is not possible, the second oldest circuit, the defensive system of mobilization or the sympathetic nervous system is activated, which enables us to fight or flee. For example, we lash out or push someone away, or we pace up and down, or run away.
- If this is not possible, the oldest circuit, the system of immobilization or the older or dorsal vagus is finally activated, which makes us freeze or collapse. We are like frozen, become unconscious or dissociate.

In a dangerous situation we cannot consciously and voluntarily decide which of the three branches is activated. It is automatically made by our autonomic nervous system due to a "reflexive mechanism" which Stephen Porges calls "Neuroception" (2019, p. 75); a "process by which the nervous system assesses danger independently of consciousness" (Porges 2018, p. 217). With the help of neuroception, our nervous system recognizes "environmental characteristics and visceral signs of safety, danger or life-threatening danger" and can "instantly change the physiological state" (Porges 2019, p. 75).

3.1.3 Immobility—Freezing and Shutdown

An immobility reaction occurs when the use of the two younger systems is not possible, i.e. "when fighting or running away does not take care of the threat" (van der Kolk 2016, p. 101). Then the phylogenetically oldest defense system is activated, the dorsal vagus "that is associated with digestive symptoms like diarrhea and nausea" (ibid.). It "slows down our heart rate and induces shallow breathing" (ibid.) At this point "we switch off" and freeze or collapse. We lose contact with our environment and with ourselves, cannot maintain our awareness and often "no longer even register physical pain" (ibid.). This state resembles a hypoarousal, i.e. an under-activation, and is also referred to as shutdown or collapse, which is expressed, among other things, in "appearing spaced out, being dissociated, lacking vitality" and "having a flat or frozen face, exhibiting facial pallor (Levine 2019a, p. 34)".

Besides this form of immobility due to under-activation, there is another in which both the sympathetic and the parasympathetic nervous system are activated; at the same time there is an over- and under-activation, i.e. a hyper- and hypoarousal. The sympathetic nervous system tries to activate our body so that it can respond to a threat or danger, while at the same time the parasympathetic nervous system tries to calm our body. It's as if we were pressing the gas and the brake at the same time while driving. The simultaneous activation of both systems triggers a physiological stalemate, which causes our body to channel the excessive energy into symptoms that are expressed both in an over-activation and in an under-activation (Levine 2019b). This state is expressed in our clients by a high-revving with strong restlessness, nervousness and tension combined with exhaustion, weakness and lack of interest. Our body is paralyzed or petrified and at the same time highly tense, as if in a frozen high-revving state.

The extent of immobility can vary greatly. For some people it is a largely constant state; they are mostly frozen or in shutdown. Often they have little or no access to their physical sensations and feelings. For others there can be a continuous alternation between high activation, immobility and a relatively balanced activation state. Again, others have temporary states of immobility activated by certain triggers, such as a smell, a sound, a touch or a look.

With his Polyvagal Theory Stephen Porges has changed our understanding of traumatization significantly. Usually, trauma is understood and treated as a stress reaction. But this only applies to those traumatic experiences that lead to a fight or flight reaction, in which the sympathetic nervous system is activated. Traumatic events that lead to a freezing reaction or shutdown, in which the dorsal vagus or both the dorsal vagus and the sympathetic nervous system are activated at the same time, are not or not purely stress reactions. Differentiating between these two types of reactions to a traumatic experience is very important for our understanding of traumatization. This enables us to respond better and more effectively to our clients. Even with the explanation of these different reaction modes we contribute significantly to their relief; so they can better understand their reactions and better comprehend their symptoms.

For effective processing of a traumatic experience, it is essential to know how our clients reacted to the event and which of their three circuits was activated and is still active. In the case of repeated or chronic traumatization, all three circuits can be activated. The immediate physical reaction—immobility or fighting respectively fleeing—is reflected in the current physiological state and in the present symptoms. As Peter Levine (2008), one of the leading US trauma experts describes, this is especially the case when the immediate impulse of the body to flee or fight is not carried out or completed or the freezing cannot be released; for instance, when someone has to remain still during a medical examination, such as an MRI, and cannot follow his impulse to flee. Or if a child resists a medical examination, such as a blood test, but is held so that it can be carried out. If she is not supported afterwards in expressing her fighting impulses, these remain in her body. Subsequently this can lead to the affected child reacting aggressively to certain triggers and, for example, hitting out. This behavior is an expression of the suppressed self-defense reaction of her body that could not be carried out. It is essential to recognize these connections, explain them to the affected child and her parents and give her the opportunity to make up for and carry out and complete the instinctive defense reaction. Like closing a circle, an action that has not yet been concluded is thus completed. If this is not possible, the child's body remains in a greatly increased level of arousal; this can, for instance, manifest in increased irritability, restlessness, tension and feelings of powerlessness, helplessness and rage.

3.1.4 The Significance of the Polyvagal Theory for Trauma Treatment

With its comprehensive understanding of traumatization the Polyvagal Theory contributes significantly to improved trauma treatment. By conveying the basics to our clients they can better understand their symptoms, emotions, body sensations and behavioral reactions and thus themselves. This also allows them to recognize the effects of their traumatic experiences as their nervous system's attempt to adapt, and no longer view them as pathological consequences that give them the feeling of being strange, sick or crazy. The Polyvagal Theory shows that safety is the basis of every trauma treatment and that we must do everything to make our clients feel safe with us (Porges 2018). Our open, appreciative presence is just as important as our open, warm gaze, as well as a pleasant voice and speech melody. Furthermore, the Polyvagal Theory points to the importance of co-regulation. This causes a mutual "linkage of oscillating emotions between different partners, contributing to the emotional stability of both" (Geller 2019, p. 129). If we are present, calm and centered our clients can also be present, calm and centered due to the resonance.

Finally, the Polyvagal Theory generally shows us the significance of the ventral vagus and the social engagement system associated with it and the necessity to support both in our clients.

In Part III, under "Our inner attitude" (chap. 17) and "Providing safety and support" (chap. 19), we will go into more detail about the importance of safety and our presence. In Part IV, we will get to know various interventions and exercises that stimulate the ventral vagus.

After this insight into our nervous system, we now want to deal with its central part, our brain.

3.2 The Triune Brain

In his model of the Triune Brain the American neuroscientist Paul MacLean (1990, cited in van der Kolk 2016) divides the human brain into three parts:

- the brain stem, also called the reptilian brain
- the limbic system, also called the mammalian brain, and
- the neocortex

Paul MacLean assumed that these three areas—similar to the branches of the autonomic nervous system described earlier—developed in different stages of evolution; phylogenetically, the reptilian brain is the oldest part of our brain and the neocortex the youngest. These three brains have large structural differences, but, according to Peter Levine (2011), they "interlock and are designed to work together as a unified ("triune") brain" (p. 313). The younger brain parts are still influenced by the older ones.

Brain stem or Reptilian Brain

The reptilian brain includes the brain stem and the cerebellum, beginning directly above the area where the spinal cord enters the skull. It enables all basic body functions such as breathing, hunger, eating and excretion, sleeping and waking, pain perception and body temperature and is responsible for our instincts. The brain stem and the hypothalamus, which lies above the brain stem, regulate the arousal level of our body together. They coordinate the functions of our heart, lungs, immune system and endocrine system. This ensures that "these basic life-sustaining systems are maintained within the relatively stable internal balance" (van der Kolk 2016, p. 70). Many traumatized people have impairments specifically in these areas; for example in the form of sleep disorders, digestive problems, loss of appetite as well as strong states of arousal and increased sensitivity to physical touch.

Limbic System or Mammalian Brain

Above the reptilian brain is the limbic system, also called the mammalian brain (van der Kolk 2016). Phylogenetically, it developed in the first mammals, which differ from reptiles in that they live in communities and feed and raise their young. The limbic system is considered the seat of emotions and our basic instincts, sexual drive and aggression readiness. It determines how we enter relationships and feel emotionally connected to other people. Furthermore, it contributes to the memory of feelings, facts and experiences. Learning only became possible through its development. The limbic system is formed based on the genetic predispositions and temperament of a child and his reaction to what he experiences. If a child grows up in a safe and secure environment, corresponding neural circuits of the feeling of safety are formed, which allow the child to explore the world and develop. If a child grows up in an insecure or violent environment, corresponding circuits of insecurity and fear are formed, which shape and control the child's perception, emotions and behavior accordingly. According to Bessel van der Kolk (2016) his brain is then "specialized" in fear. Hence, the early experiences of a child shape those structures of the limbic system that are responsible for emotions and memory.

The limbic system registers dangers, assesses whether something is pleasant or threatening, and decides what is important or unimportant for survival. Information about our environment and the state of our body reaches through our senses, skin or kinesthetic sensation our thalamus, an area in the limbic system, which takes in the inputs and forwards them in two directions.

On the one hand to the amygdala, two almond-shaped formations deep in the limbic system. This instantly estimates the emotional significance and, in case of danger, sends instructions to the hypothalamus and the brain stem to secrete stress hormones and activate the autonomic nervous system. This leads to the release of cortisol and adrenaline, which accelerate the heart rate, increases blood pressure and intensifies breathing in order to prepare the body for its defense by fight or flight. When the danger is over, the body quickly returns to its original state. However, if the ability to recover is impaired, for example by repeated traumatization, the body remains in a defensive state of fighting or fleeing.

On the other hand, the information from the thalamus is forwarded via the hippocampus and the anterior cingulum, another part of the limbic system, to the prefrontal lobe, where it reaches our consciousness and is consciously interpreted by us. The neuroscientist Joseph LeDoux (2012, cit. in van der Kolk 2016, p. 76) refers to the first path to the amygdala as the "low road" and the second to the frontal lobe as the "high road", as the processing of the information takes a few milliseconds longer here. Since the amygdala decides faster whether there is a danger than we can consciously perceive it, we often become aware of a danger only when our body has already reacted and, for instance, we run away.

The alarm function of the amygdala—van der Kolk (2016, p. 77) calls it the "smoke detector in the brain"—is in itself very reliable. However, due to repeated traumatic experiences, misjudgments can occur. That is why traumatized people frequently perceive statements, gestures or a certain facial expression or look as threatening, although they were not meant to be, and react accordingly with withdrawal (flight) or aggression (fight).

Neocortex

The neocortex is the phylogenetically youngest part of the brain. It can be divided into four areas, the so-called brain lobes (frontal, parietal, temporal and occipital lobes), each of which has different tasks. The largest part of the neocortex is taken up by the frontal lobes, which are located directly behind our forehead. They are also called prefrontal cortex. This enables us to speak, think abstractly, plan and reflect and enables us to imagine things, anticipate the consequences of our actions, make decisions and be creative (van der Kolk 2016). In addition, the frontal lobes are the seat of our empathy and thus decisive for our ability to relate to other people and to maintain harmonious relationships. The frontal lobes also prevent us from letting our impulses run free and having to express them.

Just as the amygdala can be considered a "smoke detector", the frontal lobes can be referred to as a "watchtower" that allows us to observe the events from above to determine whether a threat actually poses a danger (ibid. p. 78). In traumatized people, however, the balance between amygdala and frontal lobes is usually impaired or non existent, which is why it is often difficult for them to control their emotions and impulses.

Emotional and Rational Brain and the need for their balance

Bessel van der Kolk (2016) refers to the reptilian brain with the limbic system as the "emotional brain" and the neocortex as the "rational brain". If emotional and rational brain are in balance, then "we feel like ourselves"; if our life is in danger, this balance is no longer given and "the pathways between frontal lobes and the limbic system become extremely tenuous" (p. 80). Paul MacLean (1990) compares the relationship between emotional and rational brain to that of a "unruly" horse and its "more or less competent" rider (quoted in van der Kolk 2016, p. 80). As long as everything is going well, the rider can maintain the feeling of having everything under control. With unexpected stimuli from outside—such as a loud bang—the horse may run away. Similarly, traumatized people, who feel threatened and overwhelmed by strong emotions such as fear or anger, often have no control over their reactions. "If the interpretation of threat by the amygdala is too intense, and/or the filtering system from the higher areas of the brain is too weak", they "lose control over automatic emergency responses" (ibid., p. 76). This can lead, among other things, to "prolonged startle or aggressive outbursts".

For the overcoming and healing of trauma, the restoration of the balance between emotional and rational brain is necessary. If a balance is re-established between the two, our clients regain the feeling that they can influence themselves, their feelings and their reactions to their environment, and quite generally their life (ibid.). A key element is self-awareness, the center of which is the medial prefrontal cortex, a part of the frontal lobe, which is connected to the emotional brain. It "notices what is going on inside us" so that we "feel what we're feeling" (ibid., p. 247). Just by consciously perceiving what we feel and making ourselves aware of what is going on inside us, we can change our emotions and our experience.

The formation or restoration of this balance and hence the change of the danger warning system can take place in two ways; from top to bottom, top-down, or from bottom to top, bottom-up. The top-down regulation takes place from the medial prefrontal cortex, for example by means of self-awareness. The bottom-up regulation takes place from the reptilian brain via breathing, movement and touch. Both lead to the calming of our autonomic nervous system. There is a range of stabilization exercises for both, which we will discuss in detail in the practical section.

References

Dana D, Grant D (2019) Das Polyvagal-PlayLab: Hilfe für Therapeuten, die ihre Klienten im Sinne der Polyvagal-Theorie behandeln wollen. In: Porges SW, Dana D (Hrsg) Klinische Anwendungen der Polyvagal-Theorie. Ein neues Verständnis des Autonomen Nervensystems und seiner Anwendung in der therapeutischen Praxis. G. P. Probst, Lichtenau/Westfalen, pp 207–230 (The Polyvagal PlayLab: Helping Therapists Bring Polyvagal Theory to Their Clients. In: Porges SW, Dana D (Eds) Clinical Applications of The Polyvagal Theory. The Emergence of Polyvagal-Informed Therapies. 2018, W.W. Norton, New York, pp 185–206)

Enders G (2019) Darm mit Charme. Alles über ein unterschätztes Organ. Ullstein, Berlin (Gut: The Inside Story of Our Body's Most Underrated Organ. 2015, Scribe UK, London)

Geller SM (2019) Therapeutische Präsenz und die Polyvagal-Theorie: Prinzipien und Übungen für den Aufbau heilsamer therapeutischer Beziehungen. In: Porges SW, Dana D (Hrsg) Klinische Anwendungen der Polyvagal-Theorie. Ein neues Verständnis des Autonomen Nervensystems und seiner Anwendung in der therapeutischen Praxis. G. P. Probst, Lichtenau/Westfalen, pp 123–143 (Therapeutic Presence and Polyvagal Theory: Principles and Practices for Cultivating Effective Therapeutic Relationships. In: Porges SW, Dana D (Eds) Clinical Applications of The Polyvagal Theory. The Emergence of Polyvagal-Informed Therapies. 2018, W.W. Norton, New York, pp 106-126) Quoted from original English version (p 111)

LeDoux J (2012) Rethinking the emotional brain. Neuron 73(4):653–676. Zit. In: Van der Kolk B (2016) Verkörperter Schrecken. Traumaspuren in Gehirn, Geist und Körper und wie man sie heilen kann. G. P. Probst, Lichtenau/Westfalen (Cited in: Van der Kolk BA The Body Keeps the Score. Mind, Brain and Body in the Transformation of Trauma. 2015, Penguin Books, London)

Levine PA (2008) Vom Trauma befreien. Wie Sie seelische und körperliche Blockaden lösen. Kösel, München (Healing Trauma. A Pioneering Program for Restoring the Wisdom of Your Body. 2005, Sounds True, Boulder)

Levine PA (2011) Sprache ohne Worte. Wie unser Körper Trauma verarbeitet und uns in die innere Balance zurückführt. Kösel, München (In an Unspoken Voice. How the Body Releases Trauma and Restores Goodness. 2010, North Atlantic Books, Berkeley) Own translation

Levine PA (2019a) Polyvagal-Theorie und Trauma. In: Porges SW, Dana D (Hrsg) Klinische Anwendungen der Polyvagal-Tgheorie. Ein neues Verständnis des Autonomen Nervensystems und seiner Anwendung in der therapeutischen Praxis. G. P. Probst, Lichtenau/Westfalen, pp 19–42 (Polyvagal Theory and Trauma. In: Porges SW, Dana D (Eds) Clinical Applications of The Polyvagal Theory. The Emergence of Polyvagal-Informed Therapies. 2018, W.W. Norton, New York, pp 3-10) Quoted from original English version (pp 17–18)

Levine PA (2019b) Somatic Experiencing®. First Year. Training Material. Somatic-Experiencing Germany, Essen

MacLean PD (1990) The triune brain in evolution: role in paleocerebral functions. Springer, New York. Zit. In: Van der Kolk B (2016) Verkörperter Schrecken. Traumaspuren in Gehirn, Geist und Körper und wie man sie heilen kann. G. P. Probst, Lichtenau/Westfalen (Cited in: Van der Kolk BA The Body Keeps the Score. Mind, Brain and Body in the Transformation of Trauma. 2015, Penguin Books, London)

Porges SW (2010) Die Polyvagal-Theorie. Neurophysiologische Grundlagen der Therapie. Junfermann, Paderborn. Own translation

Porges SW (2018) Die Polyvagal-Theorie und die Suche nach Sicherheit. Traumabehandlung, soziales Engagement und Bindung. G. P. Probst, Lichtenau/Westfalen. Own translation

Porges SW (2019) Die Polyvagal-Theorie: Eine Einführung. In: Porges SW, Dana D (Hrsg) Klinische Anwendungen der Polyvagal-Theorie. Ein neues Verständnis des Autonomen Nervensystems und seiner Anwendung in der therapeutischen Praxis. G. P. Probst, Lichtenau/Westfalen, pp 67–85 (Polyvagal Theory: A Primer. In: Porges SW, Dana D (Eds) Clinical Applications of The Polyvagal Theory. The Emergence of Polyvagal-Informed Therapies. 2018, W.W. Norton, New York, pp 50–69) Quoted from original English version (pp 54, 61, 58)

Rothschild B (2017) The body remembers volume 2. Revolutionizing trauma treatment. W.W. Norton, New York

van der Kolk BA (2016) Verkörperter Schrecken. Traumaspuren in Gehirn, Geist und Körper und wie man sie heilen kann. G. P. Probst, Lichtenau/Westfalen (The Body Keeps the Score. Mind, Brain and Body in the Transformation of Trauma. 2015, Penguin Books, London). Quoted from original English version (pp 97, 64–65, 71, 72, 74, 75, 247)

Our Body and its Significance for Stabilization

4

Contents

Our body expresses trauma in various ways, manifesting symptoms such as restlessness, anxiety or tension, physical complaints such as chronic pain or digestive problems as well as certain body postures, movement patterns or behaviors.

Example from practice

Sebastian, 28, was shouted at, insulted and hit by his father from an early age, often also beaten up. He is a tall, slim young man, but he walks through life with hunched shoulders, uncertain gait and fearful look; as if he were still in danger and on the alert. ◄

At the same time, our body plays a decisive role in regaining and strengthening our stability. Firstly, for example, by reducing inner tensions through movement, by coming into the here and now through consciously using our senses, or by calming ourselves with the help of our breath. Secondly, by reinforcing and deepening the effect of stabilizing interventions and exercises, such as inner images,

R. Lackner, *Stabilization in Trauma Treatment*,
https://doi.org/10.1007/978-3-662-67480-2_4

through consciously tracking and perceiving positive body sensations evoked by them. Finally, the integration of our body is necessary in order to process and resolve traumatic experiences (i.a. Levine 1998; van der Kolk 2016).

4.1 Our Body—A Mirror of Traumatization

Example from practice

As a teenager, Markus, 21, was unexpectedly attacked and choked from behind by a classmate in school. He only managed with great difficulty to free himself from the tight grip at the last moment. Since then his throat feels very tight and he has the feeling that someone is strangling him. He repeatedly experiences great fear of not getting any air and suffocating. ◄

This is another example of how traumatic experiences can be expressed and reflected in our body. However, many times the physical signs are not as easy to trace as with Markus; like, when the underlying traumatic experience is hidden, or only vaguely or not at all pictorially retrievable.

Example from practice

For years, Valerie, 44, suffered from unexplained chronic nausea, the feeling of having to vomit and a choking sensation. She felt disgusted by some foods such as pudding or creamy soups. Only in the gradual resurfacing of memories of early sexual violence, in which she had to orally satisfy the perpetrator, did she gradually become aware of the cause of her physical symptoms and thus could comprehend and understand them. ◄

Like Valerie, traumatized people often suffer from inexplicable physical symptoms for which no medical explanation is available.

4.1.1 Physical Symptoms as a Mirror of Traumatic Events

As with Markus and Valerie, physical symptoms frequently mirror the type of traumatic event or its essential aspects. They are an expression of what has been experienced as well as an indication of where we can or should start in the treatment. For example, people who have been strangled, like Markus, or had a choking attack may have the sensation of tightness in their throat and the feeling of not getting enough air or even suffocating. People who have been forced to eat something they were unwilling to eat or, like Valerie, forced to engage in oral sex and swallowed ejaculate, may develop an indefinite nausea, the repeated feeling of having to vomit or a recurring urge to vomit.

Many people who come to my practice have already gone through a long period of suffering. Due to their symptoms, they have often visited various doctors and undergone a number of medical examinations or treatments; some have already been in psychotherapeutic or psychiatric treatment. In the course of these interventions one of the doctors will sometimes recommend a trauma therapy. Frequently, they themselves suspect or assume that their symptoms are related to earlier experiences. A trauma-specific approach is often a last resort for them and is associated with the hope that their symptoms could still experience relief or even healing. When I ask them in the first conversation about dramatic and burdensome experiences and mention various examples, there are always—sometimes several—traumatic experiences in their life stories. Many times a connection between their experiences and their symptoms appear to be plausible and accurate to me. When I share my thoughts with my clients and show the correlation between their traumatic experiences, their nervous system and their physical symptoms, these are mostly accurate for them, making previously inexplicable symptoms suddenly understandable and plausible. My clients then feel relieved and less "strange" or "crazy" and gain the feeling of being "normal" after all. Thus, even showing a possible connection between symptoms and traumatic events can have a stabilizing effect.

4.1.2 Physical Symptoms as an Expression of the Activated Defense System

Many physical symptoms can be traced back to the "survival-based behavioral and physiological (somatic and autonomic) reactions associated with" our defense mechanisms, i.e. our reactions of fight, flight and freezing (Levine 2019a, p. 39).

Traumatic experiences, especially repeated ones, can lead to a "recalibration" of our autonomic nervous system, so that our defense reactions become entrenched or chronic (Kolacz and Porges 2018). Through the chronic activation of the dorsal vagus, for instance due to repeated experiences of sexual violence, a chronic freezing reaction can lead to a number of physical complaints, mainly below the diaphragm; e.g., digestive disorders and gynecological complaints, but also chronic pain states. For example, people who have experienced physical and sexual violence in childhood and adulthood have a higher risk of developing fibromyalgia than non-affected people (Häuser et al. 2010). Women who have experienced sexual violence in childhood are significantly more likely to suffer from chronic gynecological complaints such as vaginal infections or abdominal pain, as well as sexual problems or disorders like vaginismus, than women without such experiences (Wimmer-Puchinger and Lackner 1997). If the sympathetic nervous system or our defense system of fight and flight is chronically activated, this can lead, among other things, to cardiovascular diseases such as hypertension or arrhythmias (Levine 2019a; Porges 2018). Physical symptoms, especially medically unexplained ones, can therefore have their origin in a "stress-related disorder of regulation" (Levine 2019a, p. 39).

Stephen Porges (2018) shows with his Polyvagal Theory the connections between traumatic experiences, the autonomic nervous system and physical symptoms and emphasizes that "many clinical symptoms attributed to a particular end organ by conventional medicine can be traced back to the neurological regulation of these organs" (p. 125). Therefore, they are attempts by our organism to adapt. For our clients this approach can be a very relieving explanation of their symptoms giving them hope that these can diminish and be resolved with the stabilization and the processing of their traumatic experience.

4.1.3 Physical Reactions as Diagnostic Indicators

Hence, our body expresses and reflects a traumatization; this is also shown in its reaction to a trigger that reminds of the traumatic event. Consequently, our body-also acts as a diagnostic instrument; giving us diagnostic indications showing whether and how much a traumatic experience is still in effect. When my clients mention that they have experienced something bad—and it is not obvious how much they are affected by the experience—I ask them how it is to talk about or even think about the experience and what they currently perceive in their body. Even if they do not feel any emotional burden at that moment, the experience can still be associated with unpleasant physical sensations. Many people describe feeling nausea or pressure in their chest when they think of the event. Or they feel a heaviness on their shoulders or a lump in their throat. During the naming of the body sensations, frequently feelings such as sadness, discomfort or fear appear, which they had not previously noticed. The physical reactions of our clients, which usually correspond to those in the moment of the event, show us that the experience is still affecting them.

4.1.4 Physical Reactions as an Expression of the State of Arousal

In addition to the feelings described by our clients, we can observe physical signs during their narration that indicate their body, or more precisely their nervous system, is reacting to the recalled experience and that it has not yet been (sufficiently) completed or processed. This manifests, for example, in restlessness, faster and shallower breathing, faster speaking, freezing or collapse and dissociation.

When accompanying traumatized people, it is important to pay attention to these physical signals and reactions right from the beginning, as they usually reflect the state of their autonomous nervous system. As described in chap. 3.1, this consists of two branches, the sympathetic and the parasympathetic nervous system. Both influence each other reciprocally; the more the activation of the parasympathetic nervous system increases, the more the activation of the sympathetic one decreases and vice versa. Based on different physical signs, we can recognize the respective degree of activation or an increase or decrease in the arousal of our clients' autonomous nervous system. This is important because in some states of arousal it is necessary to intervene resolutely in order to "prevent dissociation, freezing or emotional overload" or even retraumatization (Rothschild 2002, p. 163). By interrupting and taking breaks with stabilizing interventions, we can reduce and counteract the burden on our clients caused by mentioning, telling and dealing with traumatic experiences and their consequences. Thereby, the process of treatment becomes more gentle and less threatening. We will go into this in more detail in chap. 21.4.

Babette Rothschild describes six different activation states of the autonomous nervous system (2017). However, these do not quite correspond to Stephen Porges' Polyvagal Theory and Peter Levine's knowledge. If we combine these different approaches, we can distinguish the following four activation levels that are important for accompanying traumatized people:

- **Calm and relaxation**
  Recognizable signs of a relaxed state with low activation are calm, deep breathing, relaxed facial features and muscles, slightly dilated pupils, a calm look, a relaxed voice and a normal skin color. According to the Polyvagal Theory, this is an expression of the activity of the social engagement system, i.e. the ventral branch of the parasympathetic nervous system (Porges 2010). It is a state of safety and relaxation in which we are open to new things and can think clearly and learn. If our clients are in this state, we can maintain our approach.
- **Activity and vigilance**
  Signs of an active, alert state with moderate arousal are accelerated breathing, increased muscle tone, slight physical restlessness, slight sweating, slightly rosier skin color and faster speaking. This state of moderate activation of the sympathetic nervous system enables us to be attentive and alert in order to be able to react to possible stimuli. In this state we can largely maintain our approach.
- **Flight or fight**
  Recognizable signs of a stronger or strong arousal state include rapid, shallow breathing, increased muscle tone, paler skin tone, dilated pupils and/or sweat on the forehead and palms. Most of the time we can observe strong restlessness and nervousness in our clients, as well as a changed voice and speed of speech. This state of strong activation of the sympathetic nervous system allows us to respond to danger and flee or fight. It is accompanied by strong emotions such as fear or rage. If these signs are present in our clients, this may be an indication that they feel threatened or overwhelmed; for example, if a burdensome memory arises in them, if we proceed too quickly or if they talk about the traumatic events for too long. In these cases, it is necessary to "brake" using stabilizing interventions (Rothschild 2002, p. 164). We should invite our clients to take a few slow breaths, to become aware of the ground under their feet, or to look around and let their gaze rest on a pleasant or neutral impression. Likewise, we can ask our clients what they are currently perceiving in their body and then invite them to explore where it feels pleasant or neutral in their body; by staying with this sensation and consciously perceiving it, their high activation decreases (Levine 2019b). By becoming aware of their hands and/or feet, our clients can experience a sense of containment and safety, which can calm

their body (Levine 2019a). With these interrupting suggestions and interventions, we reduce the speed and intensity of the treatment process. Furthermore, we support our clients in learning to calm their body and to stabilize themselves. Through the experience that they can regulate their physical activation, they gain confidence in themselves and their ability to influence their state. By our proceeding very carefully and paying attention to dosing the process, our clients also gain a feeling of safety and trust in our joint work

Example from practice

Ursula, 67, often and quickly gets into a strongly increased arousal state. Every time this happens, I invite her to take a few slow breaths and direct her attention outward into the room. By doing so Ursula always calms down. In the meantime, she has got used to pausing, breathing slowly and observing her surroundings whenever she notices that her arousal is increasing. In this way Ursula succeeds again and again to calm down. These small interventions are now Ursula's most important tools to stabilize herself.

- **Immobility—freezing and shutdown**
  Recognizable signs of an immobility reaction include, among other things, shallow breathing, dissociation or a "remoteness," a "lack of vitality" and physical immobility or freezing as well as a rigid or expressionless, pale face (Levine 2019a, p. 34). These are signs of a collapse or shutdown, a state of hypoarousal with decreased heart rate, low blood pressure and flaccid muscels (Rothschild, 2017)
  However, there is also a form of immobility or freezing in which both the sympathetic and the parasympathetic nervous system are activated and there is both an over- and an under-activation, i.e. a hyper- and hypoarousal (Levine 2019b). This state is expressed in our clients as a high-revving with strong restlessness, nervousness and tension combined with exhaustion, weakness and lack of interest. There is also rapid, shallow breathing (Rothschild 2017). Their body is frozen/rigid and at the same time highly tense like a frozen high-revving.
  An immobilization reaction may occur in the first conversation or as part of the anamnesis when our clients tell us about threatening experiences. It can also show itself repeatedly during follow-up sessions when our clients are confronted with threatening contents. It is essential that we brake their recounting as soon as we notice they are beginning to freeze or go into shutdown. In this way we can prevent them from being overwhelmed with trauma-related stimuli, further activation and dysregulation, and running the risk of being retraumatized. We should therefore kindly interrupt our clients and invite them to pause, for example, by asking: *"As you tell me all this, how is it for you right now?"* Alternatively we can give them feedback on our perception: *"I have the impression that it burdens/stirs up/distresses you when you talk about it."* In order to reduce the activation of our clients and for them to be able to self-regulate, we must direct their attention to a resource; by asking them: *"If you look around and let your gaze wander, where does it feel good or neutral for you to linger with your gaze?"* Or by inviting our clients to take a few slow breaths in and

out, or to focus their attention to their feet and their contact with the ground, to move a bit or to change their posture.

It is essential to assure our clients that what they tell us is important and that we will continue to keep it in our focus; but that it is sensible to recount it in small stages, well dosed, so that they are not overwhelmed by it. Our body listens when we relate our trauma and reacts accordingly (Heller 2003). This may cause an increased activation, giving rise to restlessness or palpitations, which can lead to the consolidation of symptoms. By slowing our clients down in telling their story and asking them to pause, their organism can regulate and calm down again. By doing this, they experience that they can influence their state and self-regulate. Moreover, they gain confidence in our accompaniment, as they experience that we proceed considerately, protecting them from getting overwhelmed.

In order to bring our clients out of hypoarousal or hypoactivation, it is helpful to gently bring them into a slight activation, for instance, by asking them to move a bit, stand up or change their posture (Levine 2019a), to look around or change the direction of their gaze.

If our clients are in a state of simultaneous hypo- and hyperarousal, it is sensible to act calmingly first and to draw their attention to an external resource or their breathing.

Through the loosening and dissolving of the frozen state, the underlying high activation of the nervous system usually comes to light. This manifests, for example, as rage, grief or physical pain. These reactions are often experienced as irritating or threatening by our clients; many also fear the "intensity of their own energy and latent aggression" (Levine 2008, p. 38). This fear can prevent a complete discharge and restoration of normal functioning. Hence, gentle "pendulation" between these sensations or feelings on one side and a resource on the other is important (Levine 2011, p. 108). This slows down the process of dissolving the freezing and the organism can gradually regulate and calm down. Through "pendulation, slowing down, repeated pausing, tuning in ('how is it now?') and grounding or anchoring" the emerging arousal becomes "more tolerable" for our clients (Zanotta 2018, p. 131). We can support them in allowing the natural movement impulses of their body and encourage them carrying them out slowly and consciously. Thereby, the originally instinctive defense reaction, that was not expressed or completed in the moment of the traumatic event, can be made up and carried out in a controlled manner. This leads to significant relief in our clients.

We will discuss further intervention possibilities in chap. 33.

4.2 Our Body Remembers

The central burden of every traumatization lies in the uncontrolled, disturbing, confusing and/or threatening memories, emotions, body sensations, thoughts and behavioral impulses that arise. For those affected, these are mostly incomprehensible and inexplicable; they feel overwhelmed, taken over and helplessly exposed to them.

Example from practice

Margarete, 72, freezes every time someone is condescending or patronizing, or verbally attacks and devalues her. She feels helpless, paralyzed and is unable to defend herself and set boundaries for the other. Gradually she becomes aware of how much these reactions are related to her childhood experiences. As a child, Margarete was reprimanded, humiliated, shouted at and insulted by her parents almost daily. She felt completely at the mercy of them, powerless and worthless. To protect herself, she tried to be as inconspicuous as possible, withdrawing into herself, making herself invisible and allowing everything to happen to her. ◀

The connections between current stressful feelings, body sensations and behavioral impulses and traumatic experiences are based on the somatic memories of these, which are stored in our implicit memory.

Sensory information is the foundation of every experience and each memory (Rothschild 2002). It is transmitted from our body periphery and internal body to our brain. Therefore, our sensory nervous system has two branches, the exteroceptive and the interoceptive.

Exteroceptive nerves are those that receive stimuli from our environment and transmit them to our brain via our five senses. Interoceptive nerves are those that receive and transmit stimuli from our body interior. The interoceptive system is divided into viszeroception or the inner feeling that allows us to perceive body signals from our internal organs (e.g. heart palpitations), noziception, which allows us to perceive pain, and proprioception (Thieme 2020). This includes, among other things, the sense of movement or kinesthetic feeling, which plays an important role in learning activities and movements such as cycling and is essential for our implicit, procedural memory. This, also called non-declarative memory, includes our "memories of skills and habits, emotional reactions, reflex actions and classically conditioned reactions" (van der Kolk 2000, p. 222). It allows us to recall movements such as swimming or playing the piano without having to think consciously about it. It controls our behavior and thus largely determines our personality.

Explicit or declarative memory, on the other hand, stores memories of events and facts. It includes memories that we can consciously recall and easily verbalize. When we think consciously about something, we use our explicit memory. This is divided into semantic memory, which stores facts and concepts, and episodic memory, which stores events and experiences (The Human Memory 2020). Explicit and implicit memories are coded differently and stored in different brain areas.

Whether we can remember an event depends on its significance for us as well as the strength of our emotions and the degree of our arousal during the event (van der Kolk 2016). Our first love will still be remembered by us after many years or decades, whereas some flirt may not be remembered anymore. Injuries, humiliations and threatening events are particularly well remembered; this is linked to the fact that our body releases adrenaline in such situations in order to defend ourselves against the threat (ibid.). This increases the probability that we can remember these occurrences later. The more adrenaline our body releases, the more accurate is our memory. Hence, distressing or unpleasant events remain very intense and precise in our memory for a long time. However, if an event horrifies or frightens us or we are in shock, we often only remember fragments of it. Some details can remain very clear, while others are only vague or not retained at all. If there is an extremely strong arousal in our body during an experience, adequate storage and integration of incoming impressions are not possible; then they are not organized as "coherent logical narratives but in fragmented sensory and emotional traces: images, sounds, and physical sensations" (van der Kolk 2016, p. 213). These memory traces can later be activated by similar sensory stimuli. If this is the case, then "the frontal lobe shuts down, including ... the region necessary to put feelings into words, the region that creates our sense of location in time, and the thalamus, which integrates the raw data of incoming sensations"; then "the emotional brain ... takes over" (ibid.).

Example from practice

Melanie, 27, had to visit her dentist because of severe toothache. During the examination, she was put into a lying position in the dentist's chair. When her dentist bent over her to examine her, Melanie suddenly panicked due to the smell of his aftershave, and began to tremble and wriggle. She felt completely helpless, confused and exposed and was unable to communicate and put into words what was happening to her. This experience frightened and confused Melanie very much; all the more so since it left a fleeting memory of her father and the vague feeling that he had done something bad to her. In the course of our collaborative work, fragmentary memories of her father gradually emerged, including the fact that he used to use the same aftershave as her dentist. Over a period of time, Melanie gradually remembered more details, like individual puzzle pieces, which gradually formed a series of memories of various sexual assaults by her father. ◄

Different sensory stimuli can trigger memory traces and evoke flashbacks. This can be done both by exteroceptive stimuli such as a smell or a sound and by interoceptive, i.e. sensations from our inner body. For example, a rapid heartbeat, pressure in the stomach or "sensory messages from muscles and connective tissue that contain the memory of a certain posture, activity or intention" can trigger flashbacks (Rothschild 2002, p. 75). This is because our perceptions are forwarded to our brain simultaneously via two or more sensory channels. This forms a synchronous arousal pattern in our cortex, which can later be activated by just the perception via one single sensory channel (Hüther 2006). For instance, Melanie was triggered by the smell of her dentist's aftershave and by her reclining position during the dental examination. The activated implicit memory of a traumatic experience can, as with Melanie, manifest itself in feelings such as panic, helplessness or rage and disgust as well as in body sensations such as trembling, nausea or freezing, but also in instinctive behavioral reactions such as avoidance or defending oneself and attacking. These usually correspond to the immediate reactions to the traumatic event.

In this context, Antonio Damasio's (2018) Hypothesis of Somatic Markers is interesting, which he described in connection with thinking and decision-making processes. He found that these do not take place exclusively rationally; rather, our body sensations play an important role. If, for example, we think of an undesired consequence of a decision, then an "albeit very brief unpleasant sensation in the stomach" appears (ibid. p. 237). This body sensation is an expression or indication of a feeling or mental image; it marks it on a physical level. On a neuronal level, according to Antonio Damasio (2018), somatic markers are "dependent on learning in a system that links certain categories of objects or events with the unfolding of a pleasant or unpleasant body state" (p. 246). Accordingly, somatic markers are also formed through traumatic experiences, i.e. physical sensations associated with a certain experience. Sensory stimuli such as a certain sound, like a bang, or a special smell, such as the aftershave for Melanie, can reactivate the memories of a traumatic experience.

We all know this mechanism from moments when, for instance, a certain smell, like that of freshly baked cookies or freshly mown grass, or a certain song triggers a pleasant, cozy or cheerful feeling in us and we suddenly feel transported back to our grandmother's kitchen, the place of our summer holidays or to the school ski trip disco with our first love. Similarly, this happens with memories of traumatic experiences. Triggered by a sensory stimulus, we suddenly find ourselves in the former state, frequently without access to the explicit memory of the former event; often only fragments or bits of memory appear in us. This is especially true for very early and chronic traumatizations such as repeated experiences of physical and sexual violence. In these cases, mainly implicit memories in the form of certain body sensations, emotions or actions and behaviors appear later. These usually lack the reference to the original experience, to which they are connected, i.e. the explicit memory of this. Consequently, the affected people suffer from various psychological, physical or behavior-related problems, without knowing their cause or being able to establish a connection to certain experiences and conscious memories. Many times they seek our help with inexplicable or unspecific symptoms such as deep sadness, depression, anxiety or panic attacks, inexplicable physical complaints and burdensome obstructive or risky behavioral patterns.

Memories of traumatic events are stored both explicitly and implicitly, just like all other memories. However, the explicit memory, i.e. that of the course of the event or its temporal assignment, is often not accessible to traumatized people. According to Bessel van der Kolk (2016), the difference between memories of positive and traumatic experiences lies on the one hand in the way memories are organized and on the other hand in the physical reactions to the memories. Memories of positive events, such as a wedding or the birth of a child, lie in the past and are remembered as a story with a beginning, a middle and an end. They are usually not associated with physical sensations (van der Kolk 2016). By contrast, memories of traumatic events are disorganized; some details are clearly rememberable, others not at all. Likewise, the sequence and temporal assignment of the event are frequently not recalled. Moreover, memories of traumatic experiences trigger physical sensations such as nausea or pressure in the stomach. These peculiarities of traumatic memories are linked to the fact that due to the strong arousal state at the time of the trauma an adequate storage of the experiences is not possible. For example, the thalamus, which is responsible for the perception of optical, acoustic and kinesthetic stimuli and their integration into our memory, fails to do so (van der Kolk 2016).

Example from practice

Vera, 37, has an unpleasant, almost gruesome feeling when thinking about her grandfather; she feels shame and disgust and perceives a pulling sensation in her lower abdomen. Vera always has a dark memory of the attic in her grandparents' house and the vague feeling that her grandfather had done something bad to her. At the same time, Vera thinks that this can't be true and that she is just imagining it. ◀

Furthermore, traumatized people experience memories of what happened even after decades as very close, intense, alive as if it had happened only recently. Although I repeatedly encounter this in my practice when my clients tell me about their experiences, often from decades ago, and it always touches me anew, one experience particularly affected me: an interview of a man in a television documentary who survived years of Russian captivity in Siberia after World War II. His whole body reacted as he told his story: he trembled, cried, could not continue speaking for a while, his voice broke at times and he said he still suffers from nightmares almost every night and his memories of Siberia are as present as if everything had just happened recently. It was so clearly visible and tangible that this man had been living in a massively traumatized state for decades. This deeply affected me; especially the fact that he apparently had not had the opportunity to process his traumatic experiences so far. And this, although we now have therapeutic techniques that enable us to transform and resolve traumatization.

Even positive experiences, such as a new love, can evoke explicit and implicit memories in traumatized people. This is the case when associated with the same body sensations they felt during the traumatic experience, such as excitement, palpitations or a fluttering stomach. Then the positive events can trigger panic, confusion or overload and defensive reactions such as flight impulses, which appear unexpectedly and uncontrollably and are usually incomprehensible, confusing and threatening for those affected.

However, if we go after the triggers detective-like and try to identify them on the basis of specific situations, they can usually be clearly recognized. When our clients know which stimuli their body and inner self react to, they gain clarity and understanding of themselves and their reactions. This gives them a feeling of control and predictability. Moreover, our clients have the opportunity to learn to deal better with these stimuli or situations or to avoid them and thus prevent themselves from being exposed to them again. Avoidance is sensible as long as the traumatization cannot be processed sufficiently and the stimuli still act as triggers. If avoiding is not possible or would restrict their life too much, it is sensible to develop strategies with our clients and to teach them stabilization techniques with which they can better deal with the triggers or reduce their effect. For instance, the image of a protective shell as well as grounding and breathing exercises can help to cushion the effects of the triggers (see also chap. 23).

Example from practice

Eva, 48, was very afraid of her older brother since she was a child. During her childhood, he often had outbursts of rage and threw things around in her presence. He often devalued, threatened and suppressed her. The fear of him remained with her, and thus she even freezes when she receives a call from him. Imagining a ball of light surrounding and protecting her and consciously being aware of the ground under her feet, allows her to feel safer when she contacts her brother and to stay calmer. This is also supported by the fact that she remembers that she is now an adult and no longer at his mercy. This enables Eva to increasingly set boundaries with him and still feel safe. ◄

4.3 Our Body—Location and Instrument of Stabilization

The relief and healing of trauma presupposes that our body experiences that the danger of the traumatic event is over, and that it learns to live in the here and now again (van der Kolk 2016). According to Antonio Damasio (quoted in Emerson 2016), feeling our body allows us to experience fundamentally and primarily that we are alive. If we have no awareness of our body, we question our being and our existence and a deep feeling of insecurity and being lost arises in us (Emerson 2016). Therefore, perceiving our body and our body sensations as well as regaining our body awareness is a fundamental and essential element of stabilization as well as of the entire trauma healing process.

Working with our body, our body perception and our body sensations allows us (gradually):

- to be in the present moment (again)
- to (re-) experience safety and support in ourselves
- to (re-) discover our aliveness and vitality
- to find the connection to ourselves (again)
- to be completely with ourselves (again) and
- to influence and change our feelings and physical states, e.g., fear and restlessness

Bodily sensations are the basis of our self-experience and self-awareness (Damasio 2018). They are also the basis of our emotions. All feelings such as joy, fear or rage and sadness are connected with physical sensations evoked by specific patterns in our brain (Rothschild 2002). The connection between body sensations and feelings is reflected in our language; with fear we feel tightness around our heart, with rage our stomach contracts and with relief a stone falls from our heart, as we say in German, or in English a weight is taken off our mind.

As mentioned in chap. 4.2 the Hypothesis of Somatic Markers by Antonio Damasio (2018) supports the coupling of body sensation and feelings. Physical sensations make us aware of our emotions, allow us to perceive, recognize and assign them. Through stabilization exercises such as the holistic experience of inner images, i.e. the simultaneous perception of imagination, feeling and body sensation, new couplings between pleasant feelings and sensations or, to stay with Damasio's hypothesis, new somatic markers are formed. If we imagine ourselves brave and powerful like a warrior, we will probably sense strength in our body and straighten up. With some practice, the positive body sensations and feelings associated with being a warrior will be activated and felt just by thinking about it.

Some traumatized people find it easy to perceive and name their physical sensations. When I ask them what they feel in their body, they can name and describe their sensations, and allow, observe and stay with them, while others can barely do so or not at all. They sense something in their body, but cannot describe it, have no words for it, or cannot localize and assign the sensations. Again, others are hardly or not at all able to feel their body and be aware of bodily sensations.

The question why some traumatized people are able to feel body sensations and others not is still unclear. On the one hand, even those traumatized by chronic sexual and physical violence can perceive their body. On the other hand, this may be less or not even possible for others who are burdened by single traumatic experiences. In my experience, a decisive factor is whether someone was able to have positive experiences with his body during his life or whether this was not possible for him or her. I frequently see people who are traumatized by physical and/or sexual violence and yet have access to their bodily sensations due to other experiences that were positive. Yet, others chronically sexually abused and/or severely neglected during childhood who had little or no positive body experiences, find it difficult or impossible to feel their body often feeling separated from it, unable to relate to it, or as though they had no body at all.

Some, especially those traumatized by sexual and/or physical violence and those who have been defamed and devalued because of their body or gender, reject their body; they are ashamed of it, feel betrayed by it or blame it for their traumatization. Particularly for them—but also for others—physical sensations can be a threat. Their body and their body sensations are frequently a trigger for the experienced trauma and generate fear and panic, disgust or rage, so their body becomes a source of imminent threat. Therefore, they avoid feeling it, lose the reference to it, do not feel it anymore and feel separated from it or even bodiless (Levine 2011). In this way they protect themselves from "sensations and emotions that could be overwhelming" (Levine 1998, p. 81). If despite this they actually feel their body, e.g., because of physical pain, they often react with fear and panic, freezing or confusion.

Even for traumatized people who have access to their body and can feel it, this can be a source of danger and certain body sensations can be a threat. For example, sensations that they experienced as pleasant before their traumatic experience, such as increased heart rate in connection with joy or enthusiasm, can be threatening after the trauma; then their body becomes a "danger signal" (Rothschild 2002, p. 34).

Many of our clients feel abandoned or betrayed by their body because they froze during the traumatic event and since then suffer from freezing and/or physical symptoms in threatening situations, which again is burdensome and threatening for them. If this is the case, it is important to explain them first, that our body freezes to ensure our survival when neither fight nor flight is possible. Secondly, the physical reactions are an expression of the activated defense mechanisms and the symptoms are a consequence of the adaptation of their nervous system to the experience. Finally, the physical reactions associated with pleasant situations and experiences can be triggers if they are equal to those experienced by our clients in connection with the traumatic event.

By supporting our clients in being aware of their body and exploring and observing sensations, they can get in touch and (re-) familiarise themselves with it. For many this is unfamiliar at the beginning. However, some immediately find it pleasant, soothing and strengthening. Others experience it as unpleasant or threatening and sometimes react with flashbacks, dissociations, restlessness or fear and panic (van der Kolk 2016). Therefore, a slow, dosed guiding towards physical feeling through little exercises is necessary. Through simple grounding exercises, such as perceiving the ground under their feet, feeling an object with their hand, or simple movements, like opening and closing a hand, our clients can approach their body and gradually find a positive access to it. This is especially true for people who are not aware of their body and feel threatened by it. It is a slow process requiring small steps, though it is very rewarding. This way, they can eventually experience that their body is not a source of threat, but one that gives them safety, support and stability.

"When we pay attention to our body," so Peter Levine, "we use the best tool available to us to dissolve various physical, emotional and psychological symptoms" (Levine 2011, p. 352). This is about "opening up to areas of our being that are foreign to us," with which we are not familiar or feel threatened by, or which we do not want to acknowledge and have dissociated from (p. 352).

If our clients have already gained some access to their body and can feel body sensations, it is useful to take them up repeatedly in the course of stabilization and work with them. So usually, it is helpful to encourage our clients to explore where it feels pleasant or neutral in their body (Levine 1998, 2011). We can support them by inviting them to turn their attention inward and wander through their body, scanning from bottom to top (or vice versa) and look for a pleasant or neutral area. It relieves our clients if we point out that it is often only a small body area such as a little finger or the nose that feels good or neutral. When they discover a corresponding spot or sensation, we invite them to stay with their attention on it and perceive it. In general, the sensation intensifies and sometimes spreads out a bit, and their entire organism calms down.

Example from practice

Constanze, 31, was severely physically abused by her parents in her childhood and youth. She was repeatedly exposed to life-threatening situations; for example, several times she was pushed under water while bathing, so that she could no longer get air. Constanze reacts to the mere thought of her experiences with hyper and hypo arousal in the form of restlessness, tension, trembling, partial freezing and dizziness as well as fear and confusion. When I ask her where it feels neutral or maybe pleasant in her body, Constanze discovers that the tip of her nose feels neutral. While she lingers with this sensation, her organism calms down quickly. Constanze is thrilled that she can calm herself down just by feeling the tip of her nose. For her, this small intervention does not only have a stabilizing effect, she also has the important experience that she herself can calm her body and inner self. With this, Constanze has a tool that she can use in her everyday life to stabilize herself. ◀

Like Constanze, our clients can regain stability through the regulating effect of neutral or positive sensations and experience a strengthening of their self-efficacy and autonomy. Additionally, they often come into contact with their inner strength and liveliness. I am repeatedly touched by how my clients visibly blossom through exploring pleasant or neutral body sensations; they suddenly take a deep breath, their shoulders loosen, they straighten up a bit, their gaze becomes clearer and more alert and their face more relaxed. For me, becoming aware of a positive or neutral body sensation is one of the most effective and strongest ways of stabilizing.

Example from practice

Maria, 42, perceives great restlessness and trembling in her body. She feels confused and fragile. In response to my question of where in her body it feels neutral or good, Maria notices an easeing in her thighs. After spending some moments with her attention on her legs, being aware of the easeing in them, she gradually calms down, takes a deep breath and then looks more relaxed. She is quite amazed and relieved to realize that she is now much calmer. ◀

As these examples show, we can use the question of pleasant or neutral body sensations when our clients experience fear, panic or confusion or unpleasant sensations such as trembling, tension or restlessness. By exploring an area in their body that feels good or neutral and staying with it, their self-regulation is stimulated and the strong activation decreases (Levine, 1998). This is usually shown by a deep breath, a sigh, yawn, or a spontaneous movement, such as straightening up.

We can also invite our clients to stay a little bit with the unpleasant sensation at the beginning, observing it, giving it space and exploring it without judgment. By observing the sensation, it sometimes dissolves. Other times, however, it initially intensifies and then decreases. For instance, a tension in the chest may intensify, possibly spreading to the shoulders or abdomen before finally releasing. If the unpleasant sensation does not or only partially dissolve, we encourage our clients to explore where it feels neutral or pleasant in their body. When they become aware of this area, the unpleasant sensation usually decreases. If necessary, they can pendulate slowly once or at most twice between the unpleasant and the pleasant or neutral body sensation (Levine 1998, 2011). This releases some tension or charge in their body with each change, and their nervous system gradually regulates and calms down.

Felt Sense—holistic internal sensation

Besides individual body sensations, the holistic inner body sensation or the so-called felt sense plays a special role in the healing process. According to Peter Levine (1998), it helps us to "feel more natural" and "grounded", so that we are more "at home" in our body (p. 80–81).

The work with body sensation was described in detail by Eugene Gendlin (2018), an Austrian-born philosopher and psychotherapist who emigrated to the USA in the 1930s, in his approach known as Focusing. He coined the term "felt sense". It does not refer to a single body sensation, such as a pressure in the stomach, but to a holistic physical feeling. We can perceive this, for example, in relation to an experience or a memory. It is a physical experience that encompasses everything we feel and know at a particular time about a particular topic, such as an event. For instance, if we remember a traumatic incident and direct our attention to our body, we can perceive a felt sense that appears in that moment. It is a "complex whole" that includes feelings, thoughts, meanings, memories, needs and wishes (Gendlin 2018, p. 39). According to Eugene Gendlin, "relief is associated with the emergence of such an experience, as though the body were grateful to be able to form its way of being as a whole" (ibid.). By allowing and observing the felt sense, it "opens up" and allows us to recognize or feel something new (ibid.). If we think of a traumatic experience and perceive the felt sense, e. g. rage and indignation can emerge from the initial fear and threat. By staying with our attention on the felt sense it changes; a new thought, an insight, a movement impulse or a new feeling arises. This change, which Eugene Gendlin calls the "felt shift", we can also notice in our body. Through the felt shift we feel something has changed in us. If we allow the newly created felt sense to continue, it will change again. By allowing and observing this, more and more relief arises as the mere perception leads to a discharge of arousal and tension and thus to a regulation of our nervous system. We recognize this by a sigh, a yawn, a deep breath or a—sometimes only small—movement.

References

Damasio A (2018) Descartes Irrtum. Fühlen, Denke und das menschliche Gehirn. List, Berlin (Descartes´ Error: Emotion, Reason, and the Human Brain. 2005, Penguin, London) Own translation

Emerson D (2016) Healing trauma through yoga. An online e-course. The Trauma Center at the Justice Ressource Institute, Brookline

Gendlin ET (2018) Focusing-orientierte Psychotherapie. Ein Handbuch der erlebensbezogenen Methode. Klett-Cotta, Stuttgart (Focusing-Oriented Psychotherapy. 1996, Guilford Press, New York) Own translation

Häuser W, Kosseva M, Üceyler N, Kloser P, Sommer C (2010) Emotional, physical, and sexual abuse in fibromyalgia syndrome: a systematic review with meta-analysis. Arthritis Care Res 63(6):808–820. https://doi.org/10.1002/acr.20328

Heller L (2003) Somatic Experiencing®. Training, Beginner I, September 2003, Penzberg, DE

Hüther G (2006) Wie Embodiment neurobiologisch erklärt werden kann. In: Storch M, Cantieni B, Hüther G, Tschacher W Embodiment. Die Wechselwirkung von Körper und Psyche verstehen und nutzen. Hans Huber, Bern, pp 73–97

Kolacz J, Porges SW (2018) Chronic diffuse pain and functional gastrointestinal disorders after traumatic stress: pathophysiology through a polyvagal perspective. Front Med 5:145. https://doi.org/10.3389/fmed.2018.00145

Levine PA, Frederick, A. (1998) Trauma-Heilung. Das Erwachen des Tigers. Unsere Fähigkeit, traumatische Erfahrungen zu transformieren. Synthesis, Essen (Waking the Tiger. Healing Trauma. The Innate Capacity to Transform Overwhelming Experiences. 1997, North Atlantic Books, Berkeley, CA) Quoted from original English version (p 73)

Levine PA (2008) Vom Trauma befreien. Wie Sie seelische und körperliche Blockaden lösen. Kösel, München (Healing Trauma. A Pioneering Program for Restoring the Wisdom of Your Body. 2005, Sounds True, Boulder) Own translation

Levine PA (2011) Sprache ohne Worte. Wie unser Körper Trauma verarbeitet und uns in die innere Balance zurückführt. Kösel, München (In an Unspoken Voice. How the Body Releases Trauma and Restores Goodness. 2010, North Atlantic Books, Berkeley) Own translation

Levine PA (2019a) Polyvagal-Theorie und Trauma. In: Porges SW, Dana D (Hrsg) Klinische Anwendungen der Polyvagal-Theorie. Ein neues Verständnis des Autonomen Nervensystems und seiner Anwendung in der therapeutischen Praxis. G. P. Probst, Lichtenau/Westfalen, pp 19–42 (Polyvagal Theory and Trauma. In: Porges SW, Dana D (Eds) Clinical Applications of The Polyvagal Theory. The Emergence of Polyvagal-Informed Therapies. 2018, W.W. Norton, New York, pp 3-26) Quoted from original English version (p 21)

Levine PA (2019b) Somatic Experiencing®. First Year. Training Material. Somatic-Experiencing Germany, Essen, DE

Porges SW (2018) Die Polyvagal-Theorie und die Suche nach Sicherheit. Traumabehandlung, soziales Engagement und Bindung. G. P. Probst, Lichtenau/Westfalen

Porges SW (2010) Die Polyvagal-Theorie. Neurophysiologische Grundlagen der Therapie. Emotionen, Bindung, Kommunikation und ihre Entstehung. Junfermann, Paderborn

Rothschild B (2002) Der Körper erinnert sich. Die Psychophysiologie des Traumas und der Traumabehandlung. Synthesis, Essen (The Body Remembers - The Psychophysiology of Trauma and Trauma Treatment. 2000, W.W. Norton, New York) Own translation

Rothschild B (2017) The body remembers. Volume 2. Revolutionizing trauma treatment. W.W. Norton, New York

The Human memory (2020) Declarative (explicit) and prozedural (implicit) memory. https://human-memory.net/explicit-implicit-memory/. Accessed 10 May 2020

Thieme (2020) via medici. https://viamedici.thieme.de. Accessed 22 May 2020 van der Kolk BA (2000) Trauma und Gedächtnis. In: van der Kolk BA, McFarlane AC, Weisaeth L (Hrsg) Traumatic Stress. Grundlagen und Behandlungsansätze. Theorie, Praxis und Forschung zu posttraumatischem Streß sowie Traumatherapie. Junfermann, Paderborn pp 221–240 (Trauma and Memory. In: van der Kolk, BA, McFarlane AC, Weisaeth L (Eds) Traumatic Stress: The Effects of Overwhelming Experience on Mind, Body and Society. 1996, Guilford Press, New York, pp 279–302)

Van der Kolk B (2016) Verkörperter Schrecken. In: Traumaspuren in Gehirn, Geist und Körper und wie man sie heilen kann. G. P. Probst, Lichtenau/Westfalen (The Body Keeps the Score. Mind, Brain and Body in the Transformation of Trauma. 2015, Penguin Books, London) Quoted from original English version (p 211)

Wimmer-Puchinger B, Lackner R (1997) Sexueller Mißbrauch in Kindheit und Jugend und seine gynäkologischen und sexuellen Kurz- und Langzeitfolgen. BM für Umwelt, Jugend & Familie, Vienna, AT (Sexual Abuse in Childhood and Adolescents and its Gynecological and Sexual Short- and Long-term Consequences. Austrian Ministry of Environment, Youth and Family)

Zanotta S (2018) Wieder ganz werden. Traumaheilung mit Ego-State-Therapie und Körperwissen. Carl Auer, Heidelberg (Somatic Ego State Therapy™ for Trauma Healing: Whole Again. 2024, Routledge, London) Own translation

Embodiment—The Interaction Between Body and Psyche

5

Contents

Embodiment is an interdisciplinary umbrella term for a new understanding of the interplay between body and psyche or body and mind (Bermeitinger et al. 2011). It also refers to the physical expression of a certain emotion (Tschacher 2006); on the one hand as "implementation of a specific emotion" within our body (Storch et al. 2006, p. 130), i.a., through a certain posture, on the other hand as body sensation that we discern in connection with a certain feeling. Part of the research on embodiment is devoted to the so-called embodied emotions, whereby the physiological effect of our emotions on our body is researched.

The preoccupation with the interaction of body and soul goes far back in human history. In ancient times, philosophers such as Aristotle already considered the body-soul question, i.e. the connection between body and soul or body and mind. Doctors of antiquity, like those of the Middle Ages, took both, body and soul into account in their treatment. Various philosophers and scientists of the modern era, such as Rene Descartes in the 17th and Charles Darwin in the 19th century, devoted themselves, among other things, to the interaction between feelings and the body. Modern psychosomatics, whose beginnings go back to the 19th century, also deal with the interaction between body and psyche and takes into account both psychological and physical factors in the development of physical illness and psychological disorders. A sub-discipline of psychosomatics, psychoneuroimmunology, has been researching the connection between the immune system and the psyche for about 30 years and could demonstrate in numerous studies the influence of psychological factors, such as chronic stress, on the immune system (e.g. Bae et al. 2019). So, the basic idea of embodiment is not new. The knowledge

R. Lackner, *Stabilization in Trauma Treatment*,
https://doi.org/10.1007/978-3-662-67480-2_5

of the connection between body and psyche is also reflected in our everyday language. Expressions such as "the hair on the back of his neck stands up" or "she has butterflies in her stomach" are just two examples of how our feelings are expressed through our body. The approach of embodiment shows the importance of this interplay and the necessity to include the body in counseling and therapeutic accompaniment (Storch et al. 2006).

The concept of embodiment originally came from cognitive science showing that thinking without a body is not possible. Our mind is always related to our body and both, mind and body, are related to our environment, in which they are embedded (Tschacher 2006). For example, the formation of ideas, such as of an object or an abstract concept as friendship, is based on sensory experience. Only with the help of our perception by grasping, seeing, hearing and feeling can we get an idea of something (Stangl 2019). Even in decision-making processes, our body and our physical sensations play an important role (Damasio 2018). These influence our decisions: when we have a positive sensation towards an option we are more likely to accept it and when having an unpleasant one we are more likely to reject it. Since the beginning of the 21st century, the term embodiment has been gaining increasing significance in psychology and psychotherapy, although there is neither a generally valid definition nor a general theory of embodiment.

Whether external circumstances, such as shocking news, or internal ones, such as the memory of a beautiful weekend, our psychological experience always affects our physical feeling and our body expression. And our body affects our psychological experience. A number of studies confirm this. For instance, a study by Glenn Weisfeld and Jody Beresford (1982 shows that students who receive a positive grade have a more upright posture than before. Those with a negative grade have a noticeably bent posture. The reverse effect, that is, that of our body on our psyche, could be demonstrated in one of the experiments by John Riskind and Carolyn Gotay (1982). In this experiment, one group of test persons assumed a bent posture with drooping shoulders, neck and head for 8 minutes, the comparison group sat in an upright posture. Afterwards, both groups had to assemble four geometric puzzles, two unsolvable and two solvable; the first group gave up significantly faster on the unsolvable puzzles than the second. Therefore, a bent posture still has an effect even when we no longer maintain it, by reducing our perseverance in the task to be performed afterwards. Blaise Pasquarelli and Nina Bull found as early as 1951 that "a certain posture not only enables the 'appropriate' emotion, but also makes the 'inappropriate' emotion impossible" (quoted in Storch 2006, p. 48). So we can hardly be cheerful in a hunched posture and hardly sad in an upright posture.

The concept of embodiment and the knowledge of embodiment research are decisive for our accompaniment of traumatized people. On the one hand, we can increase the effectiveness of stabilizing interventions by involving their body; for example, holistically experienced inner images, in which our clients consciously become aware of their body sensations evoked by them and let these affect them, are more profound and comprehensive than mere mental images, in which arising body sensations are not taken into account and perceived. On the other hand, by incorporating certain movements and postures we can support our clients in influencing their feelings and thus gain stability. For example, we can invite them to explore the effect of an upright posture or stretching their body on a feeling of resignation. Finally, by paying attention to and involving their body our clients can experience themselves increasingly embodied and consequently gain access to their inner strength and liveliness.

References

Bae Y-S, Shin E-C, Bae Y-S, Van Eden W (2019) Editorial: stress and immunity. Front Immunol 10:245

Bermeitinger C, Koch F, Wilborn DL (2011) Embodied emotions: emotions as language of the body? LOGOS Interdisziplinair 19(4):244–259

Damasio A (2018) Descartes Irrtum. Fühlen, Denken und das menschliche Gehirn. List, Berlin (Descartes´ Error: Emotion, Reason, and the Human Brain. 2005, Penguin, London)

Pasquarelli L, Bull N (1951) Experimental investigations of the body-mind continuum in affective states. J Nerv Ment Dis 113:512–521. Zit. In: Storch M (2006) Wie Embodiment in der Psychologie erforscht wurde. In: Storch M, Cantieni B, Hüther G, Tschacher W Embodiment. Die Wechselwirkung von Körper und Psyche verstehen und nutzen. Hans Huber, Bern, pp 35–72

Riskind JH, Gotay CC (1982) Physical posture: could it have regulatory or feedback effects on motivation and emotion? Motiv Emot 6(3):273–298

Stangl W (2019) Embodiment. Online Lexikon für Psychologie und Pädagogik. http://lexikon.stangl.eu/2175/embodiment/. Accessed 23 January 2019

Storch M (2006) Wie Embodiment in der Psychologie erforscht wurde. In: Storch M, Cantieni B, Hüther G, Tschacher W Embodiment. Die Wechselwirkung von Körper und Psyche verstehen und nutzen. Hans Huber, Bern, pp 35–72

Storch M, Cantieni B, Hüther G, Tschacher T (2006) Embodiment. Die Wechselwirkung zwischen Körper und Psyche verstehen und nutzen. Hans Huber, Bern

Tschacher W (2006) Wie Embodiment zum Thema wurde. In: Storch M, Cantieni B, Hüther G, Tschacher W Embodiment. Die Wechselwirkung zwischen Körper und Psyche verstehen und nutzen. Hans Huber, Bern, pp 11–34

Weisfeld GE, Beresford JM (1982) Erectness of posture as an indicate of dominance or success in humans. Motiv Emot 6:113–131. Cited in: Storch M, Cantieni B, Hüther G, Tschacher T (2006) Embodiment. Die Wechselwirkung zwischen Körper und Psyche verstehen und nutzen. Hans Huber, Bern

Resilience

6

Contents

In the last 20 years the term resilience has gained increasing importance in psychology and gradually also in psychotherapy. Meanwhile, there is a wealth of literature on resilience and a number of programs to strengthen it. This creates the impression that it is clear what is meant by resilience and how it can be measured and promoted. Yet, this is not the case.

The term resilience was first used in psychology by the American psychologist Jack Block in 1950, in relation to our ability to adapt to life changes. He coined the term "ego-resilience" and described it as "dynamic and resourceful regulation and equilibration of impulses and inhibitions" (Block and Kremen 1996, p. 351). This means that, depending on the situation and conditions, one should be controlled emotionally as little as possible and only as much as necessary.

The word resilience comes from the Latin word "resilire" and means "to jump back" or "to bounce back" (Pons 2020). In material science, resilience refers to the property of certain materials, such as foam, to return to their original state after external influence. The Duden (2020), a dictionary of the German language, describes resilience as "psychological resistance". This meaning is also often used in professional circles, in literature and in our everyday language. However, it does not do justice to the complexity of resilience. Moreover, in this way resilience is seen exclusively as a property of the individual, as if it were up to him alone to cope with a traumatic event. But that is not the case.

Resilience research is an interdisciplinary branch of science in which researchers from various disciplines participate, including psychology, sociology,

R. Lackner, *Stabilization in Trauma Treatment*,
https://doi.org/10.1007/978-3-662-67480-2_6

neuroscience and medicine. Accordingly, there are various contexts in which resilience is investigated, like the resilience of children from families with high risk factors, of people with chronic illnesses or of war refugees. In addition, there are various theoretical concepts of resilience and numerous factors to which it is attributed, like being symptom-free, well-being or experiencing positive feelings. It is also discussed whether resilience is a property, a skill or a process (Kalisch 2017).

For example, the American Psychological Association (APA 2020) understands resilience as "the process of adapting well in the face of adversity, trauma, tragedy, threats or significant sources of stress". For Norman Garmezy, the founder of resilience research, it is both a process and a skill and, moreover, the result of successful adaptation to challenging or threatening circumstances (Masten et al. 1990). The American resilience researcher George Bonanno (2004) understands resilience as the ability of a person to remain mentally and physically healthy despite shattering experiences and to maintain a stable balance. He describes it as a complex ability in which numerous factors are involved and which we all possess: "Humans are naturally resilient" (Bonanno 2017). Raffael Kalisch, a German neuroscientist and resilience researcher, sees resilience as "the maintenance or rapid restoration of mental health during and after adversity", understanding it as a complex dynamic process (2017, p. 28). Already these few definitions show how differently resilience is described.

The beginning of resilience research goes back to Norman Garmezy, who began in the 1970s to investigate why some children whose mothers suffer from schizophrenia cope better than others. Norman Garmezy discovered that children who had a good relationship with an adult could develop and flourish despite their mother's illness. The American psychologist Emmy Werner is considered a pioneer of resilience research with her Kauai long-term study, which she conducted together with her colleague Ruth Smith from 1955 with 698 inhabitants of the Hawaiian island of Kauai. This study was followed by a series of others in different countries. They all showed that resilience is determined by individual characteristics, such as a friendly, open and active nature, and by social support and social integration (Werner 2005). Additionally, it was shown that resilient people, when under stress, actively seek support and opportunities to change their lives for the better and take advantage of such opportunities.

The latest research increasingly shows that resilience is a complex adaptation process in which a variety of different factors are involved. However, each of them determining resilience only to a small extent; hence, there is no single determinent factor (Bonanno 2015; Southwick 2014). On the one hand, resilience is shaped by the individual's ability to adapt, on the other hand it is influenced by a number of environmental conditions. Consequently, there is a variety of mutually influencing factors: psychological, genetic and epigenetic, social, cultural and economic. In childhood this may be different; repeated studies show that for the development of resilience in children, three factors are primarily decisive: a healthy, stable relationship with an adult, the ability to emotionally self-regulate and have self-awareness, and the motivation to learn and adapt to conditions (Southwick et al. 2014).

Basically, we should not only look at resilience in relation to the individual person, but rather in a comprehensive social and societal context. There is also a branch of research that deals with the resilience of families and investigates what strengthens them. Another research branch deals with the so-called socio-ecological resilience and explores the key resources of the social, economic, cultural and political environment. Researching in this area, the medical anthropologist Catherine Panter-Brick (2014) suggests thinking about structural resilience and exploring how our society should be structured to promote our resilience. This would include, among other things, access to education and a good health system as well as secure and affordable housing.

So, resilience is increasingly seen in a comprehensive context. Here, risk factors play as much of a role as protective factors. These can be present before, during and after a traumatic event, such as previous traumatic experiences, witnessing the death or serious injury of another person during the event, and social support, employment and income afterwards as well as optimism, flexibility, worries and fears (Bonanno 2015). Each of these factors contribute only a small part to resilience. However, two stand out and seem to determine resilience more strongly: firstly, the area of relationships, social support and social integration and secondly, that of optimism, self-efficacy and trust in one's own coping ability. The latest research also shows that a key factor of resilience may be flexibility (Bonanno 2015); i.e. the flexible adaptation to the respective challenges and burdens. People who are able to apply different coping mechanisms and strategies flexibly to the respective stressful events seem to cope better and are less burdened by them (Southwick et al. 2014).

Some of these factors can be stable, others can be subject to fluctuations or depend on external factors and thus be unstable. For example, if we have a good social network at home, this can support our resilience, but if we are travelling and cannot access it, we are likely to be less resilient (Bonanno 2015).

Resilience research also shows that there are not simply resilient and non-resilient people, but that we can be resilient in one area and less resilient and vulnerable in another (Southwick 2014). For instance, children who have experienced physical and/or psychological violence can achieve very good academic performance and be resilient in terms of school, but at the same time they can develop psychological symptoms and are wounded in this respect. Hence, we can assume that resilience exists along a continuum, and that it can be present to different degrees in different areas of life.

Basically, we have a high potential to cope with stress and exceptional situations and to change and adapt, but for this we need basic social and material resources (Southwick et al. 2014). These include sufficient income, secure and affordable housing and social integration. To support resilience, it is therefore important to consider that we are embedded in a social and cultural environment. Interventions in one area also support others. In order to strengthen young children, for example, it is necessary to promote the resources of their parents and schools (ibid.). Resilience must therefore be viewed in a social and political context.

Apart from the different risk factors, resilience appears to be weakened by three aspects described by Martin Seligman (2006), the founder of Positive Psychology, the so-called three Ps, namely Personalization, Pervasiveness and Permanence.

Martin Seligman refers to Personalization as an internalized attribution, i.e. the conviction of being responsible for the occurrence of bad events. This is expressed in thoughts such as "It's all my fault" or "I attract bad luck".

Under Pervasiveness, i.e. continuity or omnipresence, Martin Seligman understands the tendency to generalize and assume that a traumatic event affects or destroys the entire life. Thoughts such as "Now everything is over" or "My whole life is destroyed" reflect this.

With Permanence Martin Seligman means the conviction that the effects of a traumatization are permanent and unchangeable and that there can be no improvement. This is shown in thoughts such as "It will never be good again".

Resilience is also impaired by the experience of helplessness and powerlessness at the time of the traumatic event. If we can remain actionable in a traumatic situation and organize help or free ourselves, this reduces the risk of post-traumatic symptoms. However, if we have no possibility of action, for example if we are trapped in a car accident, and/or our body instinctively reacts with freezing or collapsing, there is a high risk of developing post-traumatic symptoms (Levine 1998).

Resilience research gives us some important suggestions for our work with traumatized people, and in particular for their stabilization:

6.1 Resilience and Empowering Our Clients

Rachel Yehuda (2014), a New York psychiatrist and trauma expert emphasizes "that some of the most resilient people, at least that I know, may have had or still have very severe PTSD that they struggle with every day. But they don't succumb to its negative effects." (p. 3). She says that for her, resilience used to be the opposite of post-traumatic stress disorder and she divided traumatized people into two groups: those who are resilient and those who develop PTSD. Gradually, she realized that traumatized people can suffer from post-traumatic symptoms or PTSD and still be resilient at the same time. Rachel Yehuda's approach and words are close to my heart; I also experience many of my clients as both very burdened and very resilient. They frequently suffer from intense symptoms for years and at the same time they have an incredible strength to deal with them, to find ways to alleviate and cope with them, and to master their lives. Many have preserved their sense of humor, their empathy for others, their love and their ability to be happy about something despite the most severe traumatization. Even with people who describe themselves as emotionally numb and empty inside, I experience moments when there is a flicker of liveliness. They all have enormous strength that allowed them to survive and master the unimaginable and that leads them to fight for a betterment of their symptoms and their lives. For Rachel Yehuda (ibid.), this forward movement is an important aspect of resilience which includes the active, recurring decision "to keep moving forward" (p. 3). With this, for me, Rachel Yehuda expresses the strength and will very aptly that many traumatized people apply to live with their traumatization, to cope and free themselves from it.

It is essential to see our clients with this comprehensive view and to perceive them both in their wounding and in their intactness and strength. Many times I experience that our clients are not aware of their struggle and all that they have already done to cope with their trauma; they are too overburdened and occupied by their symptoms and the consequences of their traumatization. It is all the more important that we convey to them that they have mastered their lives in spite of their trauma and are still mastering them. Many have achieved a lot in their lives despite the most severe abuse, neglect or other repeated traumatic experiences, although they are suffering a lot from the consequences requiring a lot of strength from them.

By honoring all this, we contribute significantly to the stability of our clients; often making it possible for them to gain a new, more comprehensive view of themselves and their lives, which also allows them to recognize their power and strength. This is an important step that forms the foundation for their stabilization and overcoming their traumatization.

Example from practice

Dora, 49, experienced psychological violence and neglect from her mother from an early age. She still has an extremely difficult relationship with her and continues to experience devaluation and humiliation. In Dora's first marriage she was also exposed to violence for years and went through a long separation process with numerous threats from her partner. A later happy partnership suddenly ended due to the life-threatening illness and sudden death of her partner. Despite all of this, Dora always pursued her profession in the health care sector with a lot of commitment and dedication; she usually worked far beyond the prescribed hours. After another serious loss, Dora fell into a state of emergency that made it impossible for her to continue her work.

In one of our first conversations, Dora reproached herself severely, saying that she was doing so badly and was unable to return to her job quickly. She experiences herself as weak and lacking resilience. I make Dora aware that she has endured a lot in her life and *despite that* she has mastered her life and achieved so much. The latest event was a further great burden for her. Due to her previous difficult life situation, her capacity to cope with difficulties was already very much stretched. With the latest loss, her capacity was exhausted; and that is completely normal. We all only have a certain "capacity" to cope. *Despite everything* Dora is coping with her current situation, facing it and mastering her everyday life with her family, and doing everything to make herself better again.

"Despite that" and "despite everything" are key words for Dora, through which she gains a different, new view of her life and of herself. The "despite that" makes her aware of what she has endured and mastered in her life. Through this recognition, Dora feels stronger, empowered and proud of what was possible for her. It forms a turning point on her path leading to more stability and self-esteem. ◀

6.2 Resilience as an Aspect of Psychoeducation

Like Dora, many traumatized people are hardly aware of their strength and previous coping and mastery of their traumatic experiences. Rather, I repeatedly experience that those affected believe themselves to be weak and have a lack of resilience, especially when they compare themselves to people who have experienced similar things but seem to suffer little or not at all. Some, who have experienced psychological and/or physical violence from their parents or have been traumatized by an accident, compare themselves to refugees who have survived war and torture. They think that what they have experienced is comparatively harmless and that they should suffer less from the consequences. Or they even deny themselves the right to feel burdened by what they have experienced. People who have survived dramatic events in which others have died often think that they should be doing well because they have survived. That always touches me very much and it affects me that even in the face of painful experiences we think in terms of performance categories and believe that we have to maintain our full performance capacity.

Traumatic experiences cannot be compared with each other; they are much too complex and multi-layered. Nor can we draw comparisons between our reaction to a traumatic event and that of someone else. How we react is determined by a multitude of factors and is therefore not comparable to the reaction of another person. In any case, even among resilience researchers, it is not quite clear what resilience really means. Are we resilient if we are mostly doing well and pushing away, repressing and ignoring what we have experienced? Are we resilient if we face up to what has happened and have to struggle with all the consequences? Probably we are resilient in both moments in different ways. And what about when our body freezes in the moment of danger because neither fight nor flight is possible and this freezing does not dissolve and continues to exist?

Once again we see how multi-layered the topic of resilience is. That is why it is so important to convey to our clients the complexity of traumatization, of its possible effects and coping processes as well as of resilience. If I make my clients aware of this complexity and emphasize that every person reacts in an individual way, that every traumatic event is unique, and that overcoming it and resilience always have to be seen in the greater context, this gives them great relief. It helps them to broaden their view, enabling them to no longer experience others as only strong or stronger than themselves and themselves as weak. Rather, despite their wounding, our clients can then perceive themselves and their traumatic experience more comprehensively and recognize their own strength and ability to overcome it.

Suggestions from resilience research for our practice

The results of resilience research can greatly enrich and support our work with traumatized people, especially in regard to their stabilization.

As we have seen, there are three main areas among the many factors that contribute more substantially to resilience: firstly self-efficacy, confidence in coping and optimism, secondly social support and social integration and thirdly flexibility (Bonanno 2015; Southwick et al. 2014).

- **Self-efficacy, confidence and optimism**
  Strengthening their self-efficacy and their trust in their ability to have an impact on something and to influence it, is particularly important for traumatized people. That is why stabilization exercises are so helpful; because our clients can discover that they can influence their well-being. We can also strengthen their self-efficacy by reinforcing their self-determination; e.g., by inviting them to check all suggested interventions and exercises, noticing whether they are suitable for them and to reject or discard them if they are not understandable, consistent or helpful.
  Among other things, our clients' confidence can be promoted by working with resources, body awareness and inner images. For example, by visualizing a pleasant image and noticing the positive feelings and body sensations it evokes, our clients can experience strength or centering and gain a lot of confidence in their healing. To support a positive view of life, we can also incorporate interventions from Positive and Prospective Psychology into the accompaniment of our clients. For instance, by suggesting they think about what went well that day every evening, we support them by focusing their attention more on positive moments in their life (Seligman 2012).
- **Social support and social integration**
  Our reliable, empowering accompaniment is a form of social support for our clients, which can reduce their feeling of isolation. Regardless of this, we can encourage them to maintain and expand social contacts or together consider new ways to find new contacts and build up a social environment in which they feel integrated.
- **Flexibility**
  We can support the flexibility of our clients, for example, by offering them various stabilizing exercises, they can try out and apply flexibly and experimentally in everyday life according to the given situation and need.

References

APA (2020) American Psychological Association. https://www.apa.org. Accessed 14 May 2020

Block G, Kremen AM (1996) IQ and ego-resiliency: conceptual and empirical connections and separateness. J Pers Soc Psychol 70(2):349–361

Bonanno GA (2004) Loss, trauma, and human resilience: have we underestimated the human capacity to thrive after extremely aversive events? Am Psychol 59(1):20–28

Bonanno GA (2015) Trauma and resilience: from heterogeneity to flexibility. Lecture. New York Teachers College, Columbia University. https://www.youtube.com/watch?v=gvxk-75brpU. Accessed 20 June 2020

Bonanno GA (2017) Human resilience in the face of loss and trauma. https://www.youtube.com/watch?v=KcZ1Zn9HjkE. Accessed 20 June 2020

Der Duden (2020) https://www.duden.de. Accessed 20 May 2020

Kalisch R (2017) Der resiliente Mensch. Wie wir Krisen erleben und bewältigen. Neueste Erkenntnisse aus Hirnforschung und Psychologie. Berliner Verlag, Berlin

Levine PA, Frederick A (1998) Trauma-Heilung. Das Erwachen des Tigers. Unsere Fähigkeit, traumatische Erfahrungen zu transformieren. Synthesis, Essen (Waking the Tiger: Healing Trauma: The Innate Capacity to Transform Overwhelming Experiences. 1997, North Atlantic Books, Berkeley)

Masten AS, Best KM, Garmezy N (1990) Resilience and development: Contributions from the study of children who overcome adversity. Development and Psychpathology 2(4):425–444

Panter-Brick C (2014) In: Southwick SM, Bonanno GA, Masten AS, Panter-Brick C, Yehuda R. Resilience definitions, theory, and challenges: interdisciplinary perspectives. Eur J Psychotraumatol 5. https://doi.org/10.3402/ejpt.v5.25338

Pons (2020) Onlinewörterbuch. https://de.pons.com. Accessed 20 May 2020

Seligman M (2006) Learned optimism: how to change your mind and your life. Vintage Books, New York

Seligman M (2012) Flourish. Wie Menschen aufblühen. Die Positive Psychologie des gelingenden Lebens. Kösel, München (Flourish. A Visionary New Understanding of Happiness and Well-Being. 2011, Free Press, New York)

Southwick SM (2014) In: Southwick SM, Bonanno GA, Masten AS, Panter-Brick C, Yehuda R. Resilience definitions, theory, and challenges: interdisciplinary perspectives. Eur J Psychotraumatol 5. https://doi.org/10.3402/ejpt.v5.25338

Southwick SM, Bonanno GA, Masten AS, Panter-Brick C, Yehuda R (2014) Resilience definitions, theory, and challenges: interdisciplinary perspectives. Eur J Psychotraumatol 5. https://doi.org/10.3402/ejpt.v5.25338

Werner E (2005) Resilience and recovery: findings from the Kauai Longitudinal Study. Res Policy Pract Child Ment Health 19(1):11–14

Yehuda R (2014) In: Southwick SM, Bonanno GA, Masten AS, Panter-Brick C, Yehuda R. Resilience definitions, theory, and challenges: interdisciplinary perspectives. Eur J Psychotraumatol 5. https://doi.org/10.3402/ejpt.v5.25338

Post-Traumatic Growth 7

Contents

Post-traumatic Growth (PTG) is a term coined by Richard Tedeschi in the 1990s. It refers to his observation that many affected people experience a positive personal transformation after a traumatic event, i.e. a positive post-traumatic development (Tedeschi and Moore 2016).

The idea of growing and maturing personally through a tragic event can be found in religious writings and in myths, legends and fairy tales, as well as in plays and novels. In religions and spiritual currents such as Christian mysticism, life crises and traumatic experiences are often described as triggers for spiritual awakening or deepening.

In the meantime, there have been a number of studies on post-traumatic growth: in connection with accidents and natural disasters, serious illnesses such as multiple sclerosis or HIV infection / AIDS, grief and war deployments (Barbir 2016). According to the studies, on average 60% of people experience a positive transformation after traumatic events (Calhoun and Tedeschi 2006, cited in Tedeschi and Moore 2016). Richard Tedeschi and Lawrence Calhoun (1996, 2004) describe five types of post-traumatic growth:

- increased appreciation of life and change in priorities
- improvement in personal relationships
- discovery of one's personal strength
- recognition of new paths and possibilities and
- spiritual change and a new understanding of life

R. Lackner, *Stabilization in Trauma Treatment*,
https://doi.org/10.1007/978-3-662-67480-2_7

Post-traumatic growth usually goes hand in hand with post-traumatic symptoms or post-traumatic stress disorder; moreover, it seems that it is possible only through this. Studies show that people who develop post-traumatic symptoms more often experience post-traumatic growth than those who remain symptom-free. PTG therefore seems to be possible only through a certain degree of inner struggle with the shock, challenge and burden that a traumatic event brings with it. Only then can the process of post-traumatic growth begin, which can ultimately lead us to a more fulfilling and conscious life. Study results suggest that people who experience PTG perceive their lives as fuller, richer and often more meaningful (Calhoun and Tedeschi 2006, cited in Tedeschi and Moore 2016). Thus, traumatization can change our view of life; like "a window into a new perspective on how you are living your life" (Tedeschi and Moore 2016, p. 3). This does not mean that we are less burdened; on the contrary, post-traumatic growth apparently presupposes a burden.

The concept of post-traumatic growth is also critically illuminated. On the one hand, the previous investigations are based exclusively on subjective assessments of the respondents and so far there are no prospective long-term studies that compare before and after a traumatic experience. On the other hand, individual studies show that a higher degree of PTG also correlates with a higher degree of post-traumatic symptoms (Engelhard et al. 2015). Hence, there are considerations that post-traumatic growth is less a consequence of coping, but rather a coping process in itself. Accordingly, the perception of having experienced a positive change due to a traumatic experience could be a form of "self-enhancing illusion", which enables those affected to bear and balance the burden (Dekel et al. 2012, p. 6). In this sense, the experience of a positive change can be a coping mechanism that needs to be supported. Regardless of these considerations, it is a fact that some people gain depth and maturity due to their traumatic experiences and live their lives more consciously and appreciatively. In this case, post-traumatic growth is likely to require a cognitive engagement with the traumatic event.

Example from practice

Thomas, 34 years old, had gone off-piste snowboarding and got caught in an avalanche. He had relied on the assessment of a friend that the slope was safe to ride. Shortly before his friend had assured him, Thomas had felt an insecure feeling. He hesitated, but then followed his friend's okay and skied off. Suddenly an avalanche set off and took Thomas with it. Thanks to his airbag, he was not completely buried by the avalanche. In processing this experience, Thomas became aware that before the descent he had strongly felt that the slope was not safe. If he had followed his feeling and not gone, he would not have gotten into the avalanche. He could have relied on his intuition. On the basis of this experience and the insight gained, Thomas decided from now on to trust and follow his intuition and his feeling for situations and people. ◄

Just like Thomas, we can retrospectively come to a realization and make a decision to change ourselves or set a certain priority through traumatic experiences. Sometimes they can make us realign our lives and live it more consciously and appreciatively:

Example from practice

Gregor, 63, survived the 2004 tsunami in Thailand with his wife. One of his legs was seriously injured at the time and he could not escape the danger zone; however, a Thai discovered him and brought him to a hill with his scooter. From there he was then taken to a nearby hospital. Only 2/3 days later, Gregor heard in a roundabout way that his wife had also survived. Gregor experienced something indescribable. The images and horror have accompanied him for a long time. However, the fact that he and his wife survived made him change his life fundamentally. He tries to live more consciously and gratefully and is involved in several aid projects. ◀

For some people, a new life task or priority triggered by a traumatic event can be a necessity in order to be able to bear the experience at all and to give it any meaning, e.g., when a loved one dies due to that event.

Example from practice

Arthur, 52, lost his 17-year-old daughter in a traffic accident caused by an alcoholized friend of hers. Afterwards he began campaigning in schools against alcohol and drugs while driving. ◀

Traumatic experiences can also leave such far-reaching and profound traces in us that a positive change and so a post-traumatic growth are not possible:

Example from practice

Anne, 74, is severely traumatized by her Second World War-traumatized parents. In her childhood and youth she was exposed to their repeated emotional breakdowns as well as physical violence, denigration, sanctions and neglect. Anne still struggles with the massive psychological and physical consequences. She has read a lot about trauma, including post-traumatic growth; in retrospect in all that she has experienced, she cannot find anything positive. For her it was all terrible. The idea of post-traumatic growth is unimaginable for her in view of her history. ◀

Like Anne, there are many people who do not experience positive post-traumatic changes. According to the study by Calhoun and Tedeschi (2006), this should be 40% (cited in Tedeschi and Moore 2016). For them, the idea of post-traumatic growth can sometimes be an imposition. In view of the intensity and massive shock that traumatic experiences can mean and the massive symptomatology that often follows, the idea of post-traumatic growth at first seems inappropriate or even cynical. Immediately after the traumatic event and in the time afterwards, many people are not able to experience positive changes or even attribute a positive meaning to what they have experienced. Yet, over time this may be possible; and so a new, deeper look at life, finding meaning or reflecting on something new can become possible.

As we can see post-traumatic growth is a complex phenomenon in which many factors play a role. First, personality factors such as openness to new experiences, optimism and self-efficacy as well as social support seem to favor its development (Slezáckovά 2019). Secondly, the type, duration and effects of traumatic experiences are likely to be determining factors. Many questions, however, remain unanswered.

Richard Tedeschi and Bret Moore (2016) describe various interventions that can stimulate the process of post-traumatic growth. They encourage different questions appropriate to the five areas in which they recognize positive changes as an expression of PTG. With regard to recognizing one's own inner strength they suggest asking: "What have you done to cope that most clearly demonstrates the strength that has gotten you through this difficult time?" (p. 73). With regard to recognizing new possibilities, they ask, e.g., about things we would like to do, regardless of whether they are feasible or not. To support a positive view of life, they suggest mindfulness exercises such as consciously being aware of our environment.

These and many other suggestions are very basic interventions that should be part of stabilization anyway. In particular, the question of what has enabled our clients to survive and cope with the traumatic experiences is very important; with it we can specifically support them in recognizing and feeling their strength. Fundamentally, it is important to reinforce our clients as soon as we notice or they tell us that they have gained an insight through their traumatic experiences, found a new aim or meaning in their life, or could change themselves or something in their life for the better. We can always pick up these changes and use them as resources. Additionally, we can support our clients in noticing more positive things in their lives, picking up interests and implementing them and/or establishing social contacts; all these are very general aspects of stabilization. However, it would be inappropriate to specifically point out the possibility of post-traumatic growth or even to specifically stimulate it without our clients addressing it themselves. After all, we cannot assume that they will experience positive changes through their traumatic experiences; this idea is inappropriate for many of them because of their experiences. It is a fact that some people gain depth and maturity through traumatic experiences and live their lives more consciously and appreciatively afterwards. Yet, it is also true that for many people this is not possible. We should be aware of and be open to both possibilities.

References

Barbir L (2016) Positive psychology and trauma: understanding and enhancing posttraumatic growth. Positive psychology. Theory Appl 11(1):21–26

Calhoun LG, Tedeschi RG (Eds) (2006) Handbook of posttraumatic growth: research and practice. Routledge, New York. Zit. In: Tedeschi RG, Moore BA (2016) The posttraumatic growth workbook. Coming through trauma wiser, stronger, and more resilient. A step-by-step guide to help you. New Harbinger Publications, Oakland

Dekel S, Ein-Dor T, Solomon Z (2012) Posttraumatic growth and posttraumatic stress: a longitudinal study. Psychol Trauma Theory Res Pract Policy 4(1):94–101. https://doi.org/10.1037/a0021865

Engelhard IM, Lomen MJJ, Sijbrandij M (2015) Changing for better or worse? Posttraumatic growth reported by soldiers deployed to Iraq. Clin Psychol J 3(5):789–796. https://doi.org/10.1177/2167702614549800

Slezáckovà A (2019) Posttraumatic Growth. Lecture, 5th Positive Psychology Tour, June, 21–23, 2019, Graz/AT

Tedeschi RG, Calhoun LG (1996) The posttraumatic growth inventory: measuring the positive legacy of trauma. J Trauma Stress 9(3):455–471

Tedeschi RG, Calhoun LG (2004) Posttraumatic growth: conceptual foundations and empirical evidence. Psychol Inq 15(1):1–18

Tedeschi RG, Moore BA (2016) The posttraumatic growth workbook. Coming through trauma wiser, stronger, and more resilient. A step-by-step guide to help you. New Harbinger Publications, Oakland

References

Part II
The Variety of Ways and Means of Stabilization

Our psychological stability can be regained, strengthened and consolidated in various ways and with different approaches and methods.

It is crucial to suggest distinct approaches and techniques to our clients and to try them out with them in order to give them the opportunity to find those that are most effective and easy to implement. It is sensible to take into account as many approaches as possible so that our clients can gain comprehensive and profound stability. Taking up and expanding existing resources, being aware of one's own body, inner images and certain movements are just a few of the many possibilities.

For some of our clients, a few exercises are enough to become or feel stable. Others need a series or variety of interventions. The initially found stabilization exercises frequently accompany them throughout the entire treatment process, often even beyond. However, they can also lose their importance or necessity in the course of the treatment or be replaced by other exercises that better correspond to the current needs of our clients. At the beginning of the treatment, generally interventions are essential, through which they can experience and regain a feeling of safety. If this grows over time, then the relevance of the original exercise decreases. Usually another important aspect for stability is then revealed, which requires support. During the treatment it frequently turns out to be necessary to deal with different possibilities of reducing tension and rage; corresponding vents that are suitable for our clients decisively contribute to their stability. Accordingly, it often requires an extension or change of the stabilization exercises. Therefore, it is important to pay attention as to whether the techniques found at the beginning are still helpful, sufficient and consistent for our clients. If this is not the case, it is necessary to explore and find other or further possibilities of stabilization. The entire stabilization is a living, dynamic process subject to change. Each individual intervention and exercise contributes a piece to the stabilization of our clients. Like different pieces of a puzzle, they complement each other over time with their different effects and thus build, promote and strengthen their stability in a comprehensive and holistic way.

In the following we will look at the variety of different ways and possibilities of stabilization.

Resources—The Heart of Stabilization

8

Contents

Resources form the heart of stabilization and the basis of any trauma treatment. They are at the beginning and build an essential part of the entire course of treatment, so to speak the ground on which it takes place. They include everything that strengthens us, is good for us, makes us feel safe and lets uns become stable; consequently, they encompass all exercises that have a stabilizing effect. Resources evoke positive feelings, body sensations and thoughts in us, strengthen us and give us support and safety. They inspire confidence and trust, and enrich us and make our life more colorful and fulfilled.

Resources represent a counterweight to traumatization and its sequelae; they counteract them, cushion them, balance them out and make it easier for us to endure, cope with and process what we have experienced. Moreover, resources support our body in its self-regulation, by balancing both an over- and an underactivation of our nervous system (Heller and Heller 2003; Wiedenmann 2019). Furthermore, they connect us with our vitality and liveliness and with our innermost self (Levine 2008; Wiedenmann 2019). The more resources we have available and the better we integrate them into our everyday life, the sooner we can gain stability and face the force of traumatic experiences and process them.

Resources are among the most effective factors of successful psychotherapy (Gassmann and Grawe 2006). Therefore, resource activation is the "primary principle of action" of any psychotherapy. Yet, stimulating resources is less a

R. Lackner, *Stabilization in Trauma Treatment*,
https://doi.org/10.1007/978-3-662-67480-2_8

technique than a "therapeutic attitude" that should run through the entire course of treatment (Grawe and Grawe-Gerber 1999, p. 63). With a resource-oriented attitude we focus on all those aspects in our clients and their lives that support and strengthen them. Our task is to help them, like a midwife or a process facilitator, to discover, use and consolidate their resources. By encouraging them to develop additional, new resources, we further expand—in the spirit of empowerment—the possibilities of our clients to influence themselves and their well-being. Moreover, this experience of being able to act on themselves and their body in a regulating, stabilizing and healing way, strengthens their self-efficacy and autonomy.

Right at the beginning of any trauma treatment it is important to show our clients the significance of resources. As with the illustration of the significance of stabilization, doing this I use the image of a balance beam with two plates: one of the two platess carries the burden of traumatization; to balance this, the second plate must be filled with resources. Working with resources is not a distraction from traumatic experiences and does not mean ignoring them at all; it is a necessary counterweight making it possible to overcome the traumatization.

A resource can be anything: a positive experience or memory, a dear person, a place where we feel comfortable, a hobby that fulfills us, a skill that we are proud of, a strengthening thought or a pleasant body sensation. Even something neutral can be a resource (Wiedenmann 2020); for example, the sight of an object that has a neutral effect on us or being aware of a body sensation that we experience as neutral. Mostly, something neutral has a calming, relieving or liberating effect on us, or evokes a feeling of openness or pleasant emptiness.

Like Peter Levine (1998) and the US trauma therapists Diane and Laurence Heller (2003), we can roughly distinguish between internal and external resources. In addition, I see our body as a special resource of its own.

8.1 External Resources

External resources include social relationships and social integration, especially people close to us, but also animals and communities such as sports clubs or religious communities. Additionally, professional activities, charitable tasks, creative activities, movement and sport can be external resources. Nature, certain places, music, literature, movies and certain objects, such as a photo or a talisman, may be resources, too, just like sensory impressions such as the view of greenery or the scent of oranges.

8.2 Internal Resources

Internal resources encompass our talents, skills, qualities and strengths such as courage, sensitivity or endurance. Our love for someone or something or our joy in someone or something are also internal resources. They include beautiful memories, positive inner images or imagining, confirming or calming thoughts, mottos and affirmations. Our goals, plans and visions can be internal resources, too. Likewise our inner connection to a deceased person or an ancestor, or to a spiritual being or power may be resources as can our spiritual accesses and faith, prayers and meditation.

8.3 Our Body—A Resource in Itself

Our body is a special resource. It can neither be assigned to the internal nor to the external ones; rather, it is connected to each resource, whether internal or external, and is involved in it. As soon as we consciously experience a resource or just imagine it, we can feel positive sensations in our body, like warmth in our stomach with a beautiful memory, a feeling of spaciousness in our chest when looking out from a mountain peak or vitality in our entire body when dancing.

Furthermore, our body is a resource in itself. On the one hand, by perceiving with our senses and so experiencing pleasant physical sensations and positive feelings; for instance, when we feel the warmth of the sun on our skin or let a piece of chocolate melt on our tongue. On the other hand, by noticing pleasant sensations in our body and experiencing positive feelings (Rothschild 2002); for example, the sensation of warmth in our stomach that gives us a feeling of safety, or of strength in our chest that evokes a feeling of power in us.

Even when we move, we can experience our body as a resource (provided we are not impaired by pain or physical restrictions), e.g., by perceiving it as alive, powerful or relaxed and feeling internally vital, strong or free.

Every resource we have is supportive; however, by consciously experiencing the positive feelings and physical sensations associated with it, it becomes an intense experience and thus even more supportive. When I talk to my clients about their resources, I always suggest that they recall one or the other and consciously experience it or imagine carrying it out. Meanwhile, I invite them to consciously perceive the feelings and physical sensations that arise. I am always amazed at the effectiveness of this simple intervention. It is clearly visible: Most of the time, my clients' facial features relax, their skin color becomes a little rosier, they often straighten up or move a little and usually they smile; overall, they generally look more relaxed, present and alive.

It makes a noticeable difference whether I merely carry out a resource, such as singing or running, or, at the same time, consciously notice the physical sensations and feelings it arouses. Similarly, it makes a difference whether I simply think of a resource, such as a beautiful memory, or envision it and thereby feel the associated feelings and physical sensations. For instance, remembering a walk on the beach may be nice. However, if we also make ourself aware of the sound of the sea, its smell, the warmth of the sun on our skin, the warm sand under our feet, the wind blowing over our skin and through our hair, the vastness we see in front of us, it is a completely different, namely a comprehensive, holistic and thus fulfilling experience. We are embedded and encompassed in our entirety, with our body, our feelings, our thoughts.

This holistic imaginative experience—that is, the conscious experiencing or imagining of a resource, the perceived feelings and the felt physical sensations—is one of the most effective interventions for stabilization. We will go into this in more detail in chap. 10. Such consciously and intensely experienced and embodied resources have a direct effect on our nervous system. Depending on the experience they have a calming effect (e.g. with the feeling of safety) or an activating one (e.g. with joy). On the other hand, by consciously experiencing a resource new neural connections are formed in our brain or existing ones are strengthened. Through the positive experience, which is equivalent to a success, "the mechanism is set in motion that makes the corresponding neural network more efficient" (Storch 2019, p. 17). By regularly allowing ourselves this success through repeating it, the positive experiences and states are gradually strengthened in us and become an important stabilizing factor.

For this reason it is important to recommend our clients to incorporate their resources into their everyday life and to experience them regularly, preferably daily, and consciously—in reality or in their imagination. Through the increasing strengthening and anchoring of the resources, they become even more effective. In addition, they are more quickly and easily accessible, even in critical moments, such as in the case of massive fear.

Caution: Sometimes resources may "flip" (Wiedenmann 2020); for example, if we stay with them for too long or if they are linked to unpleasant experiences. Therefore, it is important to pay attention to staying with a resource only as long as it is exclusively experienced as pleasant.

8.4 Notes on "Questionable" Resources

From a health perspective, some of the resources our clients mention are far from beneficial; such as cigarettes, alcohol, cannabis or intense watching television and playing computer games. Especially at the beginning of trauma treatment and stabilization, these are often the only options that at least temporarily provide them with some stability. When our clients tell us about these or similar resources, it is important to ask when and in what situations they use these means or activities and what effect they have on them. The effects, such as reduced tension and dampened emotions, reflect the burden and distress as well as the needs and desires of our clients giving us a clear indication of how we need to support them. In general, addictive substances or addictive behavior have a self-regulating effect, for instance by helping to reduce tension, enabling sleep or inhibiting intrusive thoughts. For our clients it is very relieving when we understand these means as attempts at self-regulation and coping with their traumatic experiences, and convey this to them and show understanding. Nevertheless, it is important to discuss that these are not healthy resources in the medium and long term, and that it is our task to support our clients in improving their self-care. For this reason alone, exploring different resources and integrating them into everyday life is so necessary.

It would be very problematic if we were to put pressure on our clients to stop using these means, or even make our joint work dependent on ending them. If we urge them to quit their addictive behavior before they could have processed their trauma, we take away from our clients an, albeit not positive, yet existing possibility of self-regulation. Just at the beginning of a trauma treatment this would be critical, as trauma-related content would then intrude into their consciousness and thus increase their psychological burden considerably. Therefore, it is necessary to support our clients first and foremost in finding and consolidating other suitable, stabilizing possibilities. Only then can they reduce and gradually give up unfavorable or health-endangering resources. Here too,—as always—the principle of "Trauma first" applies. Traumatic experiences must be processed first, only then can other topics such as addiction be worked on. If helpful resources and stabilization options are established and the trauma is processed, the addictive behavior often changes, too.

References

Gassmann D, Grawe K (2006) General change mechanisms: the relation between problem activation and resource activation in successful and unsuccessful therapeutic interactions. Clin Psychol Psychother 13(1):1–11

Grawe K, Grawe-Gerber M (1999) Ressourcenaktivierung. Ein primäres Wirkprinzip der Psychotherapie. Psychotherapeut 44(2):63–73

Heller DP, Heller LS (2003) Crash-Kurs zur Selbsthilfe nach Verkehrsunfällen: Vermeidung und Auflösung von traumatischen Erlebnissen. Synthesis, Essen (Crash Course: Auto Accident Recovery Breakthrough: A Self-Healing Guide to Auto Accident Trauma and Recovery. 2002, North Atlantic Books, Berkeley)

Levine PA, Frederick A (1998) Trauma-Heilung. Das Erwachen des Tigers. Unsere Fähigkeit, traumatische Erfahrungen zu transformieren. Synthesis, Essen (Waking the Tiger: Healing Trauma: The Innate Capacity to Transform Overwhelming Experiences. 1997, North Atlantic Books, Berkeley)

Levine PA (2008) Vom Trauma befreien. Wie Sie seelische und körperliche Blockaden lösen. Kösel, München (Healing Trauma. A Pioneering Program for Restoring the Wisdom of Your Body. 2005, Sounds True, Boulder)

Rothschild B (2002) Der Körper erinnert sich. Die Psychophysiologie des Traumas und der Traumabehandlung. Synthesis, Essen (The Body Remembers. The Psychophysiology of Trauma and Treatment. 2000, W.W. Norton, New York)

Storch M (2019) Das Zürcher Ressourcen Modell ZRM. http://majastorch.de/download/zrm.pdf. Accessed 1 October 2019

Wiedenmann I (2019) Somatic Experiencing®. Training, Beginner I, February/March 2019, Seitenstetten, AT

Wiedenmann I (2020) Somatic Experiencing®. Training, Intermediate II, October 2020, Seitenstetten, AT

References

9 Mindfulness and Self-Awareness

Contents

Being in the present moment is one of the most important and helpful skills for traumatized people (Fisher 1999). To acquire and develop it, mindfulness and self-awareness are necessary. Hence, both form fundamental elements of stabilization, enabling us to act on our body in a regulating way, so that our inner self can calm down. With their help we can center ourselves and come into our core. Moreover, we can gain inner distance to stirring, burdensome and threatening emotions, thoughts, memories, inner images and body sensations.

Mindfulness means being present in the here and now, perceiving what is to be perceived in this moment, whether it is inside or outside. The Vietnamese monk Thich Nhat Hanh (2005) describes mindfulness as "active awareness" (p. 16) and as the ability to "become aware of what is happening in the present moment" (p. 14). It means "truly being present" with what we do (Thich Nhat Hanh 2011, p. 16).

The interest in mindfulness began in the 1960s/1970s, on the one hand through Thich Nhat Hanh, his books and his movement of "Interbeing", on the other hand through the molecular biologist Jan Kabat-Zinn, who developed his mindfulness-based program for stress reduction (MBSR) in the 1970s. Originally designed for people with chronic illnesses and psychological challenges its effect has been scientifically researched and proven by a large number of studies. For example, based

R. Lackner, *Stabilization in Trauma Treatment*,
https://doi.org/10.1007/978-3-662-67480-2_9

on a meta-analysis of 209 studies with a total of over 12,000 participants Bassam Khoury et al. (2013) were able to show that fear, depression and stress symptoms can be treated effectively with the help of mindfulness-based therapy (MBT; among others MBSR).

Meanwhile, mindfulness has increasingly gained importance in medicine, psychology and psychotherapy. Furthermore, the interest in mindfulness and its application in everyday life is generally spreading more and more in our Western society.

Mindfulness is a core piece of Buddhism and is usually associated with it. However, it is part of every spiritual tradition and practice, such as Hinduism and yoga, or Christianity and its recently rediscovered body exercises as well as its heart prayer (Steinmetz 2018).

An essential aspect of mindfulness, which is described in particular in Buddhist teaching, is unbiased, non-judgmental perception. This is usually very difficult for us in our Western society, since we learn to judge everything and experience ourselves being evaluated from an early age. The basic attitude of mindfulness is therefore less common to the prevailing attitude in our Western world: Among other things, it means to be open, curious, unprejudiced, to accept and respect and to let go.

In our work with traumatized people this attitude is essential; with it we convey openess to our clients and a feeling of being accepted, appreciated and of normality. In this way we lay the foundation for them to feel safe with us and for stabilization and trauma processing to be possible at all.

9.1 Self-Awareness

Self-Awareness is a form of mindfulness. It refers to being aware of what we perceive inside ourselves and in our body. It means being aware of our thoughts, inner images and feelings as well as our physical sensations, our breath and our impulses to act. For Bessel van der Kolk, self-awareness and its development are "at the core of recovery" and consequently a key to healing trauma (2016, p. 249).

Now, numerous scientific studies confirm that mindfulness or self-awareness exercises can reduce the symptoms of PTSD (Thompson et al. 2011). In particular, non-judgmental perception and observation seem to be important factors. Mindfulness exercises also have a positive effect on depression and chronic pain (van der Kolk 2016); both are frequently symptoms of traumatized people. Neuroscientific studies show that, for example, attentive observation of the breath improves the regulation of our emotions (Doll et al. 2016). They reduce the activity of the amygdala, which is responsible for our emotions, including fear. In addition, they increase the integration of the amygdala and the prefrontal cortex, which is associated with improved ability to be mindful. By reducing the activity of the amygdala and increasing that of the prefrontal cortex, the risk of "reactivity to potential triggers" is reduced" (van der Kolk 2016, p. 251). Furthermore, mindfulness and self-awareness exercises calm our sympathetic nervous system, so that we are "less likely to be thrown into fight-or-flight" (ibid. p. 250). They improve our ability to perceive body sensations; "the non-judgmental observation" apparently has a positive effect "on the functioning of the brain" by using the prefrontal cortex "to support the observation of the sensumotor experience" (Ogden et al. 2010, p. 268).

However, more recently some researchers have taken a critical look at the large number of studies on mindfulness and mindfulness-based interventions and have pointed out that these are often inadequate. They usually have no control group and ignore the question of possible negative effects (e.g. Baer et al. 2019; van Dam et al. 2017). Individual studies draw attention to the fact that mindfulness exercises and meditation can, among other things, trigger and intensify fear, panic attacks and traumatic memories (Lomas et al. 2015; van Dam et al. 2017). Hence, when conveying mindfulness-based interventions and exercises, it is important to take into account the respective symptoms and focus on presence and non-judgmental perception in the here and now (Baer et al. 2019).

9.2 Mindful Exploring, Ivenstigating and Experimenting

We can promote the development and strengthening of our clients' self-awareness by repeatedly encouraging them to turn their attention inward and explore and perceive the sensations in their body and their feelings. With the help of "mindfulness-promoting questions", we support them in training their "awareness of experiencing in the present moment" (Ogden et al. 2010, p. 268). We should incorporate these questions into the entire treatment process and especially in the context of stabilization; for example, by asking our clients:

- *"How is it for you when you relate this beautiful experience?"—"What do you notice in your body?"*
- *"When you think of the first moment after the accident in which you felt safe again, what happens in your body?"*
- *"Where in your body do you feel your joy most or strongest?"*

With these and similar questions, we encourage our clients to get in touch with their inner self and their body. By accompanying and encouraging them to take on an observing position, as it were the role of an "observing self" (Ogden et al. 2010, p. 269) or an "inner observer" (Reddemann 2001, p. 39), over time they can learn to notice distressing and threatening emotions, body sensations, memories, thoughts and inner images with inner distance. This way they experience that they themselves "are" not the experience or a certain feeling, thought or sensation, but that they merely "have" a feeling, sensation or thought (Ogden et al. 2010). This separation between the "experiencing self and the observing self" is called "dual awareness" by Babette Rothschild (2002, p. 190). It is a prerequisite for processing a traumatic experience and an essential part of stabilization. Only the "simultaneous awareness of past and present" and the "distinction between both" make a "safe" trauma treatment possible (ibid. p. 189). Dual awareness enables our clients, for instance, to feel a triggered fear and at the same time be aware that they are not in danger in the present moment.

With the help of their self-awareness, our clients can experience that they gain inner distance from negative thoughts and feelings by observing and being aware of them without judgment. This way they also experience that through non-judgmental observation and acceptance, distressing feelings and thoughts lose their intensity and frequently even dissolve. For traumatized people, these are important experiences, as they counteract those of powerlessness and loss of control and give them a feeling of control and self-determination.

Through self-awareness or the perception and observation of our body sensations and feelings, we can get in touch with our liveliness and intactness, but also with our wounds and pain or other deep emotions such as grief and rage.

As already discussed in chap. 4.3., for many people who are traumatized being aware of their body and their inner self is frightening or threatening, as this often activates traumatic content. To protect themselves, they mostly avoid perceiving their feelings and physical sensations and close themselves off from their innermost self and their body. Yet, our liberation from trauma presupposes that we open ourselves up again to our inner experience (van der Kolk 2016). That is another reason why it is our task to support our clients gently in opening up to their body and inner self and noticing their feelings and physical sensations.

In doing so, it is very supportive and encouraging for our clients when we take an open, curious, exploratory and "experiment-friendly" attitude that is also characterized by a sense of playfulness (Ogden et al. 2010, p. 269).

For instance, we can pick up spontaneous movements and invite our clients to explore them: *"While you are talking, your hand keeps closing into a fist. Would you like to stay with this movement and explore what it is like when you consciously close and open your hand?—What does that do to you?—How does that feel?"* Through this exploration, both our clients and us frequently gain unexpected new insights and experiences.

Example from practice

Ricarda, 47, experienced great violence from her parents since she was a child. While she is talking about a situation at her workplace that reminded her of her childhood and made her freeze, she starts plucking at a handkerchief and rips it to little pieces. When exploring this movement, she notices that her high tension decreases and she gradually calms down. Tearing the handkerchief to bits also helps her to stay in the present. Ricarda discovers that this is a resource for her to reduce tension, calm down and stay in the moment. From then on, Ricarda uses this resource repeatedly while talking about stressful events; tearing a handkerchief is also a regulating support for her when processing her traumatic experiences using EMDR (Eye Movement Desensitization and Reprocessing). ◄

As with a movement we can also explore a feeling that arises. For example, through questions like:

- *"If you give space to your sadness and it is allowed to just be there, how is that?"*
- *"What happens when you let your tears flow?"*
- *"Where in your body do you feel your powerlessness most or strongest?"*
- *"And is there somewhere in your body an area that feels neutral or pleasant right now?"*

While exploring and investigating, it is necessary to lead our clients to a resource when threatening content, sensations, emotions and memories arise. This can be an external stimulus, such as looking out of the window or feeling the ground under their feet, or observing slow inhalation and exhalation. It can also be exploring an area within their body that our clients find pleasant or neutral (Levine 1998). Pendulating to these regulating and thus stabilizing resources is necessary throughout the entire treatment process, especially when we address stressful content and process traumatic memories.

Apart from exploring with mindful questions, we can support our clients' self-awareness also in other ways.

9.3 Body Awareness and Grounding

One way to expand and deepen self-awareness is to be aware of our body and of individual movements. With the help of different awareness and grounding exercises, we can explore the sensations in our body and their effect on our inner self. A simple exercise is, for instance, to sit and become aware of the backrest on our back, noticing how it feels, whether it is soft or hard, warm or cold. We can also suggest to our clients to rub their palms together firmly and examine how they feel during and afterwards; maybe they tingle or pulsate and feel warm or hot. Or they can focus their attention on a certain body part, e.g., one of their hands, and explore what it is like to move it, to stretch it, to close it into a fist and open it again. Or we invite them to gently turn their head back and forth and observe and explore how this movement affects them. For example, the slow turning of the head usually has a calming effect.

Another possibility is to suggest to our clients they consciously perceive with their senses; for instance, by feeling an object, stroking one hand over the other or pressing it lightly and feeling the touch.

In particular, I like to recommend to my clients that they go out into nature, if they have the opportunity, and perceive it with all their senses; consciously taking in the green of meadows and forests, seeing the sky and clouds, feeling the wind, warmth or cold, perceiving smells and consciously hearing sounds. For many people these simple perception exercises are easy to implement and mostly pleasant and beneficial. Furthermore, they are a gentle approach to their body. Since it is primarily about perceiving with their senses and not about being aware of their inner body, these exercises carry a lower risk of activating threatening contents. Additionally, experiencing with their senses leads them directly into the here and now.

Grounding exercises are another wonderful practice in self-awareness. For instance, by being aware of the seat while sitting and noticing that it carries us and we sink into it a little bit, and feeling our weight that grounds and centers us. Or by feeling the ground under our feet, our upright body and our weight while standing. Usually we notice a sensation of heaviness in our feet and legs arising, giving us a feeling of grounding, centering and strength. Doing this exercise we can suggest to our clients to imagine being rooted like a tree and to explore how this inner image affects their body and inner experience. Often a feeling of physical and inner strength and centering arises. This exercise can be combined with a small well known experiment that allows us to experience the effect of the imagination on our body. While our clients imagine having roots reaching deep into the earth from their feet, being firmly rooted in the ground, we can—after prior agreement—lightly push them on their upper arm. In general, they will remain standing firmly. If we repeat this experiment when they just stand without imagining, they will wobble when slightly pushed. For many, this experience is impressive and surprising and encourages them to trust the power of their imagination and to use it more frequently.

As with all other interventions, also concerning exercises for training their self-awareness it is necessary to find out which ones are safe and effective for our clients. If frightening or confusing contents, emotions or body sensations occur, it is important to counteract in a regulating way, for example, by asking our clients to breathe in and out slowly, to direct their attention outward and consciously perceive what they see and hear, or to move and e.g. stretch.

In addition to deepening their self-awareness, these and similar exercises for body perception generally have a calming, balancing effect on our clients´ organism. They give them a feeling of safety and are also a gentle way to (re)connect with their body. Through these excercises our clients often experience getting more in touch with themselves, being more present, and feeling themselves more alive and embodied. By the daily home practice of one or the other exercise that makes them feel good and is easy for them to do, they train their self-perception and self-awareness, and so their ability to be in the present moment. With that, they have a tool to calm down and center themselves. In turn, they experience or increasingly gain confidence in being able to influence their well-being.

9.4 Breath and Breathing Exercises

In developing self-awareness and the ability to be in the here and now, our breath has a special significance. It also plays a fundamental role in regaining and strengthening our psychological stability.

In numerous wisdom teachings and spiritual traditions and practices, the breath is regarded as life energy as well as a connection between body and soul and with a higher dimension. It supplies our body with energy and influences our physical and psychological health and well-being. Accordingly, conscious breathing also plays an important role in yoga, tai chi and Christian and shamanic body exercises.

Through our breath we can influence our autonomic nervous system and consequently affect our psychological and physical well-being. In particular, slow breathing and long exhaling stimulate the ventral vagus and thus have a regulating and calming effect on our organism (Porges 2018). They also lower our blood pressure and heart rate (e.g. Newberg and Waldman 2012; Porges 2018).

Conscious slow breathing evokes a relaxation response and allows us to relax, find our core, center ourselves and be in the present moment.

Relaxation Response

The American cardiologist Herbert Benson has been researching the effects of meditation since the 1960s. Based on his research, Herbert Benson describes the effect of meditation as a relaxation response, a state of deep relaxation, so to speak the opposite of a fight or flight reaction (Benson 2020). The relaxation response activates the parasympathetic nervous system and so has a calming effect on our nervous system. It can be brought on by meditation as well as by prayers, mindfulness and breathing exercises. Herbert Benson developed his own intervention to induce the relaxation response, which is free of spiritual or religious references. We slowly breathe in and out. After each exhalation we repeat a pleasant word that has a calming effect on us, such as peace or silence. If thoughts arise, we focus our attention again on inhaling and exhaling and the chosen word.

According to a number of studies, the relaxation response reduces tension, stress and fear as well as physical symptoms associated with stress, such as high blood pressure or gastrointestinal problems (Bensons 2020).

Our breath can therefore be an effective and yet simple "instrument" that we can always rely on.

Caution: Working with the breath is not suitable for all people in the same way. Some find breathing exercises unpleasant, frightening or even threatening. Consciously perceiving the breath can arouse fear, panic attacks or flashbacks in traumatized people and thus be a trigger that activates trauma-related content.

Example from practice

Laura, 36, was sexually abused by her tutor for several years when she was a young girl. When exploring simple exercises that allow her to be in the here and now, I suggest to her, among other things, to observe her breath and notice how her body expands a bit when inhaling and retracts when exhaling. Laura quickly feels restless, cramped and threatened. Therefore, we stop this exercise. Instead I recommend Laura feel the ground under her feet. By doing so, her organism calms down and she becomes calm and relaxed. ◀

While breathing exercises are threatening for Laura, others find them helpful and soothing. Others again, barely know what to do with them. As always, it is important to test one or the other exercise with our clients and explore whether they feel safe and comfortable with it, and experience it as supportive and strengthening.

Breath and imagination

The breath can be wonderfully combined with imagery. On the one hand, it is easier for many people to follow their breath while imagining an inner picture; this holds their attention so that they are less easily distracted. On the other hand, inner images enrich breathing exercises and make them more colorful. In addition, the simultaneous perception of breathing and inner image supports the skill of dual awareness, the development of which is particularly helpful for traumatized people (Rothschild 2002). Finally, using inner images deepen the effect of conscious breathing. It may be especially supportive to suggest our clients, for example, to connect inhaling and exhaling with the image of the wind blowing through a field of wheat; on inhalation the wind sweeps through the field from one side, on exhalation from the other side. If we invite them to try to letting the wind blow slower through the field, their breath also slows down. This allows our clients to experience being able to consciously influence their body and well-being with the help of an inner picture. This in turn strengthens their feeling of action ability and self-efficacy.

Depending on the intention and goal, we can suggest to our clients that they connect their breath with a certain image. It is helpful for some people to imagine a strengthening, calming or healing light or a pleasant color flowing into and through their body with each inbreath. For others, it is supportive to imagine releasing that which is obstructive, burdensome or painful on the outbreath and to breath in what is good, strengthening or calming. It can also be helpful for our clients to direct their breath to a certain part of their body, for instance, to an area where they feel tension or pressure or where they notice a physical sensation when they are sad or angry.

Breath and body exercises

Furthermore, conscious breathing can be combined with various body exercises, such as simple stretching; this can allow our clients to experience the feeling and sensation of expansion, becoming wider or freeing up.

Tension-reducing exercises can be combined with the breath, too. It can give our clients relief from tension or rage to shake their arms vigorously or punch alternately with their right and left clenched fist into the air on an outbreath or a hiss.

9.5 Mindful Movement—Yoga, Feldenkrais and Co.

The development and strengthening of self-awareness and mindfulness can also be supported by mindful movement. Meditative walking is probably one of the simplest forms of mindful movement to apply. While standing we focus our attention on our feet and become aware of how we slowly place one foot after the other on the ground, roll it off and lift it. By connecting our steps with our breath, e.g., three steps while breathing in and five steps while breathing out, we can get into the here and now and be in this moment (Kiehas 2020). If thoughts arise, we consciously direct our attention back to our feet, their movement and their contact with the ground.

Trauma-sensitive Yoga (TSY)

Yoga is a "fully developed and tested system" based on millennia of experience and development; its origins go back at least 5000 years (Nathschläger 2016, p. 17). In the last 20 years, interest in yoga has increased enormously in our Western world. This has led to various styles and variations as well as approaches and programs tailored to specific target groups such as pregnant women or older people.

The effects of yoga, which has an incredible wealth of experience, are increasingly being scientifically researched in recent years. Meanwhile there are a large number of studies worldwide that confirm the various effects. These show that regular yoga practice has, among other things, positive effects on high blood pressure, lung function, back pain, type II diabetes and atherosclerosis (e.g. Taneja 2014).

Interest in yoga as a support for traumatized people arose in the 1990s. David Emerson, a yoga teacher in Boston, USA, developed a form of yoga specifically for traumatized people, which he presented to Bessel van der Kolk's Trauma Center. Shortly before, he and his colleagues had come across yoga in the course of their research into ways of positively influencing heart rate variability (HRV). This led to a collaboration between the two, which resulted in a series of studies on the effects of yoga on trauma-specific symptoms and the development or further development of trauma-sensitive yoga (TSY).

One of the core elements of yoga is interoception, i.e. our ability to perceive body sensations. It enables us, for instance, to feel the backrest in our back while sitting, the ground under our feet while standing or the tension and relaxation of our muscles while moving. People who have been traumatized, especially those who have experienced complex trauma, frequently have a reduced interoception ability (Emerson 2016). Therefore, it is often difficult for them to perceive and/or assign body sensations. Trauma-sensitive yoga promotes exactly this ability through simple exercises in which we consciously direct our attention to individual body areas and explore the bodily sensations we notice. One of the exercises is the long sit. We sit on the ground with straight legs and back. First we become aware of our body in this position. Now we stretch our arms over our head and slowly bend our straight upper body as far forward as possible and become aware of our body in this position.

Another basic exercise of TSY is the so-called table (ibid.). We take up a four-legged position, support ourselves with our hands and knees from the ground, with our hands under our shoulders and our knees under our hips. Now we become aware of the contact of our hands and knees to the ground and explore the sensations we feel in our body. Then we can move slightly forward and back or to the right and left and investigate what we sense during these movements. However,

I would not use this position with clients who have experienced sexual and/or physical violence, as it could activate trauma-related content through the exposed position of the buttocks. Exercises such as the long sitting seem to me much more neutral and therefore to have a much lower risk of acting as a trigger.

For traumatized people trauma-sensitive yoga leads to an improvement in their body perception and strengthens their feeling of being able to influence and control their body. Through certain breathing exercises, which are an essential part of yoga, the parasympathetic nervous system is activated and the sympathetic one is throttled, leading to a regulation of their autonomic nervous system (e.g. Brown and Gerbarg 2009). This reduces their high level of arousal and activation and has a stress-reducing and calming effect. This effect is also helpful in emotionally stressful situations, such as flashbacks, and consequently supports self- and emotion regulation (West et al. 2017). Hence, TSY can have a comprehensive stabilizing effect.

Besides Tai Chi and Qi Gong further methods of mindful movement include forms of meditative and conscious dance (like Biodanza or Open Floor) as well as the method of Moshe Feldenkrais, which is about exploring, perceiving and experimenting with slow movements in a mindful and non-judgmental way. We can support our clients even more by incorporating elements of these or other kinds of mindful movement, giving them another tool to stabilize themselves.

Caution: Any form of mindful movement—even trauma-sensitive yoga—can trigger unpleasant or threatening sensations, emotions, inner images and flashbacks. If our clients want to attend such a workshop or course, we should inform them of this risk and recommend they choose a trauma-sensitive trainer if possible. We should encourage them to take care of themselves during the lesson, and only do those exercises that do them good and to stop them and regulate themselves with a stabilizing exercise, should unpleasant sensations occur.

9.6 Meditation

Furthermore, we can develop and deepen our self-awareness through various meditation techniques. These include the already mentioned breathing and body awareness exercises as well as mindful movements. In addition, they encompass inner images, mantras, self-observation and mindful action (Nathschläger 2016).

Numerous studies show a number of positive effects of meditation and mindfulness exercises on our physical and mental health. These include, among other things, reduction of high blood pressure, improvement in the immune response, decrease of depression and anxiety and improvement of emotion regulation (e.g. Bai et al. 2015; Hofmann et al. 2010; van der Kolk 2016).

More recently, some studies are looking into the possible negative consequences of meditation and point out that it can lead, among other things, to a worsening of fears and depression (Lomas et al. 2015).

Caution: Meditation can be a support for some traumatized people and contribute to their stabilization; however, it can also have a destabilizing effect, as it can evoke frightening or threatening body sensations, emotions, memories, inner images or thoughts. This risk is inherent in all forms of meditation, especially in those whose focus is on emptying the mind as much as possible. Attempting to stay in the present moment without focusing attention on a particular content can trigger, for instance, flashbacks. Even breathing meditation, above all certain forms such as the bellows breath in yoga, can provoke strong reactions.

Generally, caution is advised with any form of meditation. Hence, it is important to make our clients who are interested in meditation aware of the possible risks and inform them accordingly. We should better suggest movement meditation and advise them to refrain in the beginning from pure breathing meditation and such which focuses on an empty mind. In any case, we should recommend they start with brief meditation times, paying attention to themselves during meditation, and stop it as soon as they notice unpleasant or threatening sensations, feelings or inner images arise and regulate themselves with stabilizing exercises.

Regardless of this, meditating is not as easy as it is often presented; especially at the beginning of practicing, our attention span is quite short and our mind jumps from one thought to the next. Frequently we are confronted with our unresolved problems and different thoughts and feelings. Even with experience, these often appear quite intensely at the beginning of a meditation session. Therein lies the danger of the occurrence of flashbacks and other threatening content. Therefore, for traumatized people, meditation combined with movement, such as walking meditation, is safer and more to be recommended. By staying with their attention on their body and feeling the ground, they are anchored in the here and now. Thoughts or other content may appear, but they can more easily detach from them when they direct their attention back to their body and the perception of the ground. Meditation in motion also supports them to (re)connect more strongly with their body, to perceive it, to ground themselves and to feel embodied.

Examples from practice

Diana, 25, got into an extremely physically and psychologically threatening state through a mixture of marijuana and alcohol. She felt completely helpless and suffered a great fear of death for several hours. A few weeks later she took part in a yoga weekend. In one of the meditations carried out there, Diana had strong flashbacks triggering great fear and panic.

Burkhart, 44, is severely traumatized due to a serious accident with massive injuries and subsequent repeated operations, long hospital and rehabilitation stays. During one of his rehabilitation stays, he took part in a guided group meditation and had a very strengthening encounter with a power animal; thanks to this, he got in touch with his will to live and his liveliness again. ◄

As these two examples show, meditation can have very different effects, with the form of meditation playing a role. On the one hand, they can be very supportive and enriching and on the other hand they can sometimes have considerable negative effects (see also van Dam et al. 2017).

MBSR—Mindfulness-Based Stress Reduction

In recent years, the mindfulness practice developed by Jon Kabat-Zinn, the Mindfulness-Based Stress Reduction (MBSR), has gained increasing popularity. Even people who are traumatized seek help and support in MBSR courses. Often MBSR is even recommended to them. For many people and for different complaints such as high blood pressure, MBSR is a valuable support and help. Though, for traumatized people it carries some risks. One of the central exercises is the so-called body scan. In the course of this, we wander with our attention through our entire body. Starting with the toes of the left foot, we direct our perception along the leg to our buttocks, then we go from our right leg starting at the toes to the buttocks. Next we wander through our pelvis and upper body, then starting from the fingertips through our arms to the shoulders. Finally, we direct our attention from our neck to our face and back of the head. Usually the body scan takes 35–45 minutes.

Caution: Due to this long duration, the body scan carries an increased risk of triggering unpleasant or threatening feelings, sensations and inner images or flasbacks. These can already be provoked by the mere perception of the body or a physical sensation within their body. That is why it is so important for traumatized people to approach to being aware of their body and detecting body sensations with caution. MBSR also includes a daily meditation that should start with 10 minutes and be extended to 45 minutes after a few weeks (Kabat-Zinn 2019). Due to their length, they too can trigger flashbacks and anxiety states. As Babette Rothschild (2017) recommends, it would be sensible to adapt MBSR courses for traumatized people so that they carry few risks and can be a safe support and help. Accordingly, it would be advisable to significantly reduce the duration of the body scan and the meditation. In addition, traumatized people should have as much control as possible by being able to decide for themselves which exercises they want to do and for how long. And finally, it would be sensible to focus mindfulness not only inward, but also on external stimuli (ibid.).

References

Baer R, Crane C, Miller E, Kuyken W (2019) Doing no harm in mindfulness-based programs: conceptual issues and empirical findings. Clin Psychol Rev 71:101–114. https://doi.org/10.1016/j.cpr.2019.01.001

Bai Z, Chang J, Chen C, Li P, Yang K, Chi I (2015) Investigating the effect of transcendental meditation on blood pressure: a systematic review and meta-analysis. J Hum Hypertens 29:653–662

Benson H (2020) The relaxation response. http://www.relaxationresponse.org/steps/. Accessed 14 July 2020

Brown RP, Gerbarg PL (2009) Yoga breathing, meditation, and longevity. Ann N Y Acad Sci 1172:54–62

Doll A, Hölzel BK, Bratec SM, Boucard CC, Xie X, Wohlschläger AM, Sorg C (2016) Mindful attention to breath regulates emotions via increased amygdala-prefrontal cortex connectivity. NeuroImage 134:305–313

Emerson D (2016) Healing trauma through yoga. E-course. Trauma Center at JRI, Brookline

Fisher J (1999) The work of stabilization in trauma treatment. Paper presented at the Trauma Center Lection Series 1999. The Trauma Center at HRI, Boston. https://janinafisher.com/pdfs/stabilize.pdf

Hofmann SG, Sawyer AT, Witt AA, Oh D (2010) The effect of mindfulness-based therapy on anxiety and depression: a meta-analytic review. J Consult Clin Psychol 78(2):169–183

Kabat-Zinn J (2019) Gesund durch Meditation. Das große Buch der Selbstheilung mit MBSR. Knaur, München (Full Catastrophe Living. Using the Wisdom of Your Body and Mind to Face Stress, Pain, and Illness. 2013, Bantam Books, New York)

Khoury B, Lecomte T, Fortin G, Masse M, Therien P, Bouchard V, Chapleau M-A, Paquin K, Hofmann SG (2013) Mindfulness-based therapy: a comprehensive meta-analysis. Clin Psychol Rev 33(6):763–771

Kiehas C (2020) Bewegte Meditation. Yoga. Magazin für Yoga, Gesundheit und Spiritualität. YogaVision, Dechantskirchen

Levine PA, Frederick A (1998) Trauma-Heilung. Das Erwachen des Tigers. Unsere Fähigkeit, traumatische Erfahrungen zu transformieren. Synthesis, Essen (Waking the Tiger: Healing Trauma: The Innate Capacity to Transform Overwhelming Experiences. 1997, North Atlantic Books, Berkeley)

Lomas T, Cartwright T, Edginton T, Ridge D (2015) A qualitative analysis of experiential challenges associated with meditation practice. Mindfulness 6:848–860

Nathschläger AP (2016) Yoga fürs Leben. Die fünf Schätze des Yoga für den Alltag. YogaVision, Dechantskirchen, AT

Newberg A, Waldman MR (2012) Der Fingerabdruck Gottes. Wie religiöse und spirituelle Erfahrungen unser Gehirn verändern. Goldmann, München (How Good Changes Your Brain. 2009, Ballantine Books, New York)

Ogden P, Minton K, Pain C (2010) Trauma und Körper. Ein sensumotorisch orientierter psychotherapeutischer Ansatz. Junfermann, Paderborn (Trauma and the Body. A Sensorimotor Approach to Psychotherapy. 2006, W.W. Norton, New York) Own translation

Porges SW (2018) Die Polyvagal-Theorie und die Suche nach der Sicherheit. Traumabehandlung, soziales Engagement und Bindung. G. P. Probst, Lichtenau/Westfalen

Reddemann L (2001) Imagination als heilsame Kraft. Zur Behandlung von Traumafolgen mit ressourcenorientierten Verfahren. Klett-Cotta, Stuttgart (Who You Were Before Trauma: The Healing Power of Imagination for Trauma Survivors. 2020, The Experiment, New York) Own translation

Rothschild B (2002) Der Körper erinnert sich. Die Psychophysiologie des Traumas und der Traumabehandlung. Synthesis, Essen (The Body Remembers. The Psychophysiology of Trauma and Treatment. 2000, W.W. Norton, New York) Own translation

Rothschild B (2017) The body remembers. Volume 2. Revolutionizing trauma treatment. W.W. Norton, New York

Steinmetz KH (2018) Das Herzensgebet. Continuing Class. Schola Cordis, Vienna, AT

Taneja DK (2014) Yoga and health. Indian J Community Med 39(2):68–72

Thich Nhat Hanh (2005) Achtsam leben—wie geht das denn? Theseus, Berlin

Thich Nhat Hanh (2011) Versöhnung mit dem inneren Kind. Von der heilenden Kraft der Achtsamkeit. O. W. Barth, München (Reconciliation: Healing the Inner Child. 2010, Parallax Press, Berkeley)

Thompson RW, Arnkoff DB, Glass CR (2011) Conceptualizing mindfulness and acceptance as components of psychological resilience to trauma. Trauma Violence Abuse 12(4):220–235

Van Dam NT, van Vugt MK, Vago DR, Schmalzl L, Saron CD, Olendzki A, Meissner T, Lazar SW, Kerr CE, Gorchov J, Fox KCR, Field BA, Willoughby BB, Brefczynski-Lewis JA, Meyer DE (2017) Mind the hype: a critical evaluation and prescriptive agenda for research on mindfulness and meditation. Perspect Psychol Sci 13(1):36–61. https://doi.org/10.1177/1745691617709589

Van der Kolk B (2016) Verkörperter Schrecken. In: Traumaspuren in Gehirn, Geist und Körper und wie man sie heilen kann. G. P. Probst, Lichtenau/Westfalen (The Body Keeps the Score. Mind, brain and body in the transformation of trauma. 2015, Penguin Books, London). Quoted from original English version (pp 249, 250)

West J, Liang B, Spinazzola J (2017) Trauma sensitive yoga as a complementary treatment for posttraumatic stress disorder: a qualitative descriptive analysis. Int J Stress Manag 24(2):173–195. https://doi.org/10.1037/str0000040

Imagination—The Power of Inner Images

10

Contents

The term imagination (from Latin "imago", image) refers to the ability to create an inner image. Imagery, so the American psychologist Jeanne Achterberg, is a mental process that uses our senses—"vision, audition, smell, taste, the senses of movement, position, and touch"—and is directly connected to our perception, our feelings and our body (1985, p. 3). Thus, inner images have an immediate effect on our mental state and our body. For example, if we imagine being in a safe and pleasant place, our heart rate slows down, our blood pressure drops and our entire organism calms down (ibid.).

Inner images have been a universal remedy since time immemorial. For instance, they have always been used to reshape and change the course of traumatic events (rescripting) (Arntz 2012). To this day, they are an important tool in the various shamanic traditions. Consequently, shamanism is considered the oldest and most widespread method that uses imagery for healing (Achterberg 1985).

In psychology and psychotherapy, imagery has gained significance since the mid-20th century through Carl Gustav Jung and his Active Imagination and Hanscarl Leuner and his Guided Affective Imagery (Katathym Imaginative Psychotherapy, KIP). In the 1970s, Donald Meichenbaum developed some techniques using imagery to replace negative thoughts and ideas with positive ones

R. Lackner, *Stabilization in Trauma Treatment*,
https://doi.org/10.1007/978-3-662-67480-2_10

(ibid.). In 1985, Jeanne Achterberg comprehensively demonstrated the importance of imagination as a healing power in medicine and psychotherapy in her book *Imagery in Healing: Shamanism and Modern Medicine.* Since then, it has increasingly gained attention in psychology and psychotherapy as well as in some areas of medicine. For example, Arnold Lazarus (1993) describes the use of imagination to treat various psychological symptoms, such as fear. Mary Anne Layden et al. suggest using imagining to process traumatic memories (1993, quoted in Arntz and Wertmann 1999). In the early 1990s, Mervyn Schmucker developed the Imagery Rescripting & Reprocessing Therapy (IRRT), in which an altered course and outcome of a traumatic event is imagined. In the German-speaking countries Luise Reddemann (2001) established the use of imagery in trauma therapy with her book *Who you Were Before Trauma: The Healing Power of Imagination for Trauma Survivors*. She developed her own technique called Psychodynamic Imaginative Trauma Therapy (PITT). Today, inner images are an indispensable part of trauma treatment. They are of essential importance both for stabilization and for processing traumatic experiences.

With the help of their imagination, our clients can create inner images that strengthen and enable them to experience, for instance, safety, comfort, peace or strength and vitality. By imagining positive inner pictures, they also experience themselves as being capable of action and gain a feeling of mastery and control (e.g. Meichenbaum 1977; Singer 1974, quoted in Achterberg 1985).

According to neuroscientific studies, similar brain areas are active during visual perception and imagination (Ganis et al. 2004). Furthermore, imagining an emotional event can activate the autonomic nervous system and the amygdala in a similar way as experiencing the same event. Accordingly, the mere imagining of an experience also leads to similar physical reactions as the actual experience (Kosslyn et al. 2001). Imagining an experience and the actual experience therefore have a similar effect on our body and our inner self. Hence, we can make new experiences through imagining, balancing out our previous ones and "correcting" them.

10.1 Accompanying Imagery

When accompanying imagery we should consider some points:

Open questions

Basically, we should encourage our clients through open questions to discover and develop their very own inner images. For instance, by asking them: *"If everything were possible—and in our imagination everything is possible—who or what could give you a feeling of safety?"* or *"If there were a place where you felt completely safe and at ease, what would it be like?"*

A consistently positive inner image

It is important to accompany our clients in such a way that they can create a consistently positive inner image or a consistently positive inner movie. On the one hand, this means that we accompany them relatively closely giving them a secure framework and taking countermeasures if unpleasant or frightening content appears. On the other hand, it means that we still give them enough time to create their inner pictures and let them take in their effect. This relatively close accompaniment takes place firstly by means of questions about certain sensory impressions, so that our clients can develop a differentiated inner image, preferably using all their senses. Secondly, by confirming and repeating their descriptions. Thirdly, by asking them from time to time during their imagining how their inner picture or inner movie is affecting them and how they feel. In this way we can check whether the emerging imagery is completely positive for our clients and counter quickly if this is not the case.

Perceiving feelings and body sensations

We should confirm our clients´ positive feelings, encourage them to consciously be aware of them and invite them to explore where they can feel them most or strongest in their body. The intensity and effect of the imagining is significantly increased by simultaneously experiencing the inner image and the associated feelings and body sensations.

Changing threatening content

Finally, it is important to pay attention to and support our clients to change and correct unpleasant or threatening content that may infiltrate their image; e.g., by assuring them: *"You can always create everything exactly as it is right and appropriate for you."*

Introducing

Usually, guided imagery is introduced with a relaxation induction; however, this is not advisable for traumatized people (Reddemann 2001). They could feel at our mercy or experience loss of control. It is more sensible to simply invite our clients to sit comfortably and become aware of the seat or feel the ground under their feet in order to anchor themselves well in the here and now. If they wish, they can close their eyes or—if they prefer and feel more comfortable—leave them open.

10.2 The Use of Inner Images

Imagining can be incorporated into the accompanying of our clients in different ways. Often an image develops from a conversation about a certain topic, e.g., when we talk about the feeling of safety. Then it makes sense to invite our clients to imagine, for example, someone or something that gives them a feeling of safety. Or we suggest that they recall a situation in which they felt safe. Basically, we should offer our clients one or the other stabilizing image, such as the idea of something protective surrounding them, or invite them to create a supportive image in relation to a certain topic, such as boundary setting or relaxation.

10.3 The Inner Safe Place

The most common and well-known image in the context of trauma treatment is that of an inner safe place. It is not only seen as a standard image, but as a necessary prerequisite for the processing of traumatic memories (e.g. Schubbe 2006); without a safe place, trauma processing was not possible. However, this is not the case. There is a wealth of other stabilization exercises that allow our clients to cope with strong emotions, disturbing memories or physical reactions during and after processing their traumatic experiences.

Imagining an inner safe place can be a wonderful intervention; but not for everyone and for all. The goal of the inner safe place is to enable our clients to create a place in their imagination where they feel completely safe, like a so-called "Leo"[1]or a safe zone where they are protected. This inner place allows them to relax and recover as well as to regain a feeling of safety. Additionally, it enables our clients to bring their wounded and intact inner parts, especially their younger parts or inner children, to safety before or during trauma processing. Yet, many, especially severely traumatized people have great difficulty in finding or creating a safe place in their inner world. During the imagining threatening contents frequently invade the emerging picture, making it difficult or impossible to create a safe place. Even if we supportively ask our clients to imagine further safety measures such as an additional fence or a row of guards, the place often remains unsafe and/or threatening content continues to intrude into the emerging image, making it frightening or even terrifying. If this is the case, it usually leaves our clients feeling threatened and constricted. Many have the feeling that they are not up to the task and are unsettled by it. If we still try to motivate our clients to create a safe place despite their efforts and the threatening content that arises, and this succeeds after all, there is a high risk that frightening content will reappear during their independent practice at home. Then the supposedly safe place will become a threatening one. All this is exactly the opposite of what we want to achieve with our stabilizing interventions. What´s more, asking our clients to do something that is difficult for them or hardly feasible contradicts the meaning and purpose of stabilization. If it is hard for them to find or imagine a safe place and/or threatening content forces itself in during this process and cannot be resolved despite imagined protective measures, it is necessary to stop the imagining and discontinue it. Yet, it makes sense to stay in the realm of imagery and enable our clients to have a positive imaginative experience with another, easier to use image; for instance,

[1] In Austria "Leo" is the safe place when playing tag.

by picturing something protective surrounding them or a protective shell or layer. For many this image is easy to implement. It seems to be more directly and closely perceptable for our clients and so more rapidly effective; in my experience, it is very safe as it is usually not affected by threatening content.

A common argument for the need to establish an inner safe place is that we should ask our clients to go to their safe place in their inner world during the processing of their traumatic memories when they are highly stressed in order to calm down and experience a moment of safety. However, to enable this for our clients, it is not inevitably necessary to have an inner safe place. We can support them to calm down and feel safe again through a variety of other stabilizing interventions, such as orientation in the here and now, grounding exercises, memories of nice experiences, certain movements or another image that are easy for our clients to implement. Therefore, it is advisable to only use or continue the imagining of the inner safe place if this is easy for our clients to do and if no frightening content appears. Then it can be a wonderful stabilizing exercise.

Example from practice

Yara, 39, who fled from Iran as a very young woman, imagines a house by the sea surrounded by a wall and completely secluded from the outside. A wise wizard protects her and takes care that Yara is doing well, that she can follow her needs and develop freely. For her younger parts, Yara imagines a small colorful house in the garden, which is warm and cosy inside. Her inner children are taken care of and nurtured by a loving motherly figure, so that they are altogether well. ◄

As an alternative to imagining an inner safe place, Christa Diegelmann and Luise Reddemann recommend the image of a place of well-being, i.e. a place where our clients feel completely comfortable. The word safe can evoke negative associations, especially for people who have been hurt and/or abused by those who should have protected them (Reddemann 2011), or for seriously ill people who "know for sure that nothing is safe" (Diegelmann 2007, p. 153), and act as triggers for threatening content. With the invitation to imagine a place where our clients feel comfortable, we would indirectly, but not directly, address the topic of safety and reduce the risk of related negative associations. However, in my experience it makes a fine qualitative difference in the experience of our clients whether they imagine a safe or a comfortable place; the experience of safety usually has a strengthening, invigorating effect. Safety is such a major factor in the processing and healing of traumatic experiences and has a fundamental importance for traumatized people, as they felt completely vulnerable during the traumatic event. For this reason, I do use the word safe in my invitation, but I combine it with other formulations such as *"a place where you feel completely safe and at ease"* or *"a place where you feel safe and comfortable all around"*.

10.4 The Various Possibilities of the Imagination

In accompanying traumatized people we can incorporate imagery in many different ways. Apart from imagining a place where they feel safe and comfortable or something that surrounds them protectively, the image of an "inner helper" (Reddemann 2001), i.e. someone or something that is helpful, protective and strengthening, is very supportive. Likewise, imagery can be wonderfully used in working with inner parts. It is particularly healing for our clients to imagine making up for something that they would have needed in a certain situation, or what they experienced too little of or not at all in their childhood, such as comfort and safety (Arntz and Weertman 1999). It is also relieving and healing to reduce tension and rage in their imagination.

Furthermore, we can use imagery very specifically to strengthen a certain feeling or state by e.g., taking up a positive memory, such as a moment of safety. Or we can encourage our clients to a future vision by imagining, e.g., what it would be like to be internally free.

Example from practice

Matthias, 28, lost his mother at the age of 8; she died at home after a long and serious illness with numerous hospital stays. His father had little time for Matthias due to his job. Soon afterwards he entered into a new partnership. Matthias felt abandoned and withdrew more and more into himself. Since then he repeatedly suffers from great sadness and inner emptiness as well as from having the feeling of not really being alive. He longs to feel alive and be happy again. In his mind he sees himself as a vibrant, powerful young man running along a beach and jumping into the air with joy. This image revives Matthias's joy of life and vitality that he often felt as a child. ◄

We will discuss various other images in Part IV "Exercises and Interventions".

10.5 Holistically Experienced Inner Images

The full effect of an inner image does not unfold in mere imagination, but in its connection with the feelings and physical sensations consciously perceived at the same time. Therefore, it is necessary to ask our clients during imagining what they are feeling and sensing in their body. Consciously noticing the positive feelings, such as safety, strength or calm, significantly increases the effect of an inner image. This is further supported by asking our clients where they perceive this feeling most easily or strongest in their body. In this way, an embodied image is created. The coupling of imagining, feeling and body perception—that is, the holistically experienced image—has an incredibly strong effect. If we invite our clients to find a suitable word or sentence for this coupling of inner image, feeling and body sensation, such as "this safety" or "I am free", then this serves as an anchor[2], which can support our clients in recalling the state just experienced at a later time. An appropriate symbol and/or gesture or movement can be additional anchors.

10.6 A Few Hints

Imaginings have an immediate positive effect. However, in order to consolidate them, we have to train them. Only when they are "saved as an automatic response" in our implicit memory can we rely on them in challenging situations (Sachsse 2011, p. 229). For this reason, I advise my clients to practice them at least once a day, as long as it feels good to them. This can be a few minutes, but it can also be for a longer time. It is crucial that our clients feel comfortable during the imagining and experience it as positive throughout.

Sometimes inner images change; it is important though, that they remain completely pleasant for our clients. If this is not the case and threatening content appears while imagining on their own between our sessions, it is necessary for them to change their inner image so that it is again consistently positive. If this is not possible, our clients should stop imagining and take up a different stabilizing exercise. In our next session, we can then support them in developing a new helpful image.

Caution: Some people can do little or nothing with inner images, others feel uncomfortable during imagining or become restless, fearful or full of trepidation. As with all interventions and exercises, it is important to take this into account and accordingly refrain from imagining and take up other stabilizing interventions.

If our clients suffer from dissociations, we should first introduce and convey other stabilizing interventions and exercises to them, in particular interventions that support them to orient themselves in the here and now and in the outside, such as grounding and power exercises (see chap. 27). Furthermore, we should first explore with our clients in which situations or under which circumstances they dissociate. Only when they have acquired some tools to help them to regulate and stabilize themselves and know the triggers that make them dissociate, can we suggest one or the other image. While doing so, we should pay particular attention to their positive physical sensations, which can be a body ressource or anchor within their body supporting them to be in the present moment.

References

Achterberg J (1985) Imagery in healing. Shamanism and modern medicine. Shambhala, Boston

Arntz A, Weertman A (1999) Treatment of childhood memories: theory and practice. Behav Res Ther 37:715–740

Diegelmann C (2007) Trauma und Krise bewältigen. Psychotherapie mit TRUST. Klett-Cotta, Stuttgart

[2]A term from Neurolinguistic Programming (NLP).

Ganis G, Thompson WL, Kosslyn SM (2004) Brain areas underlying visual mental imagery and visual perception: an fMRI study. Cogn Brain Res 20(2):226–241

Kosslyn SM, Ganis G, Thompson WL (2001) Neural foundations of imagery. Nat Rev Neurosci 2:635–642

Layden MA, Newman CF, Freeman A, Byers Morse S (1993) Cognitive therapy of borderline personality disorder. Allyn and Bacon, Boston. Zit. In: Arntz A, Weertman A (1999) Treatment of childhood memories: theory and practice. Behav Res Ther 37:715–740

Lazarus A (1993) Innenbilder. Imaginationen in der Therapie und als Selbsthilfe. Klett-Cotta, Stuttgart (In the Mind´s Eye. The Power of Imagery for Personal Enrichment. 1984, Guilford Press, New York)

Meichenbaum D (1977) Cognitive behavioral modification: an integrative approach. Plenum, New York. Zit. In: Achterberg J (1985) Imagery in healing. Shamanism and modern medicine. Shambhala, Boston

Reddemann L (2001) Imagination als heilsame Kraft. Zur Behandlung von Traumafolgen mit ressourcenorientierten Verfahren. Klett-Cotta, Stuttgart (Who You Were Before Trauma: The Healing Power of Imagination for Trauma Survivors. 2020, The Experiment, New York)

Sachsse U (2011) Imaginationsübungen. In: Sachsse U (Hg) Traumazentrierte Psychotherapie. Theorie, Klinik und Praxis. Schattauer, Stuttgart, S 228–243

Schubbe O (Ed) (2006) Traumatherapie mit EMDR. Ein Handbuch für die Ausbildung. Vandenhoeck & Ruprecht, Göttingen

Singer JS (1974) Imagery and daydream methods in psychotherapy and behavior modification. Academic, New York. Zit. In: Achterberg J (1985) Imagery in healing. Shamanism and modern medicine. Shambhala, Boston

Reddemann L (2011) Psychodynamische Imaginative Traumatherapie PITT — Das Manual. Klett-Cotta, Stuttgart

Arntz A (2012) Imagery rescripting as a therapeutic technique: review of clinical trials, basic studies, and research agenda. J Exp Psychopathol 3(2):189–208

Inner Parts

11

Contents

Working with inner parts or self-parts or ego-states is important for stabilization. Activating and strengthening their healthy self-parts and healing their wounded ones contributes significantly to the stability of our clients.

In recent years the significance of inner parts is increasingly gaining attention in trauma treatment (e.g. Fisher 2019). There are different approaches, the most well-known being Ego-State Therapy by John and Helen Watkins and Internal Family System Therapy by Richard Schwartz.

The idea of self-parts or ego-states goes back to Paul Federn, a friend and student of Sigmund Freud. He noticed that the sense of self can vary depending on the situation and state (Peichl 2007). Consequently, he did not see the ego as a unit, but rather as a composition of different "sub-personalities" (ibid. p. 70). John and Helen Watkins picked up this idea and developed their theory of ego-states from it. These are "precipitates of distinctive interactive experiences" and "the condensate of prototypical life scenes from a certain period of development" (ibid. p. 73). Thus, they are "neuronal networks representing relationship experiences that I have made as an acting or experiencing person ..." (Peichl 2018, p. 122). Ego-states arise during childhood and adolescence; some even in adulthood (Emmerson 2015). Among other things, they develop as "defense and coping mechanisms"; through their repeated use, they evolve into "autonomous parts" of our personality (ibid. pp. 12–13). For instance, if a child is repeatedly denigrated, reprimanded and/or beaten by his parents, he may withdraw into himself in order

R. Lackner, *Stabilization in Trauma Treatment*,
https://doi.org/10.1007/978-3-662-67480-2_11

to protect himself from further attacks. From this strategy, a separate self-part can develop, which later reacts to criticism or conflicts with others by withdrawing. It gives our clients great relief to recognize that this withdrawal or not defending oneself is an expression of a self-part that was originally a protective mechanism and ensured their survival. Likewise, it can be helpful for them to discover, for example, their rage as an expression of a "fight part" and its original defensive reaction, which is now triggered by injustices (Fisher 2019, p. 47).

The idea that we all have different parts within us is easily understandable to our clients. The awareness that we always have unwounded inner parts beside wounded ones is very relieving and strengthening for them.

Example from practice

Doreen, 45, is highly stressed due to a series of traumatic experiences. Her former psychotherapist held the view that she was injured as a whole and therefore could not have an unwounded part within her. From this point of view, Doreen felt only wounded; this weakened and depressed her very much and made her feel excluded from life. The thought that she not only has injured inner parts, but also healthy ones strengthens Doreen, empowers her and gives her confidence. ◄

Understanding that we have both injured and uninjured inner parts, gives us a more comprehensive, "two-eyed" view (Fürstenau, cited in Reddemann 2011, p. 29). Similarly to how we use resources to counter traumatic experiences, we can also balance injured parts with healthy ones. By enabling our clients to recognize, revive and strengthen their healthy parts, their wounds can be balanced, cushioned and softened.

We can incorporate the work with inner parts into the accompaniment of our clients in various ways. For example, when having the impression that a younger part is active in them while they are speaking, we can ask them how old they feel right now. If a client tells us, e.g., that she repeatedly feels completely helpless and exposed in conflict situations, we could ask her how she feels while talking about it and whether she has the impression that she is her current age or younger. Often it is recognizable when our clients are in a younger "state"; something changes in their gaze, posture or voice. If they talk about a certain feeling—such as fear, rage or despair—we can ask them whether they perceive another feeling besides this one. Frequently, our clients notice that, e.g., they are not only angry, but also feel abandoned. When exploring in more detail, they often discover that these feelings are connected to different inner parts. Regarding a certain thought or conviction—such as "I'll never be able to do this"—we may inquire whether there is another thought despite that. Again, there may be different thoughts, each of them corresponding to a self-part, for instance, the courageous, self-confident or the insecure, doubting part.

Through differentiating different parts, our clients do not experience themselves as only wounded, or anxious or angry; they recognize that the wound, fear or rage is only a part of them, besides which there are others. This differentiation helps our clients to deal better with the respective feelings and states as well as with burdensome memories, thoughts and situations.

Example from practice

Susanne, 54, has great difficulty expressing her opinion, standing up for herself and setting boundaries. This is associated with great fear. As a little girl, her mother was cold and dismissive and withdrew from her when Susanne rejected something her mother liked, had a different opinion, or did not enjoy her mother's gifts. If she did something her mother did not approve of or had forbidden, her mother would not speak to her for a few days. Over time, Susanne increasingly withdrew, no longer expressed her opinion and concealed her displeasure if she did not like something that was liked by others. She recognizes that it is a younger inner part that is afraid to express her opinion and set boundaries; after all, this was threatening to her before, as it meant her mother´s withdrawal and breaking off the relationship with her. Recognizing this Susanne can relate to it, understand, and deal better with her fear. And she notices that only a part of her is taken over by fear. ◄

As with Susanne, recognizing the different parts can already lead to more clarity and inner order and thus be relieving and stabilizing for our clients. Taking up and working with these parts contributes significantly to their stability and is therefore an important element of stabilization. The work with the inner parts proceeds on an imaginative level. It is important to develop a consistently positive inner image, which either strengthens healthy parts or heals wounded ones, enabling our clients to have a positive and corrective experience. As with any other imagining, it can be useful for our clients to use it daily to deepen and consolidate its effect.

11.1 Discovering and Reviving Healthy Younger Parts

In particular, re-experiencing and reviving their healthy inner parts or inner children can be very stabilizing and strengthening for our clients.

It can be very supportive and healing to invite them to visualize a moment in their childhood, in which they felt safe and secure, alive or carefree, and to let this memory take effect on them. Many can re-experience the situation of that time and the associated feelings, often very intensely, sometimes only slightly. By perceiving them, they get into contact with, among others, their vitality and strength, and thus with the child they were. This allows them to reconnect with their innermost being, as the children we were reflect our inner and true nature.

Example from practice

Inés, 26, unexpectedly lost her father in a traffic accident at the age of 7. Her mother was in shock and fell into a severe depression, which she was only able to overcome after several years. She was physically present, but emotionally inaccessible to Inés. Since the death of her father, Inés feels empty inside, almost dead. She feels powerless, lonely and barely finds joy in anything. With great effort, Inés was able to complete school and earn a degree. She repeatedly has bad experiences with men, is exploited or cheated by them. I invite Inés to tell me something about the little girl she was before her father's death. She describes herself as a cheerful, carefree, rather wild girl. In her memory and imagination Inés sees herself playing with her friends, jumping from one foot to the other and spinning in a circle. While Inés takes in this inner image, she feels alive, powerful and free. For the first time in a long time, she feels an intense joy. She seems liberated, present and is glad and thankful to have regained access to her vitality and inner self. ◄

This reawakening of an essential inner part was decisive for Inés; it meant a significant stabilization of her overall psychological state and gave her a new or rediscovered understanding of herself.

Perceiving their unwounded inner child or childlike parts can be very touching and moving for our clients and, as with Inés, often even very blissful. Many feel more alive and complete, as if a lost part were returned to them and completed them. This contributes significantly to their stabilization and healing. However, this experience can also be associated with sadness, melancholy or rage; about the fact that they had lost these parts or they had been taken away from them. It is important to acknowledge and appreciate these feelings and at the same time encourage our clients to consciously stay with the memory and experience of the respective part and the associated positive feelings, noticing that these are now palpable and experiencable again. The healthy parts of the children we were are not lost or evaporated; they are still present in us as childlike parts, albeit often withdrawn or hidden. As soon as we discover them and turn to them we can revive them.

Some of our clients can hardly or not at all draw on positive memories, and others experience these as painful. For both, it can be very healing to imagine giving the wounded (e.g. sad or lonely) child they were all that would have been good or would be good for them.

However, some of our clients reject the child they were and meet him with reluctance or even disgust. Often they were unwanted as children, rejected, neglected and/or abused. Sometimes it is possible to support our clients to recognize a positive side or characteristic of the child they were by inquiring in more detail; for instance, by asking whether there is a part of the child that is okay, that they approve of or like in some way. This could be, for example, stubbornness that hides strength, or vulnerability that expresses sensitivity. We can pick up on this and, through questions, enable our clients to get in touch with this inner part. Occasionally it is possible to look at oneself as a child from the outside and to recognize one's own wound in a different, new light. Then we can suggest to our clients to explore what would be good for the child and what she would need. Usually this is being seen, given attention and encouragement. If they can imagine receiving this, they usually experience it as very comforting, calming, sometimes even blissful. However, often there is also pain about not having received this attention and encouragement in their childhood, perhaps even to this day. Then it is important to perceive, acknowledge and appreciate this pain and to recognize it as an important step in the healing process.

Sometimes asking whether there are advantages to not being lovable or being rejected can also enable access to the child they were and to their inner childlike parts; for instance, when it turns out that this was a protection against further injuries. Here too, it is important to see and recognize the child´s wounding and vulnerability, and have her imagine all she would have needed and that would have comforted her flowing to her.

11.2 Healing Wounded Younger Parts

If we acknowledge the injury to the child they were and express it, our clients can experience—sometimes for the first time—that they are seen and recognized in their suffering. We are like witnesses who see, recognize and testify to the bad that has happened to them. This being seen and perceived is an essential healing step. Often it enables mourning for the first time for what has happened or what was not given, such as missing love and attention. Many of our clients experience indignation or rage about what they experienced or what they had to do without. This can be very liberating and mobilize power in them; on the one hand, nudging and supporting the further healing process and, on the other hand, forming a counterforce to the frequently existing sadness, inner emptiness, hopelessness or powerlessness, strengthening our clients so that they can find their way out of it.

Hence, our clients´ wounded inner child or childlike parts may appear in connection with healthy parts or as a reaction to them as well as when talking about their traumatic experiences or other burdensome events from their childhood. Then it is helpful to ask what they would have needed then; asking this directly addresses their wounded, frightened or humiliated inner child. "Someone who would have protected me, defended me, rescued me from danger, simply been there, hugged me, comforted or encouraged me"—these are the most common answers to this question. Then we can ask our clients, e.g.: *"If you imagine that someone was there who would have protected the little one and brought her to safety, who could/should that have been?"* Some know the answer to this question immediately and have an inner image right away. Others we can further stimulate by giving a few examples: *"In our imagination everything is possible, it could be an ancestor or an ideal mother, or a spiritual being, like an angel, it could also be an animal, like a bear. Or someone completely different."*

Similarly, we can proceed whenever our clients get into contact with a wounded childlike part; for instance, when exploring fear or rage. Here too, it is useful to ask them what would be good for the respective part or the child they were and what he would need. Usually it is again to be seen and perceived as well as protection, attention, comfort and consolation.

Example from practice

Josef, 54, was neglected by his mother in many ways from an early age. Later he grew up with his grandmother, who was very strict and controlling. Josef never received recognition, praise or tenderness from her. In his mind, Josef pictures himself as a small boy being held by a big, soft bear. This bear speaks loving encouraging words to him, hugs him tightly and rocks him back and forth. During his imagining this, Josef feels increasingly soothed, his entire organism calms down and relaxes, his stomach and chest feel warm. He feels at ease, protected and held. ◀

Sometimes our clients cannot find a person, power, being or animal that appears suitable to them. For some of them, the idea that they themselves care for, comfort or hold the child they were is the most resonant.

Example from practice

Lydia, 41, was beaten, insulted and humiliated by her father from an early age. Her mother was not able to protect her and her siblings from the violence and emotional outbursts of the father. Lydia felt completely helpless in front of him. In her imagination she runs away from home and is expected and taken to a safe place by the adult she is today. The adult she is today takes her lovingly in her arms and comforts her. ◀

It is frequently necessary to convey to the inner children that the threat is over and that they are safe here and now. Many people have never been told this and often they have hardly consciously realized it themselves; so it happens that a part of them still believes they are in danger and having to re-experience something bad at any time. If this is the case, it is important that we address the inner child directly and assure her that the danger is over and that she is safe in the here and now. It is helpful to agree with our clients beforehand how we should or may address their inner children.

Example from practice

Samira, 38, was sexually abused by her uncle for several years during her childhood. When I address little Samira directly and say, "Little Samira, it's all over, you survived. It's over, you're safe," Samira takes a deep breath. Her body relaxes and tears flow down her cheeks. She looks relieved. Suddenly she became aware that the danger was over and she is safe. It was as if she had lived all those years since her youth in the belief, yes in the certainty, that she was still in danger. For the first time, she becomes aware that she has survived. With a powerful voice and determination she says: "I survived. I made it." For Samira this is a very important step, which contributes significantly to her stabilization. ◀

We can support the work with the inner children by using photos or objects from their childhood that had or have great significance for our clients. With the help of these and their stories, they can approach their inner child and get in touch with him. In addition, it is very healing for our clients to pay attention to their inner child in their everyday life, e.g., to the wounded four-year-old or the lonely eight-year-old, and consciously do something for her. Some watch a children's series like "Vicky the Viking" or "Pippi Longstocking", some go to a playground to swing, listen to fairy tales or children's songs and some eat a pudding or a Nutella sandwich. It is supportive if they do this consciously for their inner child and enjoy it. By allowing the "inner child state", "change is possible" (Sachsse 2011, pp. 214–215).

11.3 Discovering, Reviving and Strengthening Further Healthy Parts

Besides working with the inner child or childlike parts, working with other healthy self-parts such as the strong or the fighter, the confident or wise is very supporting and stabilizing, too. If we have asked our clients about their resources, about their strengths, or about qualities or abilities they are happy, proud or grateful for, then we can come back to them, pick one and invite our clients to be aware of it. Often these qualities can be recognized when they talk about their experiences, everyday life or events. Then we may pick them up directly.

I: "You have told me that you are glad that you have tried out and dared a lot. When you think about it and are aware of it, how is that?"

Karin: "Hm. Then Australia comes to my mind. I went to Australia for 3 months when I was 19."

I: "Ah, wow. And how is it when you think about it?"

K: (takes a deep breath) "That was great back then. ... I feel such a power. ... I was so fearless back then."

I: "Ah, you were so fearless. And if you think about that now and let that have an effect on you and feel the power, what happens inside of you?"

K: "Hm, everything tingles in me. … but that also makes me a bit wistful. … I'm not so fearless anymore …"

I: "And if both may be, the wistfulness and the fearlessness. … is that possible?"

K: (takes a deep breath) "Yes, that's possible. … hm, actually I'm still fearless … not quite as strong … hm, but I don't have to be that anymore."

I: "So the fearlessness is not lost at all?"

K: "No, not quite."

I: "And how is it when you notice that you are still fearless?"

K: (takes a deep breath) "Ah, yes, good. Yes, I still am. That feels good now. I wasn't aware of that. I didn't lose it."

I: "Great. You are still fearless, you didn't lose that."

K: "No … no!"

I: "Where in your body do you feel the fearlessness?"

K: "There." (puts her hand on her chest) "In the chest. And in the stomach."

I: "And how does your chest and stomach feel?"

K: "Strong. Powerful … but calm. Such a calm power."

I: "Ah, a calm power. Then be consciously aware of this calm power."

K: "I feel a lot of energy."

I: "Yes, then be aware of the energy, too. … and while you feel the power and the energy, maybe an impulse comes up in you to make a certain movement."

K: (sits up straight, clenches her fists) "Ah. Yes. Just yes. I can do it. Yep."

I: "Yep. You can do it. What is it like when you say that, Yep, I can do it?"

K: "Great. That's great, it feels really good."

I: "Then take that in consciously and enjoy it."

In this way or similarly, we can work with healthy parts using our imaginiation, picking up the healthy parts and strengthening them. Towards the end of the imagining we can ask our clients which word or sentence best expresses this experience, or whether a symbol comes to their mind that best reflects the state. Movement, word and symbol serve as an anchor that can make it easier for our clients to re-activate this state later. It can also be helpful to make a collage of the self-part and hang it up at home as an anchor in the outside or as a reminder.

Furthermore, it is useful if our clients remind themselves of their healthy parts in their everyday life and feel the physical sensation associated with them. Likewise, it is supportive if they incorporate their parts more frequently into their daily live by, for example, offering their courageous or creative self-part opportunities to express and unfold themselves.

References

Emmerson G (2015) Ego-State-Therapie. Ernst Reinhardt, München

Fisher J (2019) Die Arbeit mit Selbstanteilen in der Traumatherapie. Junfermann, Paderborn (Healing the Fragmented Selves of Trauma Survivors. Overcoming Internal Self-Alienation. 2017, Routledge, New York) Quoted from original English version (p 25)

Peichl J (2007) Die inneren Trauma-Landschaften. Borderline—Ego-State—Täter-Introjekt. Schattauer, Stuttgart

Peichl J (2018) Integration in der Traumatherapie. Vom Opfer zum Überlebenden. Klett-Cotta, Stuttgart

Reddemann L (2011) Psychodynamisch Imaginative Traumatherapie. PITT—Das Manual. Klett-Cotta, Stuttgart

Sachsse U (2011) Therapeutische Arbeit mit dem Inneren Kind. In: Sachsse U (Hg) Traumazentrierte Psychotherapie. Theorie, Klinik und Praxis. Schattauer, Stuttgart, pp 207–216

The Power of Positive Thoughts 12

Contents

Our thoughts influence how we approach life and live our lives. They are closely linked to our attitude to life, both influencing each other. Both, our thoughts and our attitude towards life, determine how we go through it, approach other people and how we maintain relationships. In addition, they determine our view of our future and whether we dare to do or shun something new. Our thoughts also interact with our feelings and mood as well as with our physical state. We can experience this interplay in everyday moments. For instance, thinking of being unable to achieve an important target is reflected in our inner self and body; we feel gloomy and powerless. However, thinking that we will make it, we feel empowered and energetic and gain energy.

Numerous studies confirm the connection between our thoughts and our mental and physical health. For example, the duration of convalescence after operations is significantly shorter in people with a positive attitude towards life than in those with a negative one (e.g. Scheier et al. 1989). People with a positive attitude who, for instance, have a higher risk of suffering from a heart disease due to their family history are a third less likely to have a heart attack or another heart disease than those with a negative attitude (Yanek et al. 2013).

Thus, with our thoughts and attitudes we have an impact on our body as well as our psyche. Accordingly, our attitude to life and our thoughts influence our coping with traumatic experiences. In chap. 6 we have learned about the three Ps of Martin Seligman (2006), which reflect attitudes that make overcoming traumatic

R. Lackner, *Stabilization in Trauma Treatment*,
https://doi.org/10.1007/978-3-662-67480-2_12

experiences more difficult, including thoughts such as "Now it's all over" or "It will never be good again". We have also seen that optimism, confidence and trust in one's own coping ability are essential for resilience (Bonanno 2015). People who hold on to their positive attitude despite their traumatic experience cope better with it (Fredrickson 2011). They have complex emotions as they do not deny "the reality of the negative" but "their positive attitude goes hand in hand with their negative feelings" (p. 132). Hence, the ability to focus on positive feelings influences our coping with traumatic experiences. The orientation towards the positive and strengthening is decisive, although it is also important to acknowledge negative feelings.

It is not about simply "thinking positive" and denying and ignoring everything burdensome or painful like in a "Lala-Land". It is more about encouraging our clients to broaden their view and despite their burdens to notice the positive. Therefore, it is advisable for them to try to pay more attention to positive impressions in their environment and pleasant moments or experiences in their everyday life, or to make themselves aware of their resources. This is often a protracted process of becoming aware, which requires us to repeatedly decide to direct our attention away from the negative and towards the positive.

Furthermore, it is useful to recommend our clients to pay attention to their thoughts, recognizing negative ones and consciously counteract them with positive ones. However, it is not beneficial to fight negative thoughts such as self-condemnation or negative expectations, which usually reinforces them. In the end, by trying to drive them away we get stuck focusing on them. "Energy flows where attention goes", a principle of Hawaiian shamanism, aptly reflects this dynamic. Numerous studies confirm the fact that by suppressing or fighting our thoughts, they are reinforced even more. One of the best known studies shows that people who were asked not to think of a polar bear thought of it much more often than those who were asked to think of one (Wegner et al. 1987). This can be explained by the Theory of Ironic Processes. When trying to control our thoughts, two processes are active: the "operative process" suppresses the thought while the "ironic process" checks if the thought returns (Wegner 2003). The more we try to suppress our thoughts, the stronger they become. Consequently, it is not about driving them away, but about allowing and acknowledging them and either dealing with them in a constructive way, noticing them and letting them pass by, or consciously dealing with something else and counteracting them with something positive.

The increased attention to positive aspects is a process that requires attention, discipline and perseverance and oftentimes means relearning long-established habits. Yet, over time, it not only enables the development and strengthening of a positive attitude and mood, but also a reduction of depressive mood, anxiety, hopelessness and inner emptiness (e.g. Fredrickson 2011).

Negative thoughts and life attitudes are usually associated with doubts, fear and/or negative expectations and frequently evoke in us a feeling of insecurity, oppression or even resignation. These, in turn, affect our physical well-being, for example, by weakening our level of physical energy.

By contrast, positive thoughts and, in particular, a positive attitude contribute to a feeling of safety and confidence and support our psychological stability and by that the process of processing traumatic experiences.

Above all, working with their resources can help our clients to gain a more positive attitude towards themselves and life. Additionally, Positive Psychology and Psychotherapy as well as Solution-focused Psychotherapy offer a number of helpful interventions, such as the "Three Blessings Exercise", "Me in My Best Form" or circular questioning, which is helpful in questioning and reviewing existing beliefs and convictions (e.g. de Shazer 1999; Seligman 2012). The latter is particularly helpful in scrutinizing and revising beliefs and convictions we have made about ourselves or taken over from other people over the course of our lives.

Example from practice

Karl, 55, was systematically mobbed by some of his colleagues over several years. After they publicly humiliated and discredited him at a team meeting, he suffered a massive panic attack. Since he had never experienced this state before, Karl believed he was having a heart attack. During the subsequent medical examination, he was diagnosed with burnout, for which he was off work for several months. At the beginning of our work, Karl feels broken, wounded and is convinced that he is completely useless, a "real wimp", as he calls it; otherwise he would have been able to deal better with his colleagues and put up with everything. In the course of talking about the events over the years and my informing him about mobbing and trauma, Karl increasingly realizes that he has endured a lot: repeated, almost daily defamation, meanness, intrigues and exclusion. In addition, he becomes aware that he had succeeded for a long time in staying firm, demarcated and unscathed and in maintaining his self-respect. Karl recognizes that the mobbing started to affect him more and more when problems arose in his marriage. These overwhelmed his capacity for coping. Realizing and becoming aware that he had endured a lot for a long time helps Karl to once again see himself as positive and resilient. This gives him back his self-esteem and a feeling of inner strength. ◀

As with Karl, our thoughts and convictions about ourselves not only influence our well-being, but also our handling of stressful events and experiences.

12.1 Trauma and the Changed View of Life

This is particularly important in the case of trauma, as it often radically changes our convictions about ourselves, life or other people.

Examples from practice

Bernhard, who as a little boy lost his best friend, believes deep down that he has no right to live. Samira, who was sexually abused by her uncle for years, is convinced that she is dirty and guilty. And Anne, who was neglected by her parents, believes she is not a valuable person.[1] ◄

These are just a few examples illustrating how chronic and early traumatizing experiences can shape, transform and reverse our attitude towards ourselves and our lives so that it is directed against us. Mostly these convictions and negative thoughts have a protective function, which we often acquire early in our lives. With them we can protect ourselves, e.g., from painful disappointments, massive feelings of guilt or unbearable feelings of shame. In this way, we can keep our parents or caregivers, who are vital to us, internally well. If children are beaten, sexually abused and/or psychologically mistreated by their parents, they usually take the responsibility for it themselves; if they were to grasp how cruel their parents are, they would feel completely unprotected and abandoned and break down. Hence, taking on guilt and responsibility is an expression of a protective mechanism that allows us to keep the people we depend on as good in our inner self and maintain the relationship with them. However, it leads to taking on responsibility for injustice or violence done to us and directing it against us in the form of self-condemnation and negative attributions. This dynamic also applies to more inconspicuous, subtle forms of violence and oppression, such as continuous denigration or the demand for "obedience".

Due to this mechanism, those affected often form negative beliefs about themselves very early in life, frequently maintaining them throughout their lives.

Regardless of this mechanism, the perpetrators usually convey to the affected persons that their behavior or statements are justified and that they deserve nothing else. That is a further reason why the affected persons usually feel responsible for the acts of violence and devaluations and are convinced that they are "guilty" themselves. Suzanne Vega (1987) expresses this very movingly in her song "Luka", which relates the story of an abused child:

I think it's because I'm clumsy, I try not to talk too loud.
Maybe it's because I'm crazy, I try not to act too proud.

In relation to sexual violence against children, the fact also plays a role that the perpetrators usually "blame" the children or adolescents for their offense; for instance, accusing them of behaving provocatively and seducing them. Often the perpetrators put the children under pressure or threaten them that they would harm them, their family or themselves if they told anyone about it. Frequently, they manipulate the children by telling them that they are very special and that the

[1] We already got to know Bernhard in chap. 2.1, Samira in chap. 11.2. and Anne in chap. 7.

sexual acts are their mutual secret. Through all this, the children are drawn into a responsibility that can never be theirs. It is particularly important in our work with sexually traumatized people to point out these dynamics and mechanisms and to make it clear to them that the responsibility lies exclusively with the perpetrators. This contributes significantly to their stabilization and to transforming and resolving their negative attributions as well as feelings of guilt and shame.

Taking on guilt and responsibility is also due to the fact that powerlessness and helplessness are unbearable feelings for us. By feeling guilty, we somehow preserve a feeling of action, influence and control within us and consequently the feeling of being able to prevent something similar in the future. Hence, it is our task to inform our clients about these different aspects and take a partisan position regarding any form of violence and neglect. This is enormously relieving for our clients and is an essential piece in the puzzle in order for them to be able to free themselves from feelings of guilt and shame.

References

Bonanno G (2015) Trauma and resilience: from heterogeneity to flexibility. Lecture. New York Teachers College, Columbia University. https://www.youtube.com/watch?v=gvxk-75brpU. Accessed 20 June 2020

Fredrickson BI (2011) Die Macht der guten Gefühle. Wie eine positive Haltung ihr Leben dauerhaft verändert. Campus, Frankfurt (Positivity. 2009, Crown Publishers, New York) Own translation

Scheier MF, Matthews KA, Owens JF, Magovern GJ, Lefebvre RC, Abbott RA, Carver CS (1989) Dispositional optimism and recovery from coronary artery bypass surgery: the beneficial effects on physical and psychological well-being. J Pers Soc Psychol 57(6):1024–1040

Seligman M (2006) Learned optimism: how to change your mind and your life. Vintage Books, New York

Seligman M (2012) Flourish. Wie Menschen aufblühen. Die Positive Psychologie des gelingenden Lebens. Kösel, München (Flourish. A Visionary New Understanding of Happiness and Well-Being. 2011, Free Press, New York)

de Shazer S (1999) Wege der erfolgreichen Kurztherapie. Klett-Cotta, Stuttgart (Keys to Solution in Brief Therapy. 1985, W.W. Norton, New York)

Vega S (1987) Luka. Solitude standing. A&M Records

Wegner DM (2003) Thought suppression and mental control. In: Encyclopedia of cognitive science. Macmillan, London, pp 395–397

Wegner DM, Schneider DJ, Carter SR 3rd, White TL (1987) Paradoxical effects of thought suppression. J Pers Soc Psychol 53(1):5–13

Yanek LR, Kral BG, Moy TF, Vaidya D, Lazo M, Becker LC, Becker DM (2013) Effect of positive well-being on incidence of symptomatic coronary artery disease. Am J Cardiol 112(8):1120–1125

Movement—Physical Activity and Sport

13

Contents

To regain and strengthen stability, any form of movement is helpful. In a traumatic experience, our body mobilizes all its strength to fight or flee, or it freezes or collapses if both are not possible. If our instinctive defense reactions are not carried out or completed and the freezing cannot be released, the enormous activation remains in our body. Consequently, it is obvious that after a traumatic experience any form of movement and physical activity supports our body to reduce this great activation and, among other things, release stress hormones. This is all the more important if the "restoring" of "core autonomic homeostasis" does not occur in time and more and more stress accumulates in our autonomic nervous system (Levine 2019, p. 40). This is particularly the case with repeated or chronic traumatization. In the long term, this can affect our health and cause various symptoms such as hypertension, arrhythmias or migraine and, among other things, lead to gastrointestinal and autoimmune diseases (McLeay et al. 2017).

The positive effect of physical activities and movement on our physical and mental health is now well known. The effectiveness of physical activity in coping with stress is well documented, too (Fuchs and Klaperski 2017). For example, an US study with 32,000 adults showes that those who jog or walk quickly for about 20 minutes a day feel significantly less stress than those who are physically inactive (Aldana et al. 1996, cited in Klaperski 2017). The positive effect of movement on our mental well-being has long been empirically confirmed (e.g. Blumenthal

R. Lackner, *Stabilization in Trauma Treatment*,
https://doi.org/10.1007/978-3-662-67480-2_13

et al. 1999). For instance, a meta-analysis of 30 studies showed that a training of 9 weeks or more leads to a significant reduction in depression; the type of activity, its frequency and intensity only played a minor role (Craft and Landers 1998). Based on these study results, the authors recommend a 20-minute training at a moderate intensity 3 times a week as an adjunct therapy for depression. It makes sense to choose an activity that brings joy and to start the training with short sessions of about 10 minutes to make it easier to integrate into everyday life (Craft and Perna 2004). Physical activity also has a positive effect on fear and anxiety disorders; both single sessions and continuous training have been shown to effectively reduce anxiety and panic disorders, with moderate training 3 to 4 times a week being the most effective (Knapen and Vancampfort 2014). On the other hand, too intensive training sessions can reinforce existing anxieties.

The effect of physical activity and sports on post-traumatic symptoms has so far only been examined in isolated cases; existing studies are usually limited to small samples without a control group. Only recently have individual studies with comparison groups been carried out for the first time. A first meta-study of 4 randomized control studies shows both the positive effects of physical activity on the symptoms of post-traumatic stress disorder and on depressive symptoms in people with PTSD (Rosenbaum et al. 2015). A comparison study with 81 inpatients suffering from post-traumatic stress disorder showed that the symptoms improved more in those patients who, in addition to conventional treatment (psychotherapy, group therapy and medication), did 0.5 h of strength training per week and walked 10,000 steps daily, than in those who did not engage in any sport (ibid.). In their small study of 33 participants with PTSD, Mathew Fetzner and Gordon Asmundson (2015) were able to show that training on an ergometer for a period of 2 weeks 3 times a week led to a significant improvement in symptoms and, among other things, reduced the fear of arousal-related body sensations (e.g. a higher heart rate). Physical sensations such as sweating, a higher pulse rate and hyperventilation can trigger fear in traumatized people; however, regular training can reduce it (Knapen et al. 2015).

We can therefore conclude that physical activity can reduce the symptoms of PTSD as well as depression, anxiety, panic and sleep disorders (Oppizzi and Umberger 2018). Accordingly, researchers suggest integrating movement and sports into every trauma treatment or recommending them in addition to it (Hegberg et al. 2019; Rosenbaum et al. 2017). We should impress upon our clients to pay attention to regular movement. As a rule, I ask my clients at the beginning of our joint work about their physical activities and make them aware of their importance for the healing process. Those who exercise regularly, I encourage to continue integrating it into their daily lives, possibly increasingly. Those who hardly or do not engage in any physical activity, I motivate to find a kind of movement that gives them pleasure or fun. I recommend they choose activities they can do easily and that don´t require much effort to integrate into their daily lives. Additionally, I advise them to start with short units.

13.1 The Positive Effects of Exercise and Sport

Physical activities, especially endurance sports such as cycling, running, walking or swimming not only reduce post-traumatic symptoms, anxieties and depression; they can also bring a number of other positive effects for our clients. For example, they reduce the increased level of arousal (Vancampfort et al. 2016); this allows our clients to experience a calming of their organism and to feel more balanced and calm inside. Moreover, they enable our clients to distract themselves from negative thoughts, feelings and flashbacks, to gain distance from them and to be in the present (Ley et al. 2017). Through movement and exercise, they can also experience mastering new movement patterns, challenges and unfamiliar situations. This strengthens their self-confidence, self-determination and their self-efficacy (Ley et al. 2014). In addition, through physical activities, our clients can also find a positive access to their body, so that it can become a resource for them. By doing so, they occasionally remember previously practiced forms of movement or games and gain access to their younger, intact inner parts. Exercise also contributes to an increased perception of control over one's own body and to an improved body image (Craft and Perna 2004; Knapen and Vancampfort 2014). Finally, physical activities as well as any kind of movement can be a vent for our clients to reduce tension, rage and aggression. Through all these possible positive effects, sport and movement can significantly support and strengthen the stability of our clients.

Examples from practice

Noemi, 36, has gotten into the habit of going for a run a few times a week. This makes her feel more balanced, stronger and more rooted in her body; giving her a feeling of safety and control. Nikolai, 56, has started going to a gym again. Through regular training, he can better cope with his strong emotions. He no longer feels so at the mercy of them and experiences himself as more centered and self-determined. Maryam, 47, has discovered skipping rope for herself. She enjoys it, it is easy to integrate into her everyday life and helps her reduce tension, to get out of thoughts and burdensome memories and calm down. ◄

13.2 Points to Consider

When exercising or practising any other form of movement, our clients should consider a few points. It is advisable that they

- avoid anything that could cause them stress, like competitive situations, lack of clarity about a course or training program, as well as places and materials that could remind them of their traumatic experiences

- refrain from sports in which they have no or only limited control or have to adhere to strict rules, as is the case with some martial arts
- make sure that they have the possibility to leave the training location and interrupt the program at any time
- make sure not to have to participate in all exercises (Ley and Rato Barrio 2019)

As with all stabilizing interventions and exercises, it is also important with physical activities that our clients pay attention to only doing those activities that they experience as supportive and strengthening or as beneficial and relaxing.

References

Aldana SG, Sutton LD, Jacobson BH, Quirk MG (1996) Relationships between leisure time physical activity and perceived stress. Percept Mot Skills 82:315–321. Zit. In: Klaperski S (2017) Exercise, stress and health: the stress-buffering effect of exercise. In: Fuchs R, Gerber M (Eds) Handbuch Stressregulation und Sport. Springer, Heidelberg, pp 227–249

Blumenthal JA, Babyak MA, Moore KA, Craighead WE, Herman S, Khatri P, Waugh R, Napolitano MA, Forman LM, Appelbaum M, Doraiswamy PM, Krishnan KR (1999) Effects of exercise training on older patients with major depression. Arch Intern Med 159(19):2349–2356

Craft LL, Landers DM (1998) The effect of exercise on clinical depression and depression resulting from mental illness: a meta-analysis. J Sport Exer 20:339–357

Craft LL, Perna FM (2004) The benefits of exercise for the clinically depressed. Primary Care Companion J Clin Psychiatr 6(3):104–111

Fetzner MG, Asmundson GJG (2015) Aerobic exercise reduces symptoms of posttraumatic stress disorder: a randomized control trial. Cogn Behav Ther 44:303–313

Fuchs R, Klaperski S (2017) Stressregulation durch Sport und Bewegung. In: Fuchs R, Gerber M (Eds) Handbuch Stressregulation und Sport. Springer, Heidelberg, pp 205–226

Hegberg NJ, Hayes JP, Hayes SM (2019) Exercise intervention in PTSD: a narrative review and rationale for implementation. Front Psychiatr 10:133. https://doi.org/10.3389/fpsyt.2019.00133

Klaperski S (2017) Exercise, stress and health: the stress-buffering effect of exercise. In: Fuchs R, Gerber M (Eds) Handbuch Stressregulation und Sport. Springer, Heidelberg, pp 227–249

Knapen J, Vancampfort D (2014) Evidence for exercise treatment of depression and anxiety. Int J Psychol Rehabil 17(2):75–87

Knapen J, Vancampfort D, Morien Y, Marchal Y (2015) Exercise therapy improves both mental and physical health in patients with major depression. Disabil Rehabil 37(16):1490–1495

Levine PA (2019) Polyvagal-Theorie und Trauma. In: Porges SW, Dana D (Hrsg) Klinische Anwendungen der Polyvagal-Theorie. Ein neues Verständnis des Autonomen Nervensystems und seiner Anwendung in der therapeutischen Praxis. G. P. Probst, Lichtenau/Westfalen, pp 19–42 (Polyvagal Theory and Trauma. In: Porges SW, Dana D (Eds.) Clinical Application of The Polyvagal Theory. The Emergence of Polyvagal-Informed Therapies. 2018, W.W. Norton, New York, pp 3-26) Quoted from original English version (p 23)

Ley C, Rato Barrio M (2019) Promoting health of refugees in and through sport and physical activity: a psychosocial, trauma-sensitive approach. In: Wenzel T, Drozdek B (Eds) An uncertain safety. Springer, Heidelberg, pp 301–343

Ley C, Lintl E, Team MK (2014) "Movi Kune—gemeinsam bewegen": bewegungstherapie mit Kriegs- und Folterüberlebenden. Spectrum 26(2):71–97

Ley C, Kramer J, Lippert D, Rato Barrio M (2017) Exploring flow in sport and exercise therapy with war and torture survivors. Ment Health Phys Act 12:83–93

McLeay SC, Harvey WM, Romaniuk MNM, Crawford DHG, Colquhoun DM, Young RMD, Dwyer M, Gibson JM, O'Sullivan RA, Cooksley G, Strakosch CR, Thomson RM, Voisey J, Lawford BR (2017) Physical comorbidities of post-traumatic stress disorder in Australian Vietnam veterans. Med J Aust 206(6):251–257. https://doi.org/10.5694/mja16.00935

Oppizzi LM, Umberger R (2018) The effect of physical activity on PTSD. Issues Ment Health Nurs 39(2):179–187

Rosenbaum S, Sherrington C, Tiedemann A (2015) Exercise augmentation compared with usual care of post-traumatic stress disorder; a randomized controlled trial. Acta Psychiatr Scand 131(5):350–359

Rosenbaum S, Stubbs B, Schuch F, Vancampfort D (2017) Exercise in posttraumatic stress disorder. In: Fuchs R, Gerber M (Hrsg) Handbuch Stressregulation und Sport. Springer, Heidelberg, pp 375–387

Vancampfort D, Richards J, Stubbs B, Akello G, Gbiri A, Ward PB, Rosenbaum S (2016) Physical activity in people with PTSD: a systematic review of correlates. J Phys Act Health 13(8):910–918

Spirituality and Religion

14

Contents

Spirituality and religion play an important role in the lives of many people. Although there is no generally accepted definition of these two terms, spirituality is usually described as an experience and devotion to a higher, spiritual world, while religion usually refers to a particular denomination and its practice.

After traumatic experiences, a spiritual or religious approach can be very supportive and helpful for those affected. As an important resource it can provide support, strength, comfort and confidence and so contribute significantly to their psychological stability. Frequently, it can provide explanations for what has happened, which can be an important help in dealing with the incomprehensible; of course, only if they are not linked to certain religious ideas or traditional convictions that interpret traumatic events as punishment. According to investigations, a condemning, punishing form of spirituality can significantly hinder the coping with traumatic experiences (National Center for PTSD 2020). However, generally, any spiritual or religious orientation free of such approaches is supportive. Meanwhile, numerous studies confirm its positive effect on overcoming traumatic experiences. For example, a national survey in the USA after the terrorist attacks of 09/11 showed that 90% of those surveyed turned to their faith to cope with the events (Schuster et al. 2001). In addition, the orientation towards spirituality also reduces the risk or extent of sequelae such as depression, alcohol consumption and physical complaints (Meichenbaum 2008). Furthermore, it seems to reduce negative self-attributions and self-condemnation as a result of traumatic experiences.

R. Lackner, *Stabilization in Trauma Treatment*,
https://doi.org/10.1007/978-3-662-67480-2_14

Many of my clients find support in their faith or spirituality in processing and overcoming their traumatic experiences. For some, it is also possible to recognize the experience as a challenge in which they can grow and mature.

People who were previously unfamiliar with spirituality or who previously described themselves as atheists or agnostics often find access to spiritual dimensions due to tragic events. Others, however, lose their faith or access to the spiritual world through traumatic incidents, especially if they are associated with the loss of a loved one. Then they doubt God or a higher power and ask themselves why He allowed this.

It is important that we are open to all these possible developments and questions of our clients—no matter in which direction they may go—and that we give them space. This is necessary as these questions and topics are important and decisive for many traumatized people and can contribute to their healing. Therefore, psychotherapy and especially trauma therapy should take into account the spiritual dimension as part of life and being and consequently of healing, provided our clients address spiritual content and questions or show openness or searching in this regard. Of course, we should take into account and accordingly exclude the area of spirituality in our accompaniment, if our clients have no access to spirituality or are rather skeptical or reject it. However, it makes sense to ask our clients at the beginning of our joint work whether religion or spirituality plays a role in their lives (National Center for PTSD 2020). In doing so, we signal our openness in this regard and might occasionally learn that spirituality is important to them. In this way we get to know of a resource we can draw on that we would not have known about without our asking.

14.1 Access to Spiritual Worlds

Many people have access to spiritual worlds and come into contact with spiritual beings or a higher power or energy, or perceive their presence.

Example from practice

Lara, 52, repeatedly feels the presence of a spiritual force with which she is connected and feels held by; it gives her strength and allows her to see her life in a larger context. After her serious accident, Lara feels strengthened and supported by this force, giving her confidence and trust in her future. ◄

If it is possible for us to meet these experiences openly and give them space, this can deepen our joint work and our clients can experience enrichment and support for their stability.

Example from practice

During our sessions Leopold, 76, repeatedly perceives the presence of a divine mother, that he experiences as incredibly healing. It leads to a clear calming of his greatly increased activation level and gives him a feeling of safety, support and comfort. These experiences are profound for Leopold and mean a turning point in his healing process. ◄

It is very precious to repeatedly pick up, draw on and use these experiences in the course of our work. Especially with regard to psychological stability, they can be incredibly strengthening, as with Leopold.

14.2 Prayers and Mantras

Prayers, prayer postures, certain body exercises and mantras can contribute to stabilization. Their positive, healing effect has been proven in a number of studies. Prayers, meditations and mindfulness exercises can support traumatized people in coping with what they have experienced (Meichenbaum 2008). For example, a study by Peter Bollens and his colleagues (2009) shows a significant improvement in anxiety states and depressive moods after those affected had prayed for 1 hour per week over a period of 6 weeks. Prayer positions or mudras can also have a stabilizing effect. The classic prayer posture of bringing our hands together in front of our hearts can be calming and centering.

Mantras can help us to relax, calm down and become more balanced, as well as center and calm our thoughts (Heitel 2007). Mohani Heitel, a physician who grew up in India and lives in Germany, describes mantras as "syllables or words with special sound properties, whose vibrations contain healing frequencies", which have a "relaxing and harmonizing effect on body, mind and soul" (2007, p. 7). Among other things, they can be supportive in anxiety, depressive moods, nightmares and sleep disorders, as well as in cases of vegetative dysregulation, stress and tension (ibid.).

The most famous and important mantra is "Om". When chanting Om, the head, chest and abdomen are put into a slight vibration, which has a calming effect on our body and psyche. According to the Polyvagal Theory, singing or toning stimulates the vagus nerve, which leads to activation of the social engagement system and relaxation (Porges 2018).

References

Bollens PA, Reeves RR, Replogle WH, Koenig H (2009) A randomized trial on the effect of prayer on depression and anxiety. Int J Psychiatry Med 39(4):377–392

Heitel M (2007) Die heilenden klänge der mantras. Südwest, München (The Healing Sounds of Mantras. 2016, Smirti, Salt Lake City) Own translation

Meichenbaum DH (2008) Trauma, spirituality, and recovery: toward a spiritually-integrated psychotherapy. Paper. https://melissainstitute.org/scientific-articles-by-author/. Accessed 10 July 2020

Porges SW (2018) Die Polyvagal-Theorie und die Suche nach Sicherheit. Traumabehandlung, soziales Engagement und Bindung. G. P. Probst, Lichtenau/Westfalen

PTSD: National Center for PTSD (2020) Spirituality and trauma: professionals working together. https://www.ptsd.va.gov/professional/treat/care/spirituality_trauma.asp. Accessed 10 July 2020

Schuster MA, Stein BD, Jaycox LH, Collins RL, Marshall GN, Elliott MN, Zhou AJ, Kanouse DE, Morrison JL, Berry SH (2001) A national survey of stress reactions after the September 11, 2001, terrorist attacks. N Engl J Med 345(20):1507–1512

Loss and Grief—Saying Goodbye and Transforming the Relationship

15

Contents

Sometimes traumatic experiences are associated with the death of a loved one. However, this can lead to trauma, too, in particular if it occurs unexpectedly and/or in a tragic way.

15.1 Saying Goodbye

Often it is not possible for the bereaved to say goodbye to a loved one; for instance, if he or she has died in another country or from an infectious disease, or if they are advised not to say goodbye, e.g., if the body of the deceased is disfigured due to an accident. However, missing a goodbye can complicate the grief process as much as the processing of trauma caused by the death of a close person.

In order to support our clients in this process and contribute to their stability, we should suggest they make up the goodbye in their imagination (Heller 2003). They can imagine in detail how they say goodbye, telling the deceased everything they wanted to tell them, and hold and embrace them once again. As with all inner images, it is helpful to invite our clients to notice their body sensations and follow their movement impulses. Many feel the proximity and embrace of their beloved person and become aware of warmth or satiety in their body. At the same time, often pain and grief emerge. Then it is supportive to ask our clients what

R. Lackner, *Stabilization in Trauma Treatment*,
https://doi.org/10.1007/978-3-662-67480-2_15

their deceased would say to them or give them as a message if they were here and experienced their pain. Mostly confirming and life-affirming words appear that give our clients comfort and confidence. Occasionally, guilt or rage about the loss emerge, too. Then it is sensible to encourage our clients to express these in an inner dialogue with the deceased, supporting them by asking what the deceased would say to our clients´ feelings and thoughts. Usually it is helpful to recommend our clients perceive and allow the different feelings at the same time—the pain and the rage, the sadness and the guilt. Commonly, this reduces the inner tension or inner conflict caused by the ambivalence of the feelings.

With the help of saying goodbye in their imagination, our clients can at least partially make up for what has remained open for them. Something in them can calm down and round off, like a wound that was still wide open and can now close a little and begin to heal.

15.2 Transforming the Relationship

It is still common to tell mourners that they have to let go of the deceased. The fact that love and the relationship to the deceased does not simply evaporate with death, but continues beyond it, is overlooked. For the German psychotherapist Roland Kachler, preserving love and transforming the relationship are the essential points of grief work. "But the love remains—the grief process as creative shaping of relationships" is the title of one chapter in one of his books, which is not about letting go, but rather about the transformation of the relationship. When urging to let their deceased go we fail to recognize the pain and struggle with the loss and the synchronicity of love and death. By affirming that love and connection remain and that it is about transforming from a relationship largely determined by physical presence and accessibility to a spiritual, emotional, internalized one, we relieve and support our clients in their grief process.

15.3 After-Death Contacts

Many people have so-called after-death contacts following the loss of a loved one, in which they suddenly and unexpectedly come into contact with the deceased. They may experience being touched by them, feeling their presence, hearing them speak and letting them know that they are doing well, or seeing the deceased in front of them.

Example from practice

Hannelore, 73, lost her son in a mountain accident. She is an independent, cheerful, down-to-earth, realistic woman. A few days after his death, Hannelore feels that "someone" is stroking her cheek, at the same time she is aware, she knows, that it is her son. This moment moves Hannelore very much; she wonders if she is just imagining this experience, if it is the product of her fantasy, an expression of her longing for her son. At the same time, she knows that she was wide awake during this experience and clearly felt the touch. In the following days and weeks, Hannelore repeatedly has similar experiences. Once she unexpectedly sees her son walking in front of her, turning and waving to her and disappearing behind a house. Hannelore has all of these experiences suddenly and unexpectedly in quite everyday situations such as waiting in a supermarket queue. In our conversations, Hannelore repeatedly questions whether she is imagining all this; at the same time, she is aware that these experiences are completely different from anything she has experienced so far. They neither resemble ideas nor wishful images or mere thoughts. They are experienced holistically, physically and emotionally and appear unannounced and without warning and disappear in the same way. With each further experience, Hannelore gains confidence that these are real. By and by, other people tell her about similar experiences. This confirms her perception and gives her comfort and the certainty that the connection to her son continues, even if he is no longer alive. ◄

Just like Hannelore, many people experience encounters with loved ones who have passed away. According to the largest study on this topic to date, more than 40% of the 2000 people surveyed had after-death experiences with deceased (Guggenheim and Guggenheim 2017). A small study with 162 grieving people shows that 68% had an after-death contact (Houck 2004, cited in Houck 2020). Bill and Judy Guggenheim distinguish twelve forms of after-death experiences. Many people feel the presence of the deceased, perceive how they are touched by them, hear their voice or see them in front of them. Often they appear to them in a dream. These experiences not only provide comfort, but also support the mourning process by helping the survivors to transform and reshape their relationship with the deceased and to preserve it in their inner self or on a spiritual level.

Even if after-death experiences may seem strange, unbelievable or unreal to us, and may not correspond to or contradict our understanding of life and death, it is very important to show our clients the greatest possible openness and to acknowledge their experience as such.

References

Guggenheim B, Guggenheim J (2017) After-death communications. Joyful contacts by deceased loved ones. www.billguggenheim.com/a-summary.html. Accessed 10 July 2020

Heller L (2003) Somatic Experiencing®. Training, Beginner I, September 2003, Penzberg, DE

Houck JA (2004) Zit. In: Houck JA (2020) The exclusive, universal, and multiple experiences of after death communication. https://www.adcrf.org/houck_research.htm. Accessed 10 July 2020

Kachler R (2005) Meine Trauer wird dich finden. Ein neuer Ansatz in der Trauerarbeit. Freiburg im Breisgau, Kreuz

References

Rage and Aggression 16

Contents

Rage and aggression are natural consequences of a threatening event. This applies to all traumatic events, but in particular to experiences of violence as well as to those in which we are endangered or harmed by other people, or in which a beloved person is injured or killed by someone else.

16.1 Rage as a Natural Reaction of Self-Protection and Defense

Rage and aggression are, on one side, an expression of our self-protection and defense mechanisms and consequently of our will to survive. On the other side, they are the result of our unfulfilled or uncompleted defense reactions (Levine 1998). For example, if we cannot follow the instinctive impulse to fight or complete a fight reaction because we are held back, then not only the enormous activation remains in our body, but also the impulse to defend. This can lead to us reacting to a trigger such as a threatening gesture, body posture or touch with rage and aggressive behavior.

R. Lackner, *Stabilization in Trauma Treatment*,
https://doi.org/10.1007/978-3-662-67480-2_16

Example from practice

Chiara, 17, was forcibly held several times as a child as part of medical examinations. Her attempts to defend herself were always prevented by holding her even tighter. Since then, Chiara reacts to touch on certain parts of her body with severe physical resistance and aggression. ◀

Last but not least, rage is an expression of our powerlessness, bewilderment, despair and pain about what has happened and its sometimes irrevocable consequences. That is why it is so important and contributes significantly to the stability of our clients to pay special attention to irritation, rage, indignation and aggressive impulses or actions. For our clients it is an enormous relief if we convey to them that these are forms of expression of their self-protection and will to live and so natural reactions to their traumatic experiences. Furthermore, for many affected people the knowledge that rage is the result of an unfulfilled or uncompleted instinctive defense reaction is very liberating. Often this enables our clients to gain a new, changed access to their rage, which allows them to acknowledge and experience it as strength and vitality and thus as a resource and expression of their empowerment (Zanotta 2018). This can also reduce their related feelings of shame and guilt.

16.2 Vents for Rage

It is therefore important to discuss with our clients how they deal with rage and whether they have vents to reduce it. Many have no way to express and resolve their rage; frequently they suppress it. However, rage does not just dissipate. Usually it remains in us and expresses itself in the form of different symptoms, uncontrolled actions and behaviors or emotional outbursts. If this happens, it often bothers our clients a lot and evokes feelings of guilt, self-accusations and feelings of helplessness and sometimes aggression against themselves. This leads to a tricky dynamic in which self-condemnation, feelings of helplessness and loss of control and rage at oneself increasingly intertwine. All this further weakens the psychological stability of our clients or makes it more difficult for them to become more stable. Hence, it is necessary to explore with them which possibilities they already have to express and reduce rage, or which other or new vents could be suitable and feasible for them. In this context, any form of movement plays an important role.

It is helpful to have both, vents that can be applied spontaneously as soon as irritability and rage occur, and possibilities to relieve tension and anger continuously. It is useful if these give our clients pleasure and can be integrated into their daily life without much effort. On one side, these can be simple gymnastic or strengthening exercises such as sit-ups or squats, skipping rope or shaking the whole body. On the other side, dancing and endurance sports such as jogging, swimming or walking are wonderful vents to reduce inner tension.

The possibility of freeing oneself from emerging rage and aggressive impulses through certain exercises contributes significantly to the stability of our clients. Thereby, they not only feel more relaxed, they also increasingly experience that they are no longer so at the mercy of their feelings, but can influence and cope with them. In addition, through these exercises they can find access to their strength and vitality and to their body.

Even short exercises for relief of tension can already be relieving, supportive and strengthening.

Example from practice

Kathleen, 52, has got into the habit of shaking her body as soon as she notices that she is irritable or angry. This happens again and again in the office where she works. She then retreats to the toilet and does her exercise there for a few minutes. Afterwards she feels freer and more centered. ◄

16.3 Expression of Rage

When we pick up and address feelings of rage, irritation and indignation in our joint work, it is useful to encourage our clients to become aware of them and to explore where they can feel them in their body. Some people sense a pressure in their chest, others tension in their hands or arms and some clenching of their teeth. Then we can suggest to our clients to observe these sensations and to feel whether they notice an impulse to do a movement. Some feel the need to hit, kick or tear something. Others would rather run away. Generally, it is very supportive for our clients to encourage them to allow these impulses and to express them in controlled and rather slow movements (Levine 1998). If we motivate them to do so, their body can carry out a reaction that it could not do or complete in the original situation of danger. Generally, this is very relieving and liberating for many.

It is also useful to invite our clients to allow themselves to vent their rage in their imagination. Many imagine saying to the person who, for example, humiliated them, all the things they wanted to say but never could. Others find a vent for their rage through the image of a volcano spewing lava and fire. And still others imagine themselves lashing out, hitting or stamping on something.

Allowing rage and indignation and expressing them on an imaginative level or in the form of attentive and controlled movements is not only relieving, but is often a necessary step in the context of a therapeutic setting in order to process traumatic experiences. By our clients allowing themselves to accept and express their respective impulses, whether in imagination, through a movement or in the connection of both, they can experience "what it would have felt like to fight back or run away" (van der Kolk 2016, p. 261). Furthermore, they can make up for and complete an action impulse that was not carried out or completed before and so experience a discharge and relief (Levine 1998). As a result, our clients usually also gain strength and self-respect.

However, allowing rage and corresponding impulses is very unfamiliar for many people, especially at the beginning. To make it easier for them, I emphasize that it is a natural and healthy reaction if we respond to a threat, to violence, humiliation, neglect or any other form of violation of our boundaries with rage or aggression. They are an expression of our natural impulse of self-protection and defense of our life. By not allowing or suppressing it, the rage does not dissipate, but remains in us, burdens us and often turns against us. Therefore, by specifically allowing it and accompaning it therapeutically it is helpful and offers relief. There are no guidelines, no right or wrong ways. The only rule is that our clients do not injure themselves or us or damage anything in our practice room. So it is a matter of supporting them to find and implement an appropriate, suitable and harmonious form of expression for them.

16.4 A Few Words about Feelings and Fantasies of Revenge

Some of our clients have feelings of revenge and feel the need to take revenge on the perpetrator, which is difficult for most of them to admit to. Many condemn this feeling, don't want to acknowledge it and want to get rid of it quickly. But revenge is a natural feeling when we have been harmed by someone. In this sense, I try to convey to my clients that justice is a fundamental need for us and that it is necessary for us to create a balance when we experience injustice. Therefore, it is often or would often be, important for those affected that the perpetrator is found guilty. Limor Goldner and her colleagues (2019) show with their study that people tend to have revenge fantasies or the need for revenge after traumatic incidents if they experience a feeling of injustice. The study participants experienced their feelings of revenge as helpful for their healing process. Yet, revenge fantasies not only counter the feeling of injustice; they also give us a feeling of control and empowerment. In this sense, they are a form of coping or a coping strategy, too (Peichl 2018). "Having revenge thoughts" can be an expression of "moving away from the place of trauma in the past to a 'safe' present" (ibid. p. 225).

In the therapeutic context, it is meaningful and healing to allow and acknowledge feelings of revenge and, in particular, their imaginative expression; they balance the injustice and the harm that was done to us. This usually has a relieving, liberating and strengthening effect; not least because it also dissolves the feelings and thoughts of revenge. Many times this is an important part of processing a traumatic experience, which supports and sometimes even enables the process of healing. Caution is advised, however, if feelings and thoughts of revenge persist over a longer period of time, repeat themselves and do not resolve. Then it is necessary to explore them more closely and to investigate the deeper causes.

It is important to support our clients in finding the most appropriate way of expressing their feelings of revenge. Sometimes it is relieving to have just talked about the thought of revenge. Otherwise, I invite my clients to allow themselves to give their feeling of revenge space in their imagination and to vent it. Some imagine, for example, that the perpetrator is condemned by a higher power or that he or she is punished for his/her deed. While doing so, it is helpful to encourage our clients to consciously be aware of their body and physical sensations and to observe how these change. For instance, an initial pressure in the heart or tension in the arms can gradually dissolve. It is also beneficial to ask our clients for movement impulses and to encourage them to actually or imaginatively carry them out (Levine 2011). Some people clench their fists, others hiss loudly or stomp on the ground. I support this by inviting them to carry out the movements in a controlled way and rather slowly or dosed and, e.g., to hit the backrest or to stamp firmly on the ground, provided they take care not to injure themselves.

Repeatedly I experience how relieving and liberating this can be for our clients. This seems to close a circle, to calm something in them that was previously unfinished, blocking energy and burdening them.

Example from practice

Ingolf, 47, was bullied and excluded in school for many years. Among other things, he suffers from severe anxiety, panic attacks, depression and is very tense. He has learned to suppress his rage and to keep it to himself. After discussing what he would like to do with his rage, Ingolf imagines telling his former classmates his opinion. And he imagines that they are bullied for a day and experience what he had to go through. By imagining this, Ingolf feels liberated, relieved and strengthened. ◄

16.5 Mindful, Controlled and Well-Dosed

For some people, though, it can be critical to allow their rage and aggression. While this can be relieving for them, it can also evoke feelings of guilt, self-condemnation and fear or feelings of punishment. I experience this especially with people who have gone through physical, psychological and/or sexual violence in their childhood through their parents or their caregivers. It is eminently relieving for them when we convey to them that their rage and aggressive impulses are natural and healthy reactions to their experiences, and expressions of their self-protection and self-defense. A careful, well-dosed approach in small steps is particularly important for them. Therefore, it is advisable to invite them to allow aggressive impulses gently and to express them, for example, through movements that are carried out rather slowly and consciously or controlled (Levine 1998). After a few moments, we should ask them to sense inside and if necessary pendulate to a balancing resource, such as feeling the ground under their feet, a few slow breaths or consciously perceiving the room. Through this dosed approach, our clients can express and channel their rage and aggression in small doses embedded in resources and so finally gain stability.

16.6 The Necessity of the Consciously Experienced Expression of Rage

It is crucial to express our rage consciously. If we do this attentively, controlled and while being aware of our body, it has a very relieving, liberating and also strengthening effect. In doing so, we experience that we can control and direct our body and our emotions. As we have discussed several times, we give our body the opportunity to make up for something that was not possible before. With this conscious, attentive and body-perceiving approach, we can channel our rage and aggression in very different ways; in our imagination, through movement, through singing and toning, making music, or through creative expression, such as painting, writing or handicrafts. Even conscious exhaling or blowing out can be helpful. Some people, however, find it less harmonious to express their rage and aggression; for them it is more appropriate to deal with them in another, rather transforming way. In accordance with the Buddhist practice of Tonglen, for some it can be helpful to inhale the rage into their heart, to accept it, to transform it and to let it out with the exhalation (Olvedi 2008). Others prefer to imagine that they shake off the rage like pitch or that it flows out of them and drains away.

References

Goldner L, Lev-Wiesel R, Simon G (2019) Revenge fantasies after experiencing traumatic events: sex differences. Front Psychol 10:886. https://doi.org/10.3389/fpsyg.2019.00886

van der Kolk B (2016) Verkörperter Schrecken. Traumaspuren in Gehirn, Geist und Körper und wie man sie heilen kann. G. P. Probst, Lichtenau/Westfalen (The Body Keeps the Score. Mind, Brain and Body in the Transformation of Trauma. 2015, Penguin Books, London) Quoted from original English version (p 261)

Levine PA (1998) Trauma-Heilung. Das Erwachen des Tigers. Unsere Fähigkeit, traumatische Erfahrungen zu transformieren. Synthesis, Essen (Waking the Tiger: Healing Trauma: The Innate Capacitiy to Transform Overwhelming Experiences. 1997, North Atlantic Books, Berkeley)

Levine PA (2011) Sprache ohne Worte. Wie unser Körper Trauma verarbeitet und uns in die innere Balance zurückführt. Kösel, München (In an Unspoken Voice. How the Body Releases Trauma and Restores Goodness. 2010, North Atlantic Books, Berkeley)

Olvedi U (2008) Mo. Das Orakel der Tibeter. Wegweisende Antworten auf alle Lebensfragen. O. W. Barth, Frankfurt/Main

Peichl J (2018) Integration in der Traumatherapie. Vom Opfer zum Überlebenden. Klett-Cotta, Stuttgart

Zanotta S (2018) Wieder ganz werden. Traumaheilung mit Ego-State-Therapie und Körperwissen. Carl Auer, Heidelberg (Somatic Ego State Therapy™ for Trauma Healing: Whole again. 2024, Routledge, New York)

Part III
Basic Conditions

Successful trauma treatment requires certain fundamental conditions; namely, taking a particular attitude, observing and ensuring safety or the feeling of safety in our clients, and considering the special significance of psychoeducation. We will discuss these factors below.

17 Our Inner Attitude

Contents

Our inner attitude and the understanding with which we take on our role as trauma therapists are the basis of our work with traumatized people. They essentially determine the effectiveness of our accompaniment. A number of factors are of great importance here.

17.1 The Significance of Our Presence

Our accompaniment can only be effective if our clients feel safe with and around us (Porges and Geller 2018). The assessment of safety or danger takes place unconsciously, but immediately leads to physiological changes that we can perceive: With safety we feel relaxed and comfortable, in case of danger we feel tense or anxious. If our nervous system registers signs of danger, then our fight or flight reactions or our immobilization are triggered. If it detects signals of safety, then these defense systems are inhibited and our system of social engagement is

R. Lackner, *Stabilization in Trauma Treatment*,
https://doi.org/10.1007/978-3-662-67480-2_17

activated (Porges 2018). This enables us to enter into relationships, to be open to new things and to learning.

Our presence as a therapist plays an important role here. With a benevolent, open, non-judgmental presence we can convey safety to our clients and have a regulating effect on their nervous system. Being present means that we are centered, grounded and in contact with our inner self and at the same time "open and receptive to the entire experience" of our clients (Porges and Geller 2018, p. 193). If we succeed in this, they can feel seen, recognized and understood by us. Through a "therapeutic situation characterized by safety" and the repeated experience of safety, not only can a trusting, healing therapeutic relationship arise, but it also favors "the development of new neural pathways" and enables our clients to make new positive experiences and to flourish (ibid. p. 191). All this is crucial for their healing.

Furthermore, a judgmental attitude would put them in a defensive state and so prevent them from feeling safe. Being judged has an effect comparable to being in danger (Porges 2018). That is why our open, understanding, non-judgmental attitude is so important.

17.2 Appreciative and Mindful

An open and understanding attitude also includes an attentive, empathetic and appreciative accompaniment of our clients. It is important to fully recognize what they entrust to us, even if, or especially if, these are vague memories, feelings and considerations regarding previous experiences and possible connections between these and their symptoms. It means acknowledging their feelings, sensations, thoughts, even if these are not immediately comprehensible to us. If we question these or even "instruct" our clients, then not only does a hierarchical difference arise—here the expert, there the ignorant client—but they also re-experience powerlessness and lack of self-determination and don't feel taken seriously and respected by us. Moreover, this activates their defense mechanisms and thus prevents them from feeling safe and being able to open up. That is why we should convey our knowledge and experience, as well as our considerations and assessments to our clients in a very respectful, prudent and understandable way that is enriching and enlightening for them and contributes to their understanding of themselves and the consequences of what they have experienced.

17.3 Transparent, Collaborative and Strengthening Self-Determination

Our transparent approach is essential in order to support our clients´ feeling of safety and trust. On the one hand, this means informing them comprehensively: about trauma and its effects, the connections between traumatizations and symptoms, possible treatment approaches and methods and the necessity and significance of stabilization. And on the other hand, explaining our respective intervention proposals and steps and their objectives and mode of action. This gives our clients a high degree of clarity and controllability counteracting their feeling of powerlessness and strengthening that of safety as well as their trust. Our transparent approach is also an expression of respect and collaboration. Transparency and collaboration presuppose that we see our clients as "competent adults" (Reddemann 2011, p. 81) and meet them on an equal footing. After all, we all want to be taken seriously and respected by others and, above all, to have someone at our side in stressful and crisis situations who, despite our distress, recognizes our competence and self-determination and treats us with respect. A collaborative attitude means that we work together with our clients, so to speak as a team, to make them feel better again. And that we support and strengthen their self-determination and autonomy. This includes, among other things, informing our clients sufficiently and making joint decisions regarding the individual treatment steps and interventions.

17.4 Open to Doubts and Criticism

This presupposes that we are open to questions, doubts and criticism from our clients; these are frequently based on insecurities, fears or lack of information. Sometimes our clients also feel irritated, insecure or hurt by a behavior, a statement or an inattention on our part. To meet all this openly and be willing to discuss it not only strengthens their trust in us and our work and thus the therapeutic relationship, it in turn also supports their feeling of safety and recognition as well as their self-determination and autonomy. In addition, our openness allows our clients—sometimes for the first time—to have the correcting experience of being able to safely express their own needs, feelings and criticism.

This open approach to questions, objections and criticism allows us to get to know our clients better, to understand them more deeply and to respond more finely tuned to them. Furthermore, this approach enables us to check our previous line of action and to possibly correct it, e.g., when we recognize that we have to take even smaller dosed steps or explain interventions more precisely.

17.5 Partiality and Solidarity

Our partiality is an important aspect in our work with traumatized people. Especially when they have experienced physical, sexual and/or psychological violence, and/or neglect, and/or have grown up in a hostile family or social environment, it is important to take a stand and express our attitude towards our clients. By clearly pointing out the responsibility for any form of violence, neglect, hostility or exclusion, we support our clients in no longer feeling guilty and ashamed for what happened to them. People affected by violence usually feel responsible for what has been done to them. Accordingly, they often suffer from feelings of guilt and shame, negative self-attributions and sometimes tendencies to self-punishment. With our clear attitude, we put the responsibility in the right place—often for the first time in the life of our clients. If we fail to express our attitude and remain neutral towards them, this would unsettle them; they would interpret our neutral attitude as a silent affirmation of their responsibility and guilt and feel abandoned by us. A pattern that many have already experienced repeatedly.

Our partiality does not in any way mean that we "badmouth" the perpetrator or join in with any insults with our clients. Our partiality means much more—and not less—than to point out the responsibility for what happened in a factual and clear way: Sexual violence against children can never be their responsibility, even if the perpetrators usually claim the opposite. Beating a woman can never be justified, even if the perpetrators want to make the affected women believe this. If parents are emotionally cold, denigrating or defamatory, this can never be the fault of their children. This clear partial attitude is an important building block for the stabilization of our clients.

Over the years some have been able to develop a good relationship with their parents or other caregivers despite the physical or psychological violence they have experienced. This can be possible if the violence has not taken place often and our clients have not experienced it as too serious (so far, I have not experienced this with massive physical and psychological violence and neglect, and above all not with sexual violence) and that their parents changed over the years, but above all if they could admit their behavior. Even if a good relationship has become possible, it is necessary to point out the responsibility and condemn the behavior of the caregivers of our clients without denouncing them as people. Investigating the possible causes of the actions of their parents, such as their own traumatization through violent experiences, can also help them to process what happened and reduce their feelings of guilt, while still maintaining their existing relationship.

17.6 Our Understanding of Trauma

Our attitude is decisively determined by our understanding of trauma and traumatization and their consequences.

The immediate reactions to traumatic events take place instinctively and cannot be influenced voluntarily; they are "adaptive reactions" , which secure our survival (Porges 2018, p. 55). By conveying this fact to our clients and telling them that our nervous system always tries to do "the right thing", we support them in recognizing and appreciating their reactions as the best possible adaptation (ibid.). This benefits their healing process. If we explain to our clients that their immediate reaction of freezing in response to a sexual assault was an instinctive, consciously uncontrollable reaction of their body that protected their life, then this gives them enormous relief. The freezing as the oldest defense system ultimately secures our survival when fighting and fleeing are hopeless (Levine 1998). Therefore, Stephen

Porges (2018) recommends assuring our clients: “In a neurobiological sense, this was the best way to react that was possible for you, and it is fortunate that you behaved in this way. Had you fought, you might be dead now.” (p. 127). We cannot fight without risking harm against a larger, stronger or more powerful perpetrator; we also cannot flee without risking being caught up and then experiencing something even worse. This information helps our clients recognize and appreciate their physical reactions as meaningful and “right” survival mechanisms and consequently to find a positive approach to themselves and their body.

It is also important that we present them with explanations for their symptoms. In general, these are expressions of the adaptation of our body and psyche and, in this sense, attempts to self-regulate and return to balance. Restlessness, palpitations, panic attacks and increased startle reactions are signs of high activation of the sympathetic nervous system (Levine 2019). Dissociations, depressions, chronic fatigue and gastrointestinal disorders such as irritable bowel syndrome are “shutdown symptoms” and indicate involvement of the dorsal vagus branch of the parasympathetic nervous system (ibid. p. 32). Rage and aggression can reflect a defense reaction not carried out or completed. Fear and obstructive beliefs or convictions can be an expression of the self-protection of a younger self-part. Feelings of guilt can arise to counter the unbearable feeling of uncontrollability. These and other explanations for various symptoms as well as pointing out the importance of triggers, implicit memories and protective mechanisms enable our clients to better understand their symptoms, reactions and behaviors and so themselves (Fisher 2019). They can also recognize a certain logic, which Janina Fisher calls “trauma logic” (ibid. p. 74) and therby gain a feeling of controllability and normality. Hence, our explanations of the various symptoms are important elements of stabilization.

17.7 Recognizing Traumatized People as Survivors with Healthy Parts

Our clients have managed to cope with the unimaginable in their own best way. By recognizing and honoring this and the strength with which they have survived and continue to live and master their lives, we support them in recognizing themselves in their strength, in their active role and as survivors. Even those who, for instance, are not able to work due to their trauma, master their lives to the best of their ability and strive to lead a “normal” life again. With this attitude we confirm our clients and contribute to them gaining a more positive self-image.

Even severely traumatized people have both injured and uninjured inner parts and are both wounded and resilient (Yehuda 2014). By recognizing this and conveying it to our clients, we direct our and their attention to their self-parts that have remained healthy despite everything. In this way they experience themselves not only as wounded, but also as unwounded. This contributes, among other things, to them no longer feeling “strange” or even “sick”, but rather “normal” and gaining strength and self-esteem. By seeing, recognizing and honoring both their injured and their healthy parts, we contribute significantly to our clients´ stability and recovery.

17.8 Leading and Guiding

Despite all the appreciative, attentive and partnership-based accompaniment, it is important to lead our clients and "gently direct the focus and pace of treatment" (Fisher 2019, p. 82). If our clients are very activated, it is necessary, for instance, ask them to orient themselves to the outside in order to regulate themselves, or to pause and feel inside in order to slow down the process. Furthermore, it is important that we stop them if they become over-activated through telling their stories to protect them from being overwhelmed or flooded with intense feelings and inner images. In this way we not only shape the process, but also convey to our clients that we are paying attention to them, thus giving them safety. And we support them in learning to self-regulate and stabilize themselves.

17.9 Taking Care of Ourselves

Just like for our clients, self-care is a necessity for us, too. By taking care of ourselves and paying attention to what is good for us, strengthens us, brings us joy and fulfillment, as well as to our limits and boundaries, we can not only better face the challenges of our work with traumatized people, but we can also be a credible model for our clients for a caring attitude towards themselves. Practicing self-care also means, among other things, paying attention to sufficient private time and our psychological capacity and resilience. This includes the question to what extent, with what kinds of trauma and which clients we want and can work with. In our field of work taking these factors and their limits into account is often only possible up to a certain extent. However, this is just as important for our psychological stability and resilience as for our ability to consistently meet our clients with presence, attentiveness and openness.

Self-care also includes our self-regulation, both generally in our lives and specifically in accompanying our clients. If we succeed in regulating ourselves in connection with them, for example, by balancing a reaction in our body during our clients telling their story, we can stay in or return to a state of safety and maintain our presence. Therefore, our self-regulation and our presence belong together; in the sense of co-regulation, they are a prerequisite for us to be able to act in a regulatory manner on our clients so that they feel safe and their organism can calm down (Geller 2019). If we are calm, our clients will be calm, too, and by being present, their presence will also increase. Conscious slow breathing, being aware of our body and grounding exercises are the most immediate effective possibilities of self-regulation. Likewise, we can use many other stabilization exercises for our regulation. It is sensible to generally pay attention to our presence and self-regulation in our lives, both regarding our own psychological stability and health and with regard to accompanying our clients.

References

Fisher J (2019) Die Arbeit mit Selbstanteilen in der Traumatherapie. Junfermann, Paderborn (Healing the Fragmented Selves of Trauma Survivors. Overcoming Internal Self-Alienation. 2017, Routledge, New York) Quoted from original English version (pp 52, 60)

Geller SM (2019) Therapeutische Präsenz und die Polyvagal-Theorie: Prinzipien und Übungen für den Aufbau heilsamer therapeutischer Beziehungen. In: Porges SW, Dana D (Hrsg) Klinische Anwendungen der Polyvagal-Theorie. Ein neues Verständnis des Autonomen Nervensystems und seiner Anwendung in der therapeutischen Praxis. G. P. Probst, Lichtenau/Westfalen, pp 123–143 (Therapeutic Presence and Polyvagal Theory: Principles and Practices for Cultivating Effective Therapeutic Relationships. In: Porges SW, Dana D (Eds) Clinical Applications of The Polyvagal Theory. The Emergence of Polyvagal-Informed Therapies. 2018, W.W. Norton, New York, pp 106-126)

Levine PA (1998) Trauma-Heilung. Das Erwachen des Tigers. Unsere Fähigkeit, traumatische Erfahrungen zu transformieren. Synthesis, Essen (Waking the Tiger: Healing Trauma. The Innate Capacitiy to Transform Overwhelming Experiences. 1997, North Atlantic Books, Berkeley)

Levine PA (2019) Polyvagal-Theorie und Trauma. In: Porges SW, Dana D (Hrsg) Klinische Anwendungen der Polyvagal-Theorie. Ein neues Verständnis des Autonomen Nervensystems und seiner Anwendung in der therapeutischen Praxis. G. P. Probst, Lichtenau/Westfalen, pp 19–42 (Polyvagal Theory and Trauma. In: Porges SW, Dana D (Eds) Clinical Applications of The Polyvagal Theory. The Emergence of Polyvagal-Informed Therapies. 2018, W.W. Norton, New York, pp 3-26)

Porges SW (2018) Die Polyvagal-Teorie und die Suche nach Sicherheit. Traumabehandlung, soziales Engagement und Bindung. Gespräche und Reflexionen zur Polyvagal-Teorie. G. P. Probst, Lichtenau/Westfalen

Porges SW, Geller SM (2018) Therapeutische Präsenz. Neurophysiologische Mechanismen, die in therapeutischen Beziehungen ein Gefühl von Sicherheit vermitteln. In: Porges SW Die Polyvagal-Teorie und die Suche nach Sicherheit. Traumabehandlung, soziales Engagement und Bindung. Gespräche und Reflexionen zur Polyvagal-Teorie. G. P. Probst, Lichtenau/Westfalen, pp 189-214

Reddemann L (2011) Psychodynamisch Imaginative Traumatherapie. PITT—Das Manual. Klett-Cotta, Stuttgart

Yehuda R (2014) In: Southwick SM, Bonanno GA, Masten AS, Panter-Brick C, Yehuda R. Resilience definitions, theory, and challenges: interdisciplinary perspectives. Eur J Psychotraumatol 5. https://doi.org/10.3402/ejpt.v5.25338.

Excursus: The View of the Positive and Strengthening

18

Contents

With regard to a strengthening, resource-oriented attitude, we can find some valuable suggestions in Positive as well as Prospective Psychology and Psychotherapy.

18.1 Positive Psychology

The idea of Positive Psychology, that is, a psychology that deals with the success of life, goes back to antiquity. Aristotle and Epicurus already asked themselves how can our life be successful and what constitates a satisfied and happy life. The term Positive Psychology was first mentioned in 1954 by Abraham Maslow, an American psychologist. He was one of the co-founders of Humanistic Psychology, which assumes that man has a high potential to recognize and change himself, and whose core topics include self-development and finding meaning. At the end of the 1990s, Martin Seligman took up the term Positive Psychology (PP). When he was elected president of the American Psychological Association (APA) in 1998, he suggested giving psychology a new goal, namely "exploring what makes life worth living and working to create conditions that enable a worthwhile life" (2012, p. 14). Since then, interest in Positive Psychology has grown enormously. In the meantime, a wealth of research projects and scientific investigations

R. Lackner, *Stabilization in Trauma Treatment*,
https://doi.org/10.1007/978-3-662-67480-2_18

have been carried out, a multitude of publications have been published and courses on PP have been established in various countries. This has changed a lot since its beginnings; originally concerned with the research of happiness, Positive Psychology now deals with well-being. According to Martin Seligman (2012), this is based on five factors, namely:

- **p**ositive emotions
- **e**ngagement
- positive **r**elationships
- **m**eaning and
- **a**ccomplishment

These five factors form the PERMA model, with the word PERMA composed of the first letters of the terms of the five factors and meaning "permanent". According to Martin Seligman, each of these factors contributes to well-being, is sought after by most people and can be defined and measured independently of other aspects. The goal of Positive Psychology is our "flourishing". A European-wide study shows people who flourish not only have positive feelings, engagement and meaning in life, but also self-respect, self-determination, optimism, resilience, vitality and positive relationships (Huppert and So 2009, cited in Seligman 2012). In contrast to conventional, predominantly deficit- and symptom-oriented psychology, Positive Psychology focuses on the promotion of strengths, positive feelings and positive relationships. It asks questions about what makes our life worth living, how we can better use our strengths and increase our life satisfaction, and how relationships can be successful (Dach-PP 2020). Over the years Martin Seligman and other representatives of PP have developed a number of interventions and researched their effectiveness in various studies. One of the best known interventions, the exercise "What went well" or "Three Blessings", was examined in a large internet study with several thousand participants. They first completed a depression and happiness test. Then every evening they wrote down three things that had gone well that day. After a week they repeated the two tests and reported their experiences with the exercise. Martin Seligman was particularly interested in the 50 participants whose depression scores were highest at the beginning and whom he classified as severely depressed. After a week, even their scores were only weak to moderate. At the same time, their happiness scores rose significantly. Martin Seligman (2012) himself admits that this study was neither randomized nor had a control group, and it can be assumed that only those people participated who hoped for an improvement in their condition. Nevertheless, he emphasizes that he has never observed comparable improvements in his long-term therapeutic work.

One element of Positive Psychology is the work with the so-called character strengths. Based on the virtues of wisdom, humanity, courage, justice, transcendence and moderation, which are valid worldwide in almost all cultures, Christopher Peterson and Martin Seligman (2004) defined twenty-four character strengths that should enable flourishing. These include creativity, optimism, discipline, humor and love. The character strengths questionnaire "Values in Action" (VIA) developed by the two can be used to measure these character strengths. Martin Seligman recommends his clients take this test, which can be accessed on the internet. In the "Exercise of Character Strengths" he then invites them to implement one or more of their strengths in a new way. If someone has creativity as a strength and has used it little so far, he could take up an artistic activity to promote it. The effect of the exercise of character strengths was examined in a multi-month internet study with 411 women and men (Seligman et al. 2005). The participants had to fill out a depression and a happiness test at the beginning and then carry out the exercise every day for a week. Immediately afterwards and at four other points in time, the participants had to take the two tests again. It was found that one month after the intervention and at all later points in time, depression was considerably reduced and well-being remarkably increased. The strongest improvement in both areas was achieved by those participants who had continued the exercise for more than the prescribed period of one week.

A meta-analysis of 51 studies with a total of over 4000 participants also showed that interventions of Positive Psychology both considerably reduce the symptoms of depression and substantially increase well-being (Sin and Lyubomirsky 2009). Based on their study results, Nancy Sin and Sonja Lyubomirsky suggest incorporating interventions of PP into the treatment of people with depression. They recommend applying them in particular in individual settings, tailored to each client, and over a longer period of time. A more recent meta-study of 39 randomized control studies shows, too, that interventions of Positive Psychology lead to a significant improvement in depressive symptoms and a distinct increase in well-being (Bolier et al. 2013).

Carmela White et al. (2019) recently reanalyzed these two meta-studies, taking into account the sample sizes of the individual studies as well as the respective effect sizes. Their results show a notably lower effectiveness of the PP interventions than the studies by Sin and Lyubomirsky (2009) and Bolier et al. (2013). The authors therefore conclude that both the duration and frequency of the intervention as well as a combination of several interventions could lead to a higher effectiveness.

A recent meta-study of 50 randomized control studies that specifically focused on the effect of the combination of various Positive Psychology interventions did indeed show a significant improvement in overall mental health, yet the effect sizes regarding the reduction of anxiety, depression and stress were only moderate to small (Hendriks et al. 2020). Although these different study results differ slightly from each other, they still reveal the significance and effectiveness of Positive Psychology interventions.

Positive feelings

Core topics of Positive Psychology include positive feelings. Barbara Fredrickson, a pioneer of PP, has made a significant contribution to this with her Broaden-and-Build Theory. While negative emotions such as fear or insecurity limit our view of our options for action, positive emotions expand our perception and thus enable us to have a greater range of thought and action (Fredrickson 2011). "Positive emotions open our hearts and our minds, so that we become more receptive and creative." (p. 36). This allows us to "discover, explore and build new skills, new bonds, new knowledge and new possibilities of being" (p. 39). If we are in a positive mood, we are more open and curious, approach other people and it is easier for us to take in new things. It has already been shown in learning research; according to this, children learn more easily in a relaxed, fear-free environment and they achieve better performance than in a tense or threatening one. This corresponds to the Polyvagal Theory, according to which we can only be open and receptive if we feel safe (Porges 2018). If we have positive feelings, we feel safe or we can only have positive feelings if we feel safe. However, if we are afraid, doubtful or angry, then our feeling of safety is reduced or even non-existent.

Strengthening and increasing positive feelings has a variety of positive effects. For example, enjoying positive emotions stimulates our reward system; this is assigned to areas of our brain whose activation leads to a reduction of stress hormones (Davidson 2015). The more intensely we enjoy positive feelings, the longer this area will be activated. This in turn leads to a reinforcement of the experience of positive feelings.

As mentioned in chap. 12, our feelings are closely linked to our thoughts; the way we interpret and judge situations, events or things influences our feelings. So, we can positively influence our evaluations and our thoughts and consequently our feelings by focusing on the positive and consciously noticing it. However, this is not always as easy as some representatives of Positive Psychology convey. Positive feelings cannot simply be "switched on whenever we want", as Barbara Fredrickson says (2011, p. 72). To be able to strengthen and increase positive feelings, attention, practice and discipline are usually required. In addition to various interventions of PP, working with resources, mindfulness exercises, inner images as well as movement and sports can be helpful.

The experience of positive feelings is dependent on our attitude towards life, both interactively influencing each other. People with a positive attitude probably find it easier to feel and enjoy positive feelings; this in turn reinforces their positive attitude. However, our attitude to life is based on numerous factors and is shaped, i.a., by our personality, our experiences, the attitudes of our parents or caregivers and social norms. All these factors influence how we perceive the world and life and how we evaluate, for instance, events and situations. These evaluations in turn shape our thoughts. Changing our attitude to life positively is therefore usually a protracted process. This involves repeatedly focusing on the positive, noticing it and bringing it to our awareness. This requires not only the conscious decision for a more positive attitude, but above all constant implementation. It also plays a role whether and what meaning we give to our life. If we cannot recognize any meaning in our life, we will probably experience burdens mainly as defeat or suffering, perhaps also as an imposition; if, on the other hand, we see life, for instance, as a process of inner growth, then we will presumably be able to recognize burdens as challenges and opportunities for learning.

A positive attitude to life is not only associated with more life satisfaction and success, but also has a positive effect on our health. Strengthening a positive attitude to life leads to a reduction in blood pressure and the release of stress hormones as well as to strengthening our immune system (NIH 2015). And it supports us in overcoming and processing burdens and traumatic experiences.

Criticism of Positive Psychology

Positive Psychology has been viewed critically since its beginnings. It is frequently equated with positive thinking. However, this criticism is too short-sighted, as Positive Psychology is not only much more complex, but also scientifically sound. Positive Psychology is not about ignoring or blocking out all burdensome or negative things like in a "Lala-Land" and smiling through life regardless of what happens. Rather, Positive Psychology is about a fundamental paradigm shift; away from a deficit- and symptom-oriented to a strength- and resource-oriented alignment. It is no longer about focusing exclusively or predominantly on diseases and problems, but rather on health and solutions. This means taking a fundamental positive attitude and conveying it to our clients.

Nevertheless, even Robert Biswas-Diener, an American representative of Positive Psychology himself, sees this critically. He emphasizes that many users of PP make themselves "slaves" of it by exclusively pursuing the strengthening of positive feelings (2019). He therefore emphasizes the need to take into account both positive and negative feelings. This is about researching the meaning of negative feelings; for example, fear caused by trauma can indicate the need for safety. Regardless, feelings such as rage or sadness are usually appropriate and should be able to be expressed; e.g., when we experience injustices or the loss of a loved one. Barbara Fredrickson (2011) emphasizes that it is not about ignoring or suppressing negative emotions; rather, it is about finding a balanced ratio between positive and negative feelings. Since we experience negatives more intensely than positives, we need to have more positive than negative feelings. The mathematician Marcial Losada, in collaboration with Barbara Fredrickson, has determined a ratio that indicates the necessary relationship between positive and negative feelings enabling a fulfilled life. According to this, we should have at least three positive emotions for every negative one; with a ratio of at least 3:1, the positive feelings become so strong that they can balance out the negatives (ibid.). Positive Psychology is thus increasingly no longer limited to positive feelings, but includes negative ones or the entire range of human feelings. In addition, it is increasingly dealing with the balance between different emotional qualities.

Another criticism of Positive Psychology is the fact that some representatives present the interventions of PP as if everything were possible with them. Although, as we have seen, they can be effective, they are by no means miracle cures. This is shown by the different studies mentioned earlier. The various studies reflect the effectiveness of PP, but also its limitation or that it is not equally effective for everyone and every symptom.

Finally, according to Robert Biswas-Diener (2019), Positive Psychology should not be presented so much, but rather be "invisible" and determine our work as a fundamental attitude and indirectly flow into it, for instance, by exploring the strengths of our clients; through questions such as, what they look forward to in their free time or when they feel brave or authentic.

18.2 Positive Psychotherapy

Martin Seligman's colleague Tayyab Rashid developed Positive Psychotherapy (PPT) from Positive Psychology for people with depression. This typically includes 14 sessions, each dedicated to a topic, whose goal is to strengthen the five PERMA factors. For example, in the first session, clients are asked to write a "positive introduction" describing a situation that shows them "at their best" (Seligman 2012, p. 68).

According to a study by Tayyab Rashid, Martin Seligman and Acacia Parks (2006), PPT significantly relieves depressive symptoms more than conventional integrative psychotherapy or conventional integrative psychotherapy plus medication with antidepressants. While 55% of PPT clients achieved improvement, this was only the case for 20% of the conventional therapy clients and 8% of the conventional therapy plus medication clients.

The Austrian Positive Psychotherapy Study, in which 92 women and men (64.1% and 35.9%, respectively) with major depression participated, compared Positive Psychotherapy with Cognitive Behavioral Therapy (CBT). Both therapy methods were applied in small groups of 6–7 participants. The participants in the PPT group not only showed a significantly greater improvement in their symptoms than those in the CBT group; the reduction in symptoms was still present at the follow-up examinations after 18 and 24 months (Laireiter 2019).

The idea of Positive Psychotherapy was not only developed by Tayyab Rashid and Martin Seligman; rather, PPT was already founded in 1986 by Nossrat Peseschkian, a German psychiatrist born in Iran. His concept of Positive Psychotherapy is based on the conviction that man is basically good and healthy and has "a wealth of abilities" that are "laid down like seeds" and can and must be "developed through education and self-education" (Peseschkian Foundation 2019). The three main principles of his Positive Psychotherapy are hope, balance and consultation. According to the principle of hope, for example, no attempt is made to immediately combat symptoms; rather, it is necessary to see them in a larger context and to recognize both their meaning and their positive aspects. With the principle of balance, it is about bringing the four life areas described by Nossrat Peseschkian (body, achievement, contact and meaning or future) into balance. If, for instance, coping with stress is mainly done in one area, such as through excessive sport (body area) or social withdrawal (contact area), it must be balanced by involving the other life areas. The principle of consultation includes five stages; one of them is the activation of resources and help for self-help.

18.3 Suggestions for Stabilization

Although there are some points of criticism about PP and PPT, they still represent a significant enrichment of our work with traumatized people. Above all, because they encourage us to focus on the intact, healthy parts as well as on the strengths and potential of our clients. It is about the "both and" that we notice both our clients´ suffering and the wounding as well as their strength and intactness. Moreover, Positive Psychology encourages us to support our clients to pay attention to the positive in their life, that is, to be aware of their abilities and potential as well as to notice positive experiences, encounters and moments as well as possibilities and positive circumstances. Collecting resources can be as helpful as keeping a diary in which our clients write down everything pleasant they experience, whether it is big, such as a professional success, or very small, such as enjoying a cup of coffee. In addition, interventions of PP and PPT, such as "Me at my best" or "Three Blessings", can be very supportive (Seligman 2012).

Example from practice

Armin, 42, has a very negative image of the world and himself due to various traumatic experiences in his childhood and youth. He tends to assume the worst, expect failure and devalue himself again and again. Armin takes up my suggestion to write down at least three positive things or experiences every day and to think about what he has contributed to them. Moreover, at the beginning of each session we talk about what was pleasant or good since our last appointment. At first Armin finds this very difficult; he interrupts himself repeatedly with "But" and makes a negative remark. Over time, however, he takes a liking to this exercise and begins to correct himself whenever he devalues himself or focuses on something negative. Gradually, Armin even enjoys recognizing when he falls into self-devaluation or negative expectations. He even gets used to consciously counter something positive: "And I managed to get my children´s crooked rabbit hutch back in order." Through these exercises, Armin's view gradually widens from the predominantly negative to the positive and he gains self-confidence and self-assurance. ◄

It is sensible to encourage our clients to have more positive experiences in their everyday life by exploring, for example, what gives them pleasure and putting it into practice. It is particularly important that they have as many positive experiences and feelings as possible in our joint work, e.g., through imagery or grounding exercises. All these are essential elements of the stabilization and healing of our clients.

18.4 Prospective Psychology and Psychotherapy

Prospective Psychology is a very young branch of psychology that arises from Positive Psychology. According to Martin Seligman et al., "prospection refers broadly to the mental representation and evaluation of possible futures." (UPenn 2020). It is both the "mental simulation of the future" (Andrews-Hanna and Arch 2019) and the ability "to pre-experience the future" (Gilbert and Wilson 2007, p. 1352). Thus it is coupled to our imagination, or our ability to imagine. When we anticipate future events, such as a goal, we visualize them in our mind´s eye. This ability is essential for our life; it enables us to make decisions, to plan, to pursue goals and ultimately to act. And it enables us to unfold and shape our lives. Our prospection ability therefore also plays a very important role for our health and life satisfaction. Prospective thinking can be both supportive and strengthening as well as burdensome and discouraging, i.e. when it is determined by worries and fear. If we have a rather negative view of the world due to our previous life experiences and personality, like Armin, we will approach our future with worries or negative expectations. This can lead to further negative experiences and thus to their consolidation. Our prospection ability or our prospective thinking is a complex process that is determined by different factors, such as our personality, previous life experiences as well as our search for meaning, attitude to life and our assumptions about life and ourselves.

As Martin Seligman et al. (UPenn 2020) have pointed out, so far social science has been focused on examining how the past shapes our present and future. By contrast, Prospective Psychology aims to explore how the future guides our actions. It seeks to answer the question of whether and how our feelings, thoughts and actions can be positively influenced by a positive vision of our future (Streit 2019). Traditional psychology and psychotherapy are largely focused on the past and on exploring the causes of our current problems, burdens and symptoms. By engaging with the past and working through it, we can achieve improvement in the present. On the contrary, Prospective Psychology and Psychotherapy see the past as a resource; we can use experiences and information from the past that are helpful or important for our future (Seligman et al. 2013). The goal of Prospective Psychology and Psychotherapy is to improve our future life, health, life satisfaction and well-being.

In particular, so-called Everest goals are useful; they serve as a kind of lighthouse, showing us where we want to develop (Streit 2019). Everest goals are characterized, among other things, by being meaningful, significant, emotional, realistic and goal-oriented and by opening up new possibilities and prospects. It is less about achieving them than about the path to them. This contributes to developing our potential and is meaningful. In a series of therapeutic sessions, the Everest goal is developed and described. Future questions, images and imaginings play a role here, as do experiences and insights from the past and from existing problems. Finally, the client is invited to describe her vision created through this process as a story; she is telling the story of herself in her future being and life (Streit 2019).

A pioneer of today's Prospective Psychotherapy and thus far ahead of his time was Viktor Frankl, an Austrian psychiatrist and holocaust survivor. In his book ... *nevertheless say yes to life: A psychologist experiences the concentration camp* (1982) he describes the necessity of being future-oriented and meaningful despite the immeasurable suffering and complete uncertainty of the end of captivity. He observed that those people who had a goal and, e.g., hoped to see a loved one again, survived more often than those who had no hope and could no longer discover any meaning in their lives. Based on his descriptions of numerous everyday occurrences in the concentration camp, it becomes recognizable and gives us an idea of how much Viktor Frankl's own future-oriented and meaningful attitude determined his survival. He describes a situation during the terrible daily march from the camp to the workplace; he escaped the tormenting constant thoughts about daily, indeed hourly survival by imagining himself standing in a large beautiful lecture hall in front of an interested audience at a lectern and lecturing on the psychology of the concentration camp. Viktor Frankl founded Logotherapy and Existential Analysis (LTEA) based on his experiences and insights. He makes three philosophical and psychological basic assumptions, namely the freedom of will, the will to meaning and the meaning in life (Batthyáni 2019). In the freedom of man, Viktor Frankl sees the "space of shaping one's own life within the limits of the given possibilities" (ibid.). However, we are not only free, but above all "free for something", namely for a meaning. This, a goal, a life task or a vision and thus the orientation towards the future are support, reinforcement and motivator in the overcoming and healing of trauma.

Prospective approaches can be found in other psychotherapeutic directions, too, such as Solution-Focused Brief Therapy or Hypnosystemic Therapy.

Solution-Focused Brief Therapy (SFBT) explores the hopes of our clients by asking what they hope to achieve and how achieving this would change their lives and daily routine (Iveson 2002). Or by asking the miracle question developed by Insoo Kim Berg and Steve de Shazer (de Shazer and Dolan 2008) and asking: "Imagine a miracle happens overnight and your problem is gone; how do you know the next morning when you wake up that your problem is solved?" This question encourages us to imagine a future in which we have already left the current problem behind. It helps us to find out what a "solution image" can look like (Greenberg et al. 2001). This brings us into contact with our intact parts, our resources and our strength and strengthens our hope and motivation.

The Hypnosystemic Therapy is also goal- and thus future-oriented. One of its important steps is the "differentiated development of goal descriptions" and the "visions associated with them" (Schmidt 2018). By describing our goals and visions in detail, we visualize and anticipate them. It is about picturing what will be or begin; for example, we imagine what it is like to be relaxed and relieved. When we imagine our goal achieved, it becomes tangible. This makes "something of the desired accessible" to us and we experience that "something can be changed in the desired direction" (ibid. p. 103). This confirms our hope and confidence and strengthens our trust in ourselves and our ability to change ourselves or our lives.

18.5 Suggestions for Stabilization

A prospective approach or the use of future-oriented interventions is very supportive for the development and strengthening of our clients´ stability and healing. For example, it can be very helpful to invite them to develop an inner image of themselves in their future life (after overcoming their traumatic experiences). We can also suggest to our clients to see themselves free of symptoms or in a state that they hope and wish for.

Example from practice

Stephanie, 22, lost her younger sister in a traffic accident when she was 8 years old. Her parents were in shock. Despite their efforts, they were emotionally unavailable to Stephanie due to their great grief. Stephanie felt completely alone with her shock and pain. She withdrew to not burden her parents. The death of her sister overshadowed her family for years. Stephanie has been increasingly depressed and lonely since then. In one of our first sessions we talk about Stephanie's goals and hopes; she longs to feel alive again. Therefore, I suggest to her to beam herself into the future and imagine that she is fully alive. Stephanie sees herself as a lively young woman, wearing a colorful summer dress, running over a meadow of flowers and jumping over a small stream. She perceives an intense feeling of vitality, strength and joy; she feels tingling in her body and a lot of energy. Imagining this puts Stephanie in touch with her vitality and strength again. She regains a feeling of who she truly is in her innermost being. Imagining this daily, supports Stephanie to revive and gradually unfold her true nature and vitality. ◄

With the miracle question of Solution-Focused Brief Therapy, we can also encourage our clients to imagine a future, improved state and so get in touch with their resources, strengths and potentials. By anticipating and imagining a future state, they orient themselves inwardly to this and focus their attention and energy to achieve it. This promotes their motivation and confidence and their entire healing process. Likewise, discussing and exploring their life goals, visions and dreams can be very supportive for our clients. Together we can consider whether and how these can be implemented, even if only to some extent; in doing so, our clients can discover and strengthen their resources, strengths and potentials and unfold them.

References

Andrews-Hanna J, Arch J (2019) Large-scale momentary experience sampling and neurocognitive mechanisms of functional and dysfunctional prospective thought. https://www.prospectiepsych.org/content/projects. Accessed 20 May 2020

Batthyáni A (2019) Was ist Logotherapie/Existenzanalyse? Logotherapie und Existenzanalyse. Viktor Frankl Institut, Universität Wien. https://www.univie.ac.at/logotherapy/logotherapie.html. Accessed 15 October 2019. Translated quote from https://viktorfrankl.org/logotherapy.html. Accessed 30 December 2023

Biswas-Diener R (2019) Positive coaching tools. 5. Positive Psychology Tour. 21–23 June 2019, Graz, AT

Bolier L, Haverman M, Westerhof GJ, Riper H, Smit F, Bohlmeijer E (2013) Positive psychology interventions: a meta-analysis of randomized controlled studies. BMC Public Health 13:119. https://doi.org/10.1186/1471-2458-13-119

Dach-PP (2020) Deutschsprachiger Dachverband für Positive Psychologie. https://www.dach-pp.eu. Accessed 18 May 2020

Davidson R (2015) In: Positive emotions and your health. Developing a brighter outlook. NIH. www.https://newsinhealth.nih.gov/2015/08/positive-emotions-your-health. Accessed 20 May 2020

De Shazer S, Dolan Y (2008) Mehr als ein Wunder. Lösungsfokussierte Kurztherapie heute. Carl Auer, Heidelberg (More than Miracles: The State of the Art of Solution-Focused Brief Therapy. 2021, Routledge, New York)

Frankl V (1982) Trotzdem ja zum Leben sagen. dtv, München (Yes to Life in Spite of Everything. 2020, Riders Book, London)

Fredrickson BI (2011) Die Macht der guten Gefühle. Wie eine positive Haltung ihr Leben dauerhaft verändert. Campus, Frankfurt (Positivity. 2009, Crown Publishers, New York) Own translation

Gilbert DT, Wilson TD (2007) Prospection: experiencing the future. Science 317:1351–1354

Greenberg G, Ganshorn K, Danilkewich A (2001) Solution-focused therapy counseling model for busy family physicians. Can Fam Physician 47:2289–2295

Hendriks T, Schotanus-Dijkstra M, Hassankhan A, de Jong J, Bohlmeijer E (2020) The efficacy of multi-component positive psychology interventions: a systematic review and meta-analysis of randomized controlled trials. J Happiness Stud 21(1):357–390. https://doi.org/10.1007/s10902-019-00082-1

Huppert FA, So T (2009) What percentage of people in Europe are flourishing and what characterizes them? IX ISQOLS Conference, July, 1–7. Cited in: Seligman M (2014) Flourish. Wie Menschen aufblühen. Die Positive Psychologie des gelingenden Lebens. Kösel, München (Flourish. A Visionary New Understanding of Happiness and Well-Being. 2011, Free Press, New York)

Iveson C (2002) Solution-focused brief-therapy. Adv Psychiatr Treat 8(2):149–156

Laireiter A (2019) Positive Psychotherapie in Österreich (Positive Psychotherapy in Austria). 5. Positive Psychology Tour. 21–23 June 2019, Graz, AT

NIH (2015) Positive emotions and your health. Developing a brighter outlook. https://www.newsinhealth.nih.gov/2015/08/positive-emotions-your-health. Accessed 20 May 2020

Peseschkian Stiftung (2019) Die Methode. https://www.peseschkian-stiftung.de. Accessed 15 October 2019

Peterson C, Seligman MEP (2004) Character strengths and virtues: a handbook and classification. Oxford University Press, Oxford. Cited in: Seligman M (2012) Flourish. Wie Menschen aufblühen. Die Positive Psychologie des gelingenden Lebens. Kösel, München (Flourish. A Visionary New Understanding of Happiness and Well-Being. 2011, Free Press, New York) Own translation

Porges SW (2018) Die Polyvagal-Theorie und die Suche nach Sicherheit. Traumabehandlung, soziales Engagement und Bindung. G. P. Probst, Lichtenau/Westfalen

Rashid T, Seligman M, Parks AC (2006) Positive psychotherapy. Am Psychol 61(8):774–788

Schmidt G (2018) Einführung in die hypnosystemische Therapie und Beratung. Carl-Auer, Heidelberg

Seligman MEP (2012) Flourish. Wie Menschen aufblühen. Die Positive Psychologie des gelingenden Lebens. Kösel, München (Flourish. A Visionary New Understanding of Happiness and Well-Being. 2011, Free Press, New York)

Seligman MEP, Steen TA, Park N, Peterson C (2005) Positive psychology progress. Empirical validation of interventions. Am Psychol 60(5):410–421

Seligman MEP, Railton P, Baumeister RF, Sripada C (2013) Navigating into the future or driven by the past. Perspect Psychol Sci 8(2):119–141. http://www.pps.sagepub.com/content/8/2/119

Sin NL, Lyubomirsky S (2009) Enhancing well-being and alleviating depressive symptoms with positive psychology-interventions: a practice-friendly meta-analysis. J Clin Psychol 65(5):467–487

Streit P (2019) Prospektive Psychotherapie (Prospective Psychotherapy). 5. Positive Psychology Tour. 21–23 June 2019, Graz, AT

UPenn (2020) About prospection. Prospective psychology. University of Pennsylvania. http://www.https://www.prospectivepsych.org/content/about-prospection. Accessed 20 October 2020

White CA, Uttl B, Holder MD (2019) Meta-analyses of positive psychology interventions: The effects are much smaller than previously reported. PLoS ONE 14(5). http://www.org/10.1371/journal.pone.0216588

19 Providing Safety and Support

Contents

The experience of safety is the prerequisite for processing traumatic experiences and healing from trauma. Hence, safety is the basis of any trauma treatment. As already mentioned, the development of a healing therapeutic relationship requires the experience of safety; this is necessary for our clients to make new positive experiences, learn new things and develop. We should therefore do everything to enable them to feel safe with us. Certain conditions are required for this, which go beyond the elimination of real threats (Porges 2019). Essential here are signals of safety that have a calming effect on our clients´ autonomic nervous system.

19.1 Signals of Safety

We can evoke a feeling of safety in our clients by using a melodious, pleasant voice, a friendly facial expression, a warm open look as well as positive mimic and gesture (Porges 2018). Furthermore, the aspects of our attitude described above, including our presence, mindfulness and appreciation as well as partnership and partisanship, are essential for our clients to feel safe.

R. Lackner, *Stabilization in Trauma Treatment*,
https://doi.org/10.1007/978-3-662-67480-2_19

19.2 External Conditions

Our clients´ feeling of safety can be influenced by external conditions. The certainty of being in a protected room that no one enters unannounced is important for everyone, but especially for traumatized people. Likewise, a silent room, as noises in the low frequency range, such as those from fans, elevators, traffic or MRI machines, are a danger signal to our nervous system and activate our defense systems (Porges 2018). Accordingly, we should reduce low-frequency noises in our practice or clinic rooms as far as possible. If disturbances still occur, it is important to inform our clients of their cause and possible duration; such clarity contributes to their feeling of safety. In addition, it is helpful to assure our clients that they are safe here and now.

19.3 Basic Guidelines

Basic guidlines that apply in conventional psychotherapies should be particularly taken into account with traumatized people. These include in particular:

- our reliability, i.e. that we only announce what we can certainly keep, or point out if we cannot promise something for definite, like a quick contact with a treating psychiatrist or our availability between individual appointments
- continuity, constancy and punctuality of our accompaniment, so that our clients can rely on this and us
- clarity regarding the duration of our respective appointments or units and our cancellation policy
- transparency regarding costs and any refund or financial support options
- the assurance and emphasis of our duty of confidentiality; this is particularly important for traumatized people and contributes to their feeling of safety

19.4 External before Internal Safety

Trauma-therapeutic accompaniment presupposes that our clients are not currently exposed to danger, for example, from a violent partner. We can only work trauma-specifically, if this is guaranteed. If external safety is not ensured, it is important to support and advise our clients accordingly, to take steps to establish their safety, or to refer them to an appropriate facility. It is imperative to explain to our clients why a trauma-therapeutic approach is only possible when their external safety is guaranteed.

References

Porges SW (2018) Die Polyvagal-Teorie und die Suche nach Sicherheit. Traumabehandlung, soziales Engagement und Bindung. Gespräche und Reflexionen zur Polyvagal-Teorie. G. P. Probst, Lichtenau/Westfalen

Porges SW (2019) Die Polyvagal-Theorie. Eine Einführung. In: Porges SW, Dana D (Hrsg) Klinische Anwendungen der Polyvagal-Theorie. Ein neues Verständnis des Autonomen Nervensystems und seiner Anwendung in der therapeutischen Praxis. G. P. Probst, Lichtenau/Westfalen, pp 67–85 (Polyvagal Theory: A Primer. In: Porges SW, Dana D (Eds) Clinical Applications of The Polyvagal Theory. The Emergence of Polyvagal-Informed Therapies. 2018, W.W. Norton, New York, pp 50–69)

The Significance of Psychoeducation

20

Contents

Psychoeducation plays a crucial role in stabilization. By informing our clients about trauma, showing them the effect of traumatic experiences on our body and psyche, providing them with different explanatory approaches to various symptoms and explaining the significance of triggers, implicit memories and protective mechanisms, they can better understand their symptoms, reactions and behaviors as well as their feelings and bodily sensations—and so themselves (Fisher 2019).

As already mentioned, it is important, among other things, to convey to our clients that the immediate reaction to a traumatic event is instinctive and cannot be voluntarily influenced by us; it is the best possible reaction of our body under the given circumstances to ensure our survival (Porges 2018). Furthermore, it is essential to explain to our clients that the consequences of a traumatic experience are attempts of our body and psyche to self-regulate and come back into balance. They are therefore not an expression of a disorder or illness, but rather an expression of the adaptation of our organism to an overwhelming event with which we try to cope as best we can. All this information relieves our clients and helps them to feel less "strange" and to lose their fear of "going crazy". Moreover, it gives them a feeling of control and strengthens their self-determination and autonomy.

Part of the psychoeducation should be the information that traumatization is treatable and curable, and that there are now some very effective techniques and methods to treat trauma, such as Eye Movement Desensitization and Reprocessing (EMDR) by Francine Shapiro (1999), Somatic Experiencing by Peter Levine (1998) and Brainspotting by David Grand (2013).

R. Lackner, *Stabilization in Trauma Treatment*,
https://doi.org/10.1007/978-3-662-67480-2_20

Finally, educating our clients about stabilization and its necessity, benefits and effects is an important part of psychoeducation; here we should inform them about the different possibilities and approaches to stabilization and the importance of resources as well as about the goal and the effect of the respective stabilizing intervention or exercise that we recommend to them.

References

Fisher J (2019) Die Arbeit mit Selbstanteilen in der Traumatherapie. Junfermann, Paderborn (Healing the Fragmented Selves of Trauma Survivors. Overcoming Internal Self-Alienation. 2017, Routledge, New York)

Grand D (2013) Brainspotting. The revolutionary new therapy for rapid and effective change. Sounds True, Louisville

Levine PA (1998) Trauma-Heilung. Das Erwachen des Tigers. Unsere Fähigkeit, traumatische Erfahrungen zu transformieren. Synthesis, Essen (Waking the Tiger: Healing Trauma. The Innate Capacitiy to Transform Overwhelming Experiences. 1997, North Atlantic Books, Berkeley)

Porges SW (2018) Die Polyvagal-Teorie und die Suche nach Sicherheit. Traumabehandlung, soziales Engagement und Bindung. Gespräche und Reflexionen zur Polyvagal-Teorie. G. P. Probst, Lichtenau/Westfalen

Shapiro F (1999) EMDR. Eye Movement Desensitization and Reprocessing. Grundlagen & Praxis. Handbuch zur Behandlung traumatisierter Menschen. Junfermann, Paderborn (Eye Movement Desensitization and Reprocessing (EMDR) Therapy: Basic Pinciples, Protocols, and Procedures. 2018, Guilford Press, New York)

Part IV
Exercises and Interventions

Stabilization is the foundation and the heart of every trauma treatment. It plays an important role not only at the beginning, but throughout the course of treatment, significantly contributing to the improvement of our clients´ symptoms, well-being and quality of life. To be able to support it as best as possible, we need a wide range of different stabilizing exercises and interventions from which we can offer them different ones according to their symptoms and depending on the respective needs and goals.

Explaining Stabilization—Selecting, Explaining and Applying Exercises and Interventions

21

Contents

Right from the start of our joint work, we should inform our clients about the significance and necessity of stabilization. The previously mentioned image of a balance beam with two plates can illustrate the importance of stabilization: one of the plates carries the burden of the traumatic experience, the other the balancing force of stability and stabilization. The greater the burden of trauma, the greater the force of stability and stabilization must be in order to counteract it.

It is advisable to take the first stabilizing step right from our first conversation and to discuss their resources with our clients. Tailored to their mental and physical condition and existing resources, individual stabilizing exercises and interventions should then be proposed. In the spirit of our partnership approach and respect for the self-determination of our clients, it is important to inform them about the goal and mode of action of the respective exercise. By trying them out, they can find out whether they are easy to implement, suitable and helpful for them.

Depending on their burden, some of our clients may only need individual or few stabilizing interventions, while others may need several or a variety. To support them in the best possible way, often a number of different stabilizing exercises have to be incorporated gradually into our accompaniment. It is sensible to consider different approaches so that our clients can gain stability in a comprehensive way. Individualized to the respective aspect of their stabilization, such as

R. Lackner, *Stabilization in Trauma Treatment*, https://doi.org/10.1007/978-3-662-67480-2_21

the experience of safety or the reduction of rage, each individual intervention and exercise contributes with its mode of action to their stability.

21.1 Tailoring Exercises and Interventions Individually

We have a wealth of possibilities for working with our clients in a stabilizing manner. It is decisive that together we find those interventions and exercises that are comprehensible, appealing, easy to implement and most effective for them. We should discontinue interventions that are laborious, unpleasant or even threatening to our clients, as well as those that are incomprehensible, or do not appeal to them or those they experience as ineffective; even if they are helpful for other clients, recommended as standard interventions or described as necessary in the literature. The processing and healing of trauma and its consequences is in any case a process that requires a lot of courage, strength and frequently endurance from our clients; it is all the more helpful and relieving for them if they can discover beneficial and effective exercises for themselves that can be implemented as easily as possible.

Moreover, it is necessary for our clients to decide for themselves which of the interventions suggested they want to carry out. By giving them the freedom of choice, we convey appreciation and recognition and support their self-determination; all this contributes to their feeling of safety, which is the basis of every trauma treatment. "When safety and choice are paramount, the evolutionarily newer ventral vagal branch of the parasympathetic system ... is activated." (Ogden 2019, pp. 55–56). This leads to the calming of our clients´ organism and the activation of their system for social engagement (Porges 2018). Both are a prerequisite to have new experiences and learn new things, which in turn is essential for stabilization. Regardless of this, the exercises chosen by our clients are usually particularly effective, as they appeal to them and so increase their motivation to use them regularly. In contrast, it makes little sense to prescribe interventions in a standardized way to all clients. Not every intervention is equally helpful for all people; some are very effective for some people, yet, only a little or not at all for others, and even contraindicated for some; for instance, if they evoke fear or increase their restlessness. That is why it is so important to tailor the interventions to the individual.

Last but not least, it is a significant experience for our clients that they can decide for themselves which interventions they want to use; this is essential especially for those repeatedly, chronically and complexly traumatized, whose self-determination was severely violated and often hardly or not at all given.

With the interventions tailored to them, our clients can not only experience an improvement in their stability and so a relief and strengthening, but also a reinforcement of their self-efficacy and autonomy; and finally they can often have moments of lightness and joy as well. Again and again I see that even highly stressed people experience moments in which they feel lighter and experience joy through appropriate, appealing exercises.

Example from practice

Livia, 51, is still very burdened and traumatized by her experiences during the Bosnian war. She is highly activated and suffers from a number of psychological and physical symptoms. When exploring possibilities to calm down, Livia discovers that it feels good to her to breathe in and out slowly while imagining sitting on a swing, swinging back and forth. She gradually relaxes, feels increasingly relieved and senses a light joy rising in her. ◄

21.2 Compiling a Repertoire of Different Exercises

Basically, it is important that we compile a repertoire of various exercises with our clients so that they have different possibilities to act on themselves and their condition according to their needs and circumstances; this in itself strengthens our clients ability to act and their autonomy, which contributes to improving their stability. Furthermore, not all exercises are always equally effective and under all conditions; for example, a breathing exercise may be very helpful in one moment, less useful or even contraindicated in another.

In the course of the treatment process, besides the already explored, mostly further stabilizing interventions are necessary. Especially in the case of chronic, complex and attachment trauma new stabilizing exercises are always useful and necessary. This is also the case when symptoms change or a new theme appears, like an emerging rage, feelings of guilt or the longing for more self-expression. Likewise, if the previous exercises are no longer appropriate or sufficiently effective. It may well be that an intervention was very helpful at the beginning, but lost its effectiveness over time. Then it is necessary to change it or replace it with another. Apart from this, it is frequently necessary and sensible to offer our clients additional exercises and so expand their repertoire.

Many of the following interventions can contribute to a fundamental improvement in our clients´ stability; for some even to the extent that processing their traumatic experiences is no longer necessary. Other interventions are more of an additional support that offers them another possibility of self-help.

All interventions can be used directly in the setting with our clients to cushion and regulate, e.g., their high activation, flashbacks or dissociations. At the same time they can use them as exercises for themselves at home and as self-help tools between our appointments. Especially at the beginning of our collaboration, it is often necessary to find several interventions with our clients in order to initiate their stabilization as comprehensively as possible. However, we should be careful not to suggest too many exercises at once so that our clients do not feel overwhelmed; in my experience, there should be a maximum of 3 or 4 exercises per session.

21.3 Strengthening with Bilateral Stimulation

With the help of bilateral stimulation we can strengthen and consolidate many of the stabilizing exercises and interventions.

Bilateral stimulation is the basic technique of EMDR (Eye Movement Desensitization and Reprocessing), as well as part of other methods, such as Wingwave.

While rapid bilateral stimulation allows the processing of traumatic memories, slow bilateral stimulation can be used to fortify and consolidate positive feelings, sensations and states. We can set optical, tactile or acoustic stimuli; by moving our hand horizontally back and forth at eye level of our clients and they follow this movement only with their eyes, by lightly tapping alternately on their right and left knees or back of their hands, or by snapping alternately with our right and left hand. It is crucial to set slow, almost slow motion stimuli (about one tap per second). If our clients, for instance, imagine a beautiful, pleasant memory and experience it holistically, as an inner image with the associated positive feeling and body sensation, we can reinforce and consolidate this image at the end with bilateral stimulation (Shapiro 1999). Thereby it is important that the respective experience is continuously positive. Our clients can also use slow taps by themselves; many like the butterfly hug, in which they alternately tap their left upper arm with their right hand and their right upper arm with their left hand (fig. 21.1).

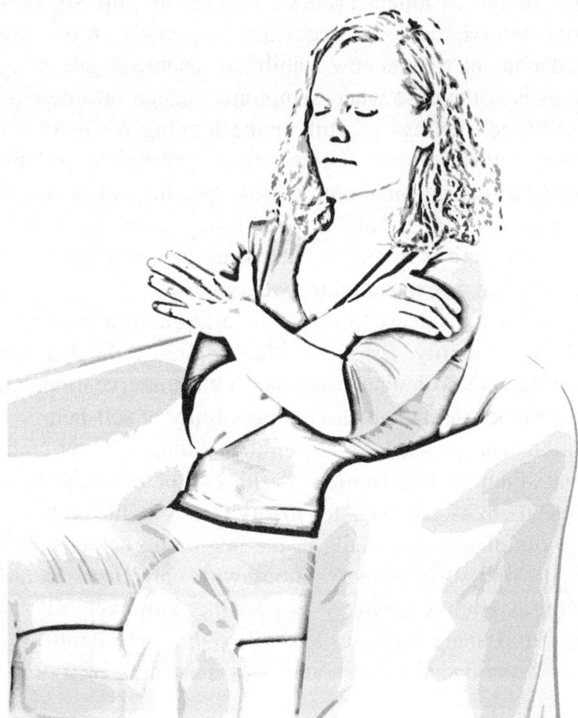

Fig. 21.1 Butterfly Hug—alternately tap slowly on the right and left upper arm

21.4 Considering the Window of Tolerance—Observing, Dosing and Braking

Any stabilizing intervention or exercise can occasionally lead to a higher or high activation of our clients, sometimes to an under activation. This is due to our "window of tolerance", that is, the "range of arousal" within which we can function well (Siegel 2012, p. 212). So it can happen that we exceed our window of tolerance through an exercise and then become confused, restless or frozen. A stabilizing exercise or parts and elements of it can, for example, touch and activate an experience or memory in us that is burdensome or threatening. This often happens without us being aware of it. Even positive feelings and states that are evoked by a stabilization exercise can be linked to unpleasant or threatening memories and feelings; this can be the case, for instance, if we received the news of the death of a close person in a moment of great exuberance. Therefore, we should observe our clients attentively during every intervention and exercise

- and pay attention to their physical reactions (i.a. their breathing) and
- always ask them during the exercise how they experience it and how they feel.

In this way, we can recognize as early as possible if our clients are over activated by an intervention or exercise and exceed their tolerance window, and counteract by "braking" (Rothschild 2002, p. 164) and dosing; e.g., by asking our clients to pause and sense inside, to focus their attention outside of themselves, to breathe in and out slowly or to move. If our clients find an intervention or exercise unpleasant or threatening and feel uncomfortable during it, we should stop it and take other stabilizing steps. It is important to convey to our clients on the basis of the model of the window of tolerance, that it is normal for some exercises or interventions to be too activating, threatening or unpleasant.

References

Ogden P (2019) Die Polyvagal-Theorie und die Sensumotorische Psychotherapie. In: Porges SW, Dana D (Hrsg) Klinische Anwendungen der Polyvagal-Theorie. Ein neues Verständnis des Autonomen Nervensystems und seiner Anwendung in der therapeutischen Praxis. G. P. Probst, Lichtenau/Westfalen, pp 49–65 (Polyvagal Theory and Sensorimotor Psychotherapy. In: Porges SW, Dana D (Eds) Clinical Applications of The Polyvagal Theory. The Emergence of Polyvagal-Informed Therapies. 2018, W.W. Norton, New York, pp 34–49) Quoted from original English version (p 40)

Porges SW (2018) Die Polyvagal-Theorie und die Suche nach Sicherheit. Traumabehandlung, soziales Engagement und Bindung. G. P. Probst, Lichtenau/Westfalen

Rothschild B (2002) Der Körper erinnert sich. Die Psychophysiologie des Traumas und der Traumabehandlung. Synthesis, Essen (The Body Remembers. The Psychophysiology of Trauma and Treatment. 2000, W.W. Norton, New York) Own translation

Shapiro F (1999) EMDR. Eye Movement Desensitization and Reprocessing. Grundlagen & Praxis. Handbuch zur Behandlung traumatisierter Menschen. Junfermann, Paderborn (Eye

Movement Desensitization and Reprocessing (EMDR) Therapy: Basic Principles, Protocols, and Procedures. 2018, Guilford Press, New York)

Siegel DJ (2012) Mindsight. Die neue Wissenschaft der persönlichen Transformation. Goldmann, München (Mindsight. The New Science of Personal Transformation. 2010, Bantam Books, New York) Own translation

Exploring, Activating, Strengthening and Expanding Resources

22

Contents

Besides the first information about traumatization and it effects, the first stabilizing step is to explore the resources of our clients. As described in chap. 8, resources can be anything that is strengthening, supportive, relaxing or pleasant for us, giving us a feeling of safety, leading us out of our circling thoughts or relieving us from tensions and aggression.

22.1 Simple but Effective

The following suggestions for exploring and expanding existing resources are very simple, almost obvious, and yet—and sometimes precisely because of this—very effective. They can be used in an initial conversation, as part of a crisis intervention or in a single contact, as well as at the beginning or during the course of a longer therapeutic process. Their effectiveness depends very much on the intensity of the feelings that the respective resource evokes in us and on the physical

R. Lackner, *Stabilization in Trauma Treatment*,
https://doi.org/10.1007/978-3-662-67480-2_22

sensations that we notice during it. The key to the effectiveness of our resources—as with all other stabilization exercises—lies in their conscious and most holistic experience possible. With a suitable word or sentence as well as a gesture or movement, we can set an additional anchor that strengthens our experience and helps us to remember and recall it later.

Caution: As already discussed in chap. 8.3, resources can sometimes "flip" (Wiedenmann 2020); for example, our clients can become restless or feel fear if they stay with a resource for too long. Therefore, it is important to make sure that they only stay with a resource as long as they experience it exclusively positive. Sometimes it turns out that a resource is linked to unpleasant memories or negative associations; then it is necessary to discard it and together find another one.

22.2 Collecting Current Resources

In general, I ask my clients in our first conversation about their resources and recommend that they have a think about them until our next appointment. I suggest they pay attention to what does them good, brings them joy and helps them to relax, switch off and reduce tension or rage in their everyday life. I recommend they get a special notebook or book to record their resources. In our follow-up appointment we then discuss these in more detail; I encourage them to integrate these more and more into their everyday life and we clarify whether they need more resources. Through engaging and writing down, our clients concentrate their attention intensively on their resources and bring them to their conscious awareness. Their resource book can help them at times or moments in which they have no or hardly any access to their resources; by reading their collection, they can bring them back to mind, pick them up and use them again.

Already just by dealing with our resources usually has positive effects. This directs our attention to what is positive in our life. Thus our view, which was possibly mainly directed to the burdensome, bad, widens and we can again see life in a greater diversity; as if a color spectrum, which was previously limited to dark tones, were now to be enhanced by a few or even several bright nuances. To recognize that there is something or some, perhaps even a lot, that is good in our life has a positive effect on our well-being and so on our psychological stability and lets us (again) see our life (a bit) more positively.

Example from practice

Emma, 32, experienced a lot of physical and psychological violence between her parents from an early age. She has suffered from fear, panic attacks and depression since her youth. Nevertheless, she was able to finish school and complete an apprenticeship. Due to her fear and inner tension she experienced both as very stressful. She works in a large company, in which she often feels exploited.

After some difficult relationships, she is currently single. Emma looks like she is electrified; she can hardly switch off and has little that gives her pleasure. When asked if there is something that does her good, she says after considering for a while that she likes to be in nature. She loves to walk through the forest. She always feels free and safe in nature. While talking about it, Emma increasingly relaxes and becomes more alive. During our conversation she discovers a lot more that does her good: listening to music, meeting friends, cooking, watching old movies with Hans Moser (a famous Austrian actor), Pilates and swimming, taking a long warm shower, reading poems. We agree that Emma might take time at least once a day for one or more of her resources. ◀

As with Emma, we often observe a positive change in our clients when they tell us about their resources; be it in their voice, their look or their posture. We can pick up on our observation and give them feedback. Regardless of this, we should ask our clients how it is for them when they think of their individual resources and talk about them. If they have a good feeling about it, it is sensible to invite them to consciously take it in and to encourage them after a few moments to explore where they can feel it most easily or strongest in their body.

I: "Fully feel the joy … and let it work on you. … and while you take in the joy, where in your body do you feel the joy most or strongest?"

Emma: "In my stomach, it's very warm … and in my chest, it's freer." (takes a deep breath in and out)

I: "Then consciously take in that your stomach feels very warm and your chest freer. … how is that right now?"

E: "Nice …" (takes a deep breath)

I: "Then just keep taking in the joy, and that your stomach is very warm and your chest freer and let it work on you … and if you like, imagine that every cell of your body takes in this state of joy, stores it and realigns itself."

With this short intervention, resources and the positive feelings they evoke can be strengthened. It is very supportive for our clients, if they use the resource as often as possible or envision it and re-experience it in their imagination and consciously take in and enjoy the positive feelings and body sensations associated with it.

22.3 Drawing on Previous Resources

As an extension, it is useful to explore with our clients what did them good in the past, before the traumatic event. This question is especially important if they currently have few or no resources. The following questions can be helpful:

- *"What helped you in the past?"*
- *"What did you used to like to do? What gave you enjoyment or fun?"*

- *"Which hobbies did you have in the past?"*
- *"What helped you to relax in the past?"*
- *"What helped you clear your head in the past?"*
- *"Were there moments when you were exuberant or felt free?"*
- *"Was there something that helped you to reduce tension, anger or rage?"*

22.4 Drawing on Childhood Resources

In addition, it can be very helpful to explore with our clients what used to make them feel good or bring them joy as a child, or which hobbies they had then. It is certainly worthwhile to consider whether one or the other of the former resources could be supportive now. We can encourage our clients to take up something that used to do them good in order to find out whether it is still or again beneficial for them.

Example from practice

Leopold[1], 76, has been suffering from great fear and severe depressive states for decades. There is hardly anything that does him good. When asked what used to give him enjoyment, he spontaneously remembers that as a boy he liked to build model boats and often immersed himself for hours in a book about model boats. He immediately agreed when I asked him as to whether he would still find pleasure in model boats, maybe even building them; he decides to look for his old book at home. In our next session Leopold reports enthusiastically that he found his book and enjoyed flipping through it. Meanwhile he has bought a model boat kit and has already started to assemble it. While talking, Leopold's eyes sparkle and his joy is clearly palpable. He himself notices this with surprise and is happy and wonders if his severe depression and fear may even improve after all. I invite Leopold to perceive and enjoy his joy. After a few moments I ask him where he senses the joy in his body. He answers: "In my heart … it feels light." So I ask Leopold to consciously feel his joy and light heart. When I ask him if a word or gesture comes to mind that reflects this state, Leopold puts his left hand on his heart and says: "carefree".—"While you sense that your heart feels light and your left hand is on your heart, and you say 'carefree', maybe you have an inner image that best reflects this state. That can be, but does not have to be."—"Yes, a boy, about 8 or 9, playing with a small boat by a creek … that's me and my best friend Hannes … in summer, in the countryside."—"Then consciously perceive this picture of you and Hannes, … feel that your heart feels light, and that your left hand is on your heart, … take the joy in, and if you like, you can say the words 'carefree' aloud or silently. … Take all this in consciously and into

[1] We already got to know Leopold in chap. 14.1.

yourself. … You know, you can always re-experience this state of joy, your picture, your hand on your heart and the words 'carefree' will support you." ◄

Leopold does this exercise every day. It improves his well-being within a few weeks; he experiences positive moments repeatedly, gains confidence and finds interest and joy in other things, too.

22.5 Positive Memories as Resources

When asking questions about positive events in the life of our clients, we focus on what was good, strengthening or safe and healing in their previous or earlier life. In reference to the idea of the joy biography of the Swiss psychologist Verena Kast (2014) we can suggest our clients collect and write down everything they have experienced that was beautiful, successful, precious, great or blissful up to now. The following questions can be supportive:

- *"If you look back, what was particularly beautiful/blissful/fulfilling in your life up to now?"*
- *"What are you proud of?"*
- *"Were there moments when you felt really good, when you were carefree/happy/unburdened?"*
- *"Were there moments when you felt completely comfortable?"*

Example from practice

Anna, 62, has experienced a lot of physical and psychological violence from her long-term partner. After several attempts to end this partnership, she finally succeeded in separating from her husband and building a new life. The effects of the violence experiences still burden Anna very much. However, she has numerous beautiful memories of her life before she met her husband. She particularly likes to think back to a trip with her best friend through Spain. At that time she was footloose and fancy-free, enjoyed life, lived from one day to the next, was adventurous and curious about what would come to her. ◄

We can invite our clients to think of a specific, particularly beautiful memory, to re-experience it inwardly and to feel and enjoy the feelings it evokes.

Example from practice

While Anna recalls her trip through Spain, she feels her vitality, freedom and curiosity. She perceives these as strength and life force in her body. By consciously enjoying them, they become even more tangible. Annas memory is a resource she can always access and so re-experience and reinforces her vitality and strength. ◄

By consciously and repeatedly experiencing a positive memory, the corresponding positive feelings and sensations are intensified and strengthened as well as the entire organism of our clients can calm down; in this way they can experience moments of recovery and refueling.

22.6 Enabling New Resources

If our clients have only few resources it is helpful to jointly investigate which further resources could be added to support them. With this or one of the following questions we open the space for possible new resources:

- *"What would you (still) need?"*
- *"What would (still) do you good?"*
- *"What could strengthen you?"*
- *"What could give you support/safety?"*
- *"What would (still) give you joy/fun?"*

To these or similar questions our clients can collect ideas and wishes—as free as possible from any mental limitations. Then we can jointly consider which of these can be implemented. It can also be helpful to ask what our clients have always wanted to learn or try out.

Example from practice

Tobias, 53, has a great need to reduce his tension and calm down. He says he has been thinking a long time about doing some kind of sport. It would do him good to be fitter and have more strength; then he would feel stronger and firmer overall. For a long time he wanted to start a martial art. So far he has not dared to do so. Tobias decides to finally realize this wish and see whether a martial art suits him. We discuss that he should choose a studio and arrange a trial session by our next appointment. ◀

Sometimes accompanying our clients is simply about encouraging them, occasionally even gently nudging them, to try something new, in order to support their stabilization process.

22.7 The Three Blessings

The "Three Blessings", which we already got to know in chap. 14.3, reduces depression and anxiety and strengthens general well-being when used daily over a longer period of time (Seligman 2012). Consequently, it can contribute to the stabilization of our clients. By writing down three things that went well during the day, they focus their attention on the positive and successful. By answering the question of what led to the "blessing" or made it possible, they focus more intensively on the positive aspects of their lives. If we modify the question and encourage our clients to ask themselves what contribution they have made so that the "three blessings" could happen, they become aware of their strengths and abilities without which the "blessing" would not have happened. For example, if they had a friendly encounter with their neighbor, they will be able to see that it was their open and friendly manner that made the pleasant conversation possible.

22.8 Dreams and Visions as Resources

As already described in connection with the Prospective Psychology, it can be very beneficial to invite our clients to develop an inner image of themselves in their future life—after having processed their traumatic experiences. We can also suggest they imagining being free of symptoms or in the state that they hope for.

Or we can encourage our clients to imagine a future state by asking the already mentioned miracle question of the Solution-Focused Brief Therapy. Imagining a desired state can be a very supportive, empowering resource. In this way, our clients orient themselves internally to their goal and focus their attention and energy to achieve it.

Discussing and exploring their life goals, visions and dreams can be very helpful for our clients, too. Together we can consider whether and how these can be implemented—perhaps only as a beginning; by doing so, they can discover, develop and reinforce their resources, strengths and potential and so gain stability.

22.9 Strengths and Abilities as Resources

A very effective support for our stability is the collection of our strengths and abilities. Similarly to collecting their resources, it is helpful to recommend our clients get a special notebook in which they only write their strengths, abilities, talents and any positive feedback they have received from others. Engaging with their strengths creates a counterweight to our clients´ burden and supports their stabilization. As with all other exercises, it is useful when discussing their strengths to ask our clients about their feelings and physical sensations associated with them and invite them to consciously perceive them.

Besides feelings of strength, joy, confidence, courage or pride, while talking about their own strengths, often feelings of shame, insecurity, doubt or presumption and bad conscience interfere. If this is the case, it is helpful to invite our clients to notice these feelings, too. And then ask if it is possible to allow both their strengths and their doubts to exist concurrently, so that both can be present at the same time. This allows our clients to find it easier to recognize and name their strengths. Then they are more likely to focus their attention on them and be aware of them.

22.10 Resource Portfolio and Resource Collage

In line with Barbara Fredrickson's (2011) portfolios of the ten basic emotions, such as love, gratitude and cheerfulness, we can suggest our clients create a resource portfolio or a resource collage. It is about collecting everything they associate with their resources: photos, drawings, poems or sayings, words and symbols, scents and objects. Our clients can paste or write all of this into a book or arrange it on a poster. The advantage of a poster is that they can hang it up visibly at home, so they can see it easily and are reminded of their resources and the associated feelings as often as possible.

Example from practice

Tessa's poster of her resources includes photos of herself as a happy little girl and of her favorite people, the text of a song from her favorite band that gives her a lot of strength, a few sayings, a drawn dumbbell that she associates with power and strength, the words "be free" and "be in my center", the symbol of a sun, the sketch of an arrow pointing steeply upwards, a rainbow and a prayer. Tessa hung this resource poster in her kitchen so that she can see it from her dining table. The poster always reminds her of everything that is good for her and important and reinforces and strengthens her. ◄

References

Fredrickson BI (2011) Die Macht der positiven Gefühle. Wie eine positive Haltung ihr Leben dauerhaft verändert. Campus, Frankfurt/Main (Positivity. 2009, Crown Publishers, New York)

Kast V (2014) Was wirklich zählt ist das gelebte Leben. Die Kraft des Lebensrückblicks. Kreuz, Zürich

Seligman M (2012) Flourish. Wie Menschen aufblühen. Die positive Psychologie des gelingenden Lebens. Kösel, München (Flourish. A Visionary New Understanding of Happiness and Well-Being. 2011, Free Press, New York)

Wiedenmann I (2020) Somatic Experiencing®. Training, Intermediate II, October 2020, Seitenstetten/AT

Feeling Safe and Protected 23

Contents

Experiencing feeling safe is the basis of any trauma treatment and the heart of stabilization. Therefore, at the very beginning of our joint work we should explore with our clients whether and when they feel safe. By pursuing this question, we can find moments, situations or conditions that have a regulating and balancing effect on our clients and let them relax and refuel. For some people, these are quite long periods of time, such as from the moment they arrive at home; for others, these can be shorter times, e.g., when they take a bath, drink a glass of wine or listen to certain music. Others tell us that they never feel completely safe and always feel a certain tension or threat. If we pursue the question together whether and when there are even very short moments in which they feel safe, however, most people will find one or the other corresponding situation. We can pick up on these and use them as a resource.

R. Lackner, *Stabilization in Trauma Treatment*,
https://doi.org/10.1007/978-3-662-67480-2_23

Basically, it is important to make our clients aware of consciously paying attention to their feeling safe or compromised or lack of safety in their everyday life. They should consciously use the factors and moments that give them a feeling of safety and integrate, strengthen and increase them in their daily life; however, if possible, they should avoid or largely reduce any that compromise their feeling of safety and cause feeling unsafe or threatened.

23.1 Exploring and Integrating Moments of Experienced Safety

It is particularly helpful for our clients to discover everyday moments in which they feel safe, such as their morning breakfast, as well as moments that they can easily and often integrate into their everyday life, such as listening to certain music. It makes sense to recommend that they allow themselves these moments as often as possible and consciously perceive the feeling of safety and the associated physical sensations and let them have an effect on them.

23.2 Recalling and Activating Moments of Experienced Safety

We can also invite our clients to recall a moment in which they felt safe and to re-experience it in their memory.

Example from practice

Nora, 36, has been suffering from great fear, strong general activation and a feeling of permanent insecurity and danger since she was raped after being drugged. In exploring moments of safety, Nora remembers that she felt safe when she was visiting her mother and sitting in the warm afternoon sun in the garden, cuddling up to her on a Hollywood swing and drinking cocoa. ◄

I: "When you recall this moment you were sitting with your mother in the afternoon sun on the Hollywood swing, cuddling with her and drinking cocoa, how is that?"

Nora: "That's good. … it is all good there."

I: "Hm, it is all good there. Then let that take effect on you. … and while you do that, where in your body do you feel that it is all good there?"

N: "Hm, there … in my stomach …" (takes a deep breath in and out)

I: "How does that feel?"

N: "It feels calm, and warm."

I: "Then consciously take note that your stomach feels calm and warm."

N: "Hm …" (takes a deep breath in and out)

I: “How is that now?”
N: “That makes me calm.”
I: “Then take note of that too; and stay with the memory of how you are sitting with your mother on the Hollywood swing and it is all good. And feel that your stomach feels calm and warm and you become calm.”

Nora was able to re-experience feeling safe through the memory of being with her mother; by consciously searching for and feeling the body sensations perceived (calm, warm stomach), her experience of safety intensified and deepened. During the daily use of this image, Nora always experiences moments of feeling safe. Her high activation can decrease and her organism can calm down. Through repeating this experience, Nora’s feeling of safety gradually increases.

23.3 Something Protective that Surrounds Us

Imagining something protective that surrounds them is very helpful for most traumatized people. As in the following, we can suggest our clients try out an exercise that can enable them to re-experience feeling safe:

I: “It is often helpful if we imagine something that surrounds us and protects us, so that we feel safe all around. Like a protective shell or a protective cloak or a protective mantle; it can also be a beam of light or even something completely different that surrounds us protectively. In our imagination, everything is possible. If you allow this idea and give your imagination free rein, is there something that comes to your mind?”
Konstantin: “Hm … a shell maybe … like a second skin.”
I: “Ah, a shell like a second skin.”
K: “Yes, it’s all around me.”
I: “Ah, what is this second skin like?”
K: “… it’s like rubber, but permeable.”
I: “Aha, like rubber, but permeable.”
K: “Yes, exactly. But still tear-resistant.”
I: “Ah, so it can’t tear. And does it cover you from top to bottom, or are there areas it doesn’t cover?”
K: “No, it covers me completely. From top to bottom.”
I: “And when this skin covers you completely, how is that?”
K: “Good. … it mustn’t be too close to me, not so close to my body.”
I: “And is it possible for it not to be so close to your body?”
K: “Yes, that’s possible. A few centimeters distance. That’s good. That’s enough air for me.”
I: “Aha, that’s enough air for you. And how is that?”
K: “Yes, that feels good.”

I: "Would you like to check if you feel safe all around with this skin ... or does something have to be changed so that you feel completely safe?"

K: "I already feel safe. But if something threatening were to come, it would have to be thicker."

I: "And is it possible for it to become thicker if necessary?"

K: "Yes, actually it is. Yes, it can become thicker … and also thinner, just as I need it!"

I: "Ah, that's really great, it can become thicker and thinner, just as you need it."

K: "Yes, exactly. That's really great!"

I: "Yes, that's great. If you let this take effect on you, this second skin, getting thicker and thinner, just as you need it … how is that for you?"

K: "Great. That really feels good, I feel really safe, almost invulnerable." (laughs, straightens up and breathes deeply in and out)

I: "That´s great. And when you notice that you feel really safe and almost invulnerable ... how is that for you?"

K: "Really good!" (takes a deep breath in and out) "I feel strong now." (straightens up a bit)

I: "Where in your body do you feel that?"

K: "In my shoulders and back; they are stronger now, somehow firmer." (straightens up completely)

I: "Then really become consciously aware of it."

K: (breathes out strongly) "… yes, and here." (points to his chest) "It is wider now." (takes a deep breath in and out)

I: "Then become aware of that too, that your chest is wider now."

K: "Yes, that's good."

As in this example, we can directly lead from the conversation to an inner image; but we could also discuss with our clients what it could be that surrounds them protectively after having explained the exercise and then guiding their imagery:

I: "Then I would like to invite you to sit comfortably and feel the seat you are sitting on and the backrest in your back. … take a few slow breaths in and out leaving everything behind and focusing completely on this exercise. … you can close your eyes if you like or leave them open, whatever is comfortable for you. If you leave your eyes open, it is helpful to focus your gaze on a certain point so that you can do this exercise more easily. … and if it suits you, I would like to invite you to imagine that you have a second skin around you. … is that possible?"

K: "Yes, that works."

I: "What does your second skin look like?"

After our explanation of the exercise we could also invite our clients directly to imagining without discussing anything beforehand:

I: "And if it suits you, I would like to invite you to imagine something protective surrounding you so that you feel safe all around. … that can be a protective shell or a protective layer or a cloak, a certain light or a color that surrounds you, or something completely different. … and describe what you perceive so that I can accompany you in your imagining."

K: "… that is a shell … like a second skin."

With the image of something protective surrounding them, our clients can have a calming effect on their body and experience a feeling of safety. Through regular, ideally daily practice, they can gradually build it up, strengthen and consolidate it. Furthermore, they can specifically draw on this image before or in situations in which they feel anxious, insecure or threatened; this can counteract these feelings and cushion them.

Example from practice

Amina, 24, has a protective cover in the shape of a Barbapapa. It surrounds her whole body, adapts to every movement and can become thicker or thinner, bigger or smaller according to Amina's needs. The idea of a Barbapapa protective cover is not only helpful for Amina because she feels safe with it; it is also relieving because the thought of the Barbapapas amuses her. In situations that make Amina afraid or that are threatening for her, she imagines her Barbapapa protective cover and feels safer and less vulnerable. ◀

Luise Reddemannn (2011) suggests very specific inner images for experiencing protection, such as an "egg of light" or a "protective mantle" (p. 153). These can also be very supportive images. However, I do not find it useful to give our clients a specific suggestion; after all, we are prescribing something for them in which they may not recognize themselves or with which they may not know what to do. In my view, it is more meaningful and supporting to invite our clients openly and without prescription to imagine something that surrounds them protectively; trusting that in their inner self that which is the most helpful and healing for them will be revealed. With our open and free invitation, we stimulate the deepest impulses, ideas and images of our clients, and thus their inner wisdom and self-healing. Though, if it is difficult for them and no inner images or ideas emerge, then it is meaningful and important to support them with some exemplary ideas, such as the "egg of light" or the "protective mantle" to find and create an inner image of protection. I would, however, mention these suggestions as just two of several ideas to stimulate the imagination of our clients.

23.4 Safety and Security through Someone or Something

In order to experience a feeling of safety, it is very helpful for many people to imagine someone or something that stands by their side, is there for them, or embraces and holds them. Here too, it is important not to give our clients any prescriptions, but to invite them to give free rein to their imagination. By making them aware that anything is possible in our imagination, we stimulate the world of their inner images. To support them, we can mention a few examples, such as an ancestor or a spiritual figure, like an angel, who stands by their side. Or it can be a fantasy figure, an animal, a mythical creature or a historical personality or someone or something entirely different.

It is sensible if our clients do not imagine real people or animals as they can easily be disappointed or hurt by them or they can be lost or even die. Using this argument, we can also explain to those clients who choose a real person or a living animal that it is better to find someone or something else.

Example from practice

Kevin, 32, imagines a granny; she is powerful, funny and loving. She not only provides him with pasta and lasagna, but also holds Kevin tightly in her arms. His granny feels soft and comfortable and has a fragrant smell. Imagining her, Kevin feels completely secure, safe and accepted. He feels how his entire body gradually calms down and relaxes, and he can let go. ◄

Examples from practice

Rita, 59, imagines an eagle that holds her warmly and protectively under its wings. And Philipp, 27, imagines his deceased grandfather standing behind him protecting him and strengthening his back. ◄

23.5 Safety and Security for a Younger Inner Part

When dealing with early traumas, it is very healing to explore with our clients what they would have needed as a child or what would have been good for them at that time. Mostly it is about someone being there who would have protected them or brought them to safety, held them and comforted them. Similar to what we discussed earlier, we can invite our clients to imagine someone or something that gives their younger part or the child they were, all that it needs or would have needed. Before that, it is useful to discuss with our clients how we may name and address their younger part.

I: "Who or what could give little Sonja safety and security?"

Sonja: "Hm … I can't think of anything."

I: "If everything is possible, and in our imagination everything is possible, could it perhaps be an ideal mother who gives little Sonja everything she needs, or a granny or a caregiver or maybe a paternal figure?"

S: "Hm … yes, maybe such a motherly woman … my best friend had such a lovely grandma. Someone like her, a woman like her it could do, such a dear grandma."

I: "Ah, a dear grandma?"

S: "Yes."
I: "And what is she like, this dear grandma?"
S: "Hm, she is a bit chubby and has a lovely, round face with bright blue eyes. She is very kind and is so calm and peaceful, you can really feel safe there … and she laughs so heartily."
I: "If you see this dear grandma in front of you, with her lovely face and her bright blue eyes, and imagine that she gives little Sonja everything she needs. … is that possible?"
S: "Yes, she hugs me and rocks me back and forth." (smiles)
I: "How is that?"
S: "Hm, that's really nice." (rocks back and forth gently)
I: "Yes, then consciously take that in how nice it is … and also notice that you are rocking back and forth gently. … and what happens while you do that?"
S: "I become very calm."
I: "Then take that in consciously. … and where in your body do you feel that you become very calm?"
S: "Everywhere … especially in my upper body, it's all warm now." (takes a deep breath in and out)
I: "Then also become aware that your upper body is all warm now."
S: "Yes" (keeps rocking back and forth) "… that's nice."
I: "Enjoy that and take it all in."

23.6 A Place where We Feel Completely Safe and Comfortable

We can also invite our clients to imagine a place where they feel completely safe and comfortable and where they feel good all around. As an incentive, we can give a few examples or paraphrases.

I: "This can be a real place or a place in your imagination, which you imagine exactly as you want it to be. … for example, a beautiful garden or a tree house, an island or a spaceship or a completely different place."
Max: "It should be warm, like in summer in the late afternoon."
I: "So that it's warm, but no longer hot?"
M: "Yes, exactly, pleasantly warm. And the sun should be shining."
I: "And if it's so pleasantly warm and the sun is shining, a summer afternoon, and you look around, what do you see?"
M: "Hm … a blooming poppy field and meadows and individual trees, further away a forest."

In order to deepen the experience of their inner image, it is helpful to ask our clients how this or what they perceive affects them and where they feel it in their body.

I: "And when you see this landscape in front of you and let it take effect on you, how is that?"
M: "Good" (breathes deeply in and out) "something in me expands."
I: "Ah, and how is it when something in you expands?"
M: "That makes me freer … and calmer."
I: "And while you notice that it makes you freer and calmer, where in your body do you feel that?"
M: "Hm, here" (points to his chest) "it feels wider, freer."
I: "Then consciously notice that your chest now feels wider, freer."
M: "It's now expanding, my stomach also feels freer now."
I: "Ah, then consciously take that in that your stomach now also feels freer."

By addressing all perception channels as much as possible with our questions, our clients can experience a very vivid inner image.

I: "And when you look around again, where are you in your picture right now?"
M: "I'm standing in the meadow in front of the poppy field and looking out into the landscape."
I: "Ah, and are you barefoot or do you have shoes on?"
M: "Barefoot."
I: "How does it feel when you stand barefoot in the meadow?"
M: "Good. I can feel the earth. … it's wet in some places and then dry in others. A bit strawish sometimes."
I: "And what is it like when you feel the earth, sometimes wet, then dry again?"
M: "Good. My feet start to tingle. But pleasantly, so full of energy."

In general, it is very supportive to ask our clients for movement impulses. These are usually expressions of vitality that can be expressed by allowing and carrying out the emerging impulse—whether in the imagination or in reality.

I: "And as you feel the tingling in your feet, so full of energy, what would your feet like to do?"
M: "Hm, run, yes, they really want to run."
I: "Ah, they want to run. And do they?"
M: "Yes, I'm running across the meadow now."
I: "What is it like when you run across the meadow?"
M: "Great, I feel so full of energy, so alive."
I: "Then consciously notice that you feel full of energy and so alive."

We can also invite our clients to actually carry out the movement impulse; some gladly accept this invitation, others prefer to carry out the movement in their imagination. Both are usually a deepening, strengthening experience.

Dealing with threatening content

For every inner image it is important to accompany our clients in such a way that they can imagine a safe, all-round soothing and thus consistently stabilizing inner image. If threatening content still arises from their inner self, we must counteract this by asking our clients to imagine special or additional protective measures, like a guard, a wall or a defense system, or to assign the threatening content a limited place or location.

Olivia: "There is this dark shadow that is somehow scarry."
I: "You know, you can always create your picture so that it is all around good and harmonious for you. ... if everything is possible, who or what could be helpful?"
O: "Hm ... maybe a shield, a defense shield."
I: "Ah, a defense shield. What does it look like?"
O: "It's very big, made of gold. And it radiates so strongly that the shadow retreats and disappears."
I: "Ah, it radiates so strongly that the shadow disappears. How is that when you see it like that?"
O: "That's good."

...

O: "The shadow comes back. It creeps up on me."
I: "Would you like to try assigning the shadow a place where it is allowed to be? Maybe somewhere in a corner of the garden or further away, maybe even very far away. So that it´s okay for you and you feel safe. Is that possible?"
O: "... yes ... at the compost heap, that's his place ... in a small tin box."
I: "And how is it for you when the shadow has its place in the tin box at the compost heap?"
O: "Good. He's safely locked up there. And I can always see that he's there. I have him under control. And the defense shield is also nearby and shields the corner of the garden well, but so that I can see the box."

Assigning a place for threatening content is often a necessary and usually very relieving intervention. If we try to banish, fight or ignore frightening content instead, it appears more and more vehemently. By accepting frightening, threatening content and assigning it a limited place at a safe distance, it generally loses power and influence. This enables our clients to influence even threatening content in their inner images and not to be at its mercy. This strengthens their self-efficacy and self-confidence. If the emerging content is persistent and cannot be easily controlled, it is important to break off the imagining and acknowledge that it is not a helpful exercise at the moment. Then it is necessary to suggest another stabilizing exercise to our clients, such as the imagining of something protective that surrounds them, which in my experience usually does not evoke any threatening content.

23.7 Becoming Aware that the Danger is over

For some of our clients, it is essential to emphasize that the danger is over, they have survived and they are now safe.

Example from practice

For Sheila, 23, who had been repeatedly sexually abused by her stepbrother as a child, it was an essential step in her processing to become aware that his sexual assaults are over and that she is now safe. ◄

I: "If you become aware that your stepbrother's assaults are long gone and you are now an adult and standing on your own feet, how is that?"
Sheila: "Yes, that's right, that's long gone."
I: "Yes, that's long gone."
S: "… strange, I never thought of that before. … but that's how it is, that's long ago. Hm … somehow I still believed it continues. But it's over." (takes a deep breath in and out and smiles)
I: "And as you now become aware of this, that it's over, how is that for you?"
S: "That´s like a load off my mind. Like a heavy weight lifted off. ... yes, it is really over."
I: "Yes, it´s really over. Really be aware of that."
S: (takes a deep breathe in and out) "... yes, it´s as though I only just now really get it. I was never aware of it." (takes a deep breath out and begins to move her shoulders and stretch her arms)
I: "And as you become aware that it is over and as you keep inhaling and exhaling deeply and stretching, what happens?"
S: (takes a deep breath out) "… yes, I survived it, I made it. … I (emphasizes) survived it!"
I: "Yes, exactly, you made it, you survived it."

Examples from practice

Sheila consciously recognizes and grasps for the first time that her stepbrother's assaults are over and she has survived and made it through. This relieves and eases her tremendously; and she experiences an inner liberation and a sense of safety and strength. ◄

For some of our clients, the recognition that the danger is over comes by itself. If this is the case, it is important to pick it up, reinforce it and support our clients in becoming aware of this recognition and feeling the associated feelings and body sensations.

23.8 Grounding Oneself

Grounding or body exercises in which we feel the contact with the ground or the surface on which we are sitting or lying, can give us a feeling of safety. These exercises, which Stephen Porges (2019) counts among the "neural exercises", help us to regulate our physiological state, to calm our organism and to center ourselves. One possibility is, for instance, to invite our clients to direct their attention to their buttocks and the contact with the seat and to stay there with their awareness, and then to ask how that is for them. Many sense their buttocks and their lower body clearly, often with the sensation of a pleasant heaviness or warmth. This is frequently experienced as centering or as being more with oneself and in one's own center. With this feeling, a sense of safety usually arises. It is also supportive to invite our clients to stand and direct their attention to their feet and notice the contact with the ground. Many feel a sensation of centering heaviness or a pulsation or tingling. By staying with it, this feeling usually spreads to their lower legs and up to their upper thighs. Meanwhile, they often experience an inner strength, centering and stability and with that safety.

For some people it is agreeable to connect this exercise with the inner image of a tree. It is also supportive to first allow the inner image of a tree or the idea of being a tree; with that, some find it easier to sense their body and the contact with the ground and so to feel grounded, stable and safe. The idea of having roots that reach into the earth and are anchored there can also be supportive. For some of our clients, however, this idea is unpleasant, as they feel too pinned down and restricted.

23.9 Perceiving Body Sensations

Another way to support our clients in regaining a feeling of safety is to invite them to recall a situation in which they felt completely safe. If they have a feeling of safety during a memory, it is useful to encourage them to explore where they can perceive it most easily or most strongly in their body. This can be, for instance, a fullness in the stomach or a pleasant heaviness in the lower abdomen. As they let the feeling take effect on them, it can be helpful to ask if an inner image, a word or a body posture, movement or gesture comes to mind. By simultaneously perceiving feeling, body sensation and an inner image or movement, their experience of safety is further strengthened. Furthermore, the image, movement or gesture becomes an anchor making it easier for them to recall the feeling of safety later and feel it again.

Examples from practice

When experiencing safety for Astrid, 59, the inner image of a large, old lime tree appears. Manfred, 45, thinks of the word "held" and puts his hand on his heart. And Leonhard, 32, has the inner image of a rock and says to himself, "safe as a rock". ◀

23.10 Taking up a Body Posture that Conveys Safety

We can also invite our clients to take up a body posture that they associate with safety and to let it work on them. If an image, word or symbol comes to their mind, they can simultaneously perceive it with the body posture and the feeling of safety thus linking them together.

Example from practice

Franziska, 62, stands upright with feet hip-width apart, looking straight ahead, her hands lie on top of each other on her heart. ◄

Certain postures such as mudras can also create a feeling of safety, e.g., the "Mudra for Self-Confidence and the Feeling of Inner Safety" (Mesko 2001, p. 130). We sit upright and bring our back of hands together in front of the breastbone at the height of our heart. We breathe slowly in and out. After 1.5 minutes we change our hand position and take a prayer posture; we press our palms lightly against each other, with our thumbs touching our chest or breastbone. Again, we breathe slowly in and out. After 1.5 minutes we can return to the first posture.

Caution: Meditative exercises such as holding mudras can sometimes evoke unpleasant sensations, feelings and inner images or flashbacks. It is important to inform our clients about this and to suggest that they take the respective posture at the beginning only for a short time, and to discontinue it as soon as threatening feelings, sensations or inner images arise and to regulate themselves with other stabilizing exercises.

23.11 Touching, Embracing and Cuddling

Touch is an essential factor when it comes to our experience of safety. In particular, hugs and being held by people with whom we feel safe can contribute to strengthening our inner safety. Together with our clients we can, for instance, consider whether there might be someone in their social environment from whom they could consciously and deliberately receive hugs and be held in order to experience and nurture feeling safe. It is important that they clearly define the hug and being held as a mindful exercise of experiencing safety and holding and consciously perceive and let it take effect on them. It is advantageous to agree on a time frame. Even in the position of those who embrace or hold the other, our clients can experience safety and often also inner strength.

Example from practice

Pia, 41, agrees with her husband that they will take turns holding each other and giving each other safety and security a few times a week, when it suits them both. ◄

Many people have no one to hug them or who is close or familiar enough to hold them. For many, the thought of such an exercise is inappropriate. However, the idea of being hugged and held is possible for many. Usually it is very healing and strengthening for our clients if we invite them to allow the imagining of a hug and to feel safe and secure. By exploring what they sense in their body and by letting the corresponding body sensation take effect on them, they can experience the feeling of safety and security intensified and more deeply.

Sometimes this image can evoke nostalgia, sadness or grief in our clients, for example, that there is currently no one in their life whom they can hug. As always, it is important to acknowledge these feelings and suggest our clients allow both, the nostalgia as well as the support in the hug. If they are able to do this, we could invite them after a few moments to focus their attention more on being held and experiencing safety.

If it is difficult for our clients to imagine someone hugging them, we should stimulate their imagination with a few ideas and make them aware that in our imagination everything is possible; e.g., it can even be a bear, a fairy or an angel who hugs them.

For some of our clients it is also helpful to wrap themselves in blankets or to build a nest with them in which they can snuggle up and feel safe and secure (Wiedemann 2020).

Example from practice

Hubert, 55, is highly traumatized due to a series of violent experiences in his family of origin. He is highly strung with simultaneous exhaustion and lethargy. When exploring possibilities that could give Hubert a feeling of safety, he discovers that his body gradually calms down when he wraps himself in a blanket and snuggles into his sofa. Doing this Hubert relaxes and feels safe. ◀

23.12 See-sawing, Swinging and Rocking

Steven Porges (2018) points out that one of the "simplest ways to calm down and self-regulate" is to "carry out swinging movements" (p. 158). Rocking in a rocking chair or on an exercise ball can activate the parasympathetic nervous system in the area of the coccyx, leading to the calming of our body and thus contribute to us feeling safe. Accordingly, we can recommend our clients to regularly see-saw, swing or rock back and forth while sitting, especially in moments of insecurity, fear or panic. Apart from rocking chairs and exercise balls, swings and swing chairs are also wonderful for this.

Example from practice

Due to the restrictions on going out during the Covid-19 pandemic, Nicole, 31, experiences a reactivation of her traumatization experienced from an early age. From a young age, Nicole was repeatedly locked up by her parents and forbidden to have any contact with her friends. She was exposed to great deprivations and considerable restrictions of her freedom of movement and scope of action. Through the reactivation, Nicole experiences extreme insecurity, tension, threat and fear. Besides paying special attention to everything that brings her joy, it helps Nicole to regularly see-saw and rock; this allows her to calm down immediately and feel safe. ◄

23.13 Singing and Toning—Hearing and Listening

Singing, humming, toning and playing a wind instrument have a calming effect on our organism and consequently on our inner self and contribute to us feeling safe. On the one hand, we automatically breathe out longer, which leads to stimulation of the vagus nerve (Porges 2018). On the other hand, "the chest (heart and lungs), mouth and throat" open up when we "tone, sing or hum from the resonance space of the lower abdomen", which also "stimulates the many intertwined branches of the vagus nerve" (Levine 2011, p. 164).

Moreover, when singing and whistling, as well as when toning vowels or mantras such as OM, not only does our body quieten but also our thoughts, which has an additional calming effect and supports our feeling of safety.

Listening to soothing music in a frequency range, that is not too low, or to a pleasant, not too deep, melodic voice stimulates the ventral vagus via the inner ear (ibid.). Therefore, we should recommend our clients listen to pleasant music and sing, tone or whistle and hum regularly.

23.14 Prayers, Mantras and Affirmations

People who have access to the spiritual world can experience a feeling of safety through prayers or mantras. Above all, the connection of prayer or mantra to an inner image can be very supportive.

We could encourage those clients, who we know have a spiritual access, to consider whether a prayer could give them a feeling of safety.

Example from practice

Through this question, Richard, 40, becomes aware that the heart prayer gives him a feeling of security and support. While praying he imagines a warm, yellow light flowing through him when he inhales. ◄

For other people, personally formulated sentences and affirmations give a feeling of safety and have a supportive effect.

References

Levine PA (2011) Sprache ohne Worte. Wie unser Körper Trauma verarbeitet und uns in die innere Balance zurückführt. Kösel, München (In an Unspoken Voice. How the Body Releases Trauma and Restores Goodness. 2010, North Atlantic Books, Berkeley) Own translation

Mesko S (2001) Heilende Mudras. Das „Yoga der Hände" für Gesundheit, Lebensenergie und Erfolg. Goldmann, München (Healing Mudras: Yoga for Your Hands. 2000, Ballantine Books, New York) Own translation

Porges SW (2018) Die Polyvagal-Theorie und die Suche nach Sicherheit. Traumabehandlung, soziales Engagement und Bindung. G. P. Probst, Lichtenau/Westfalen

Porges SW (2019) Die Polyvagal-Theorie: Eine Einführung. In: Porges SW, Dana D (Hrsg) Klinische Anwendungen der Polyvagal-Theorie. Ein neues Verständnis des Autonomen Nervensystems und seiner Anwendung in der therapeutischen Praxis. G. P. Probst, Lichtenau/Westfalen, pp 67–85 (Polyvagal Theory: A Primer. In: Porges SW, Dana D (Eds) Clinical Applications of The Polyvagal Theory. The Emergence of Polyvagal-Informed Therapies. 2018, W.W. Norton, New York, pp 50-69) Quoted from original English version (p 62)

Reddemann L (2011) Psychodynamisch Imaginative Traumatherapie. PITT – Das Manual. Klett-Cotta, Stuttgart

Wiedemann I (2020) Somatic experiencing®. Training, Intermeditate I, February/March 2020, Seitenstetten, AT

24 Gaining Inner Strength

Contents

We can strengthen our sense of safety and consequently our stability by becoming aware of our inner strength and deepen it.

24.1 Becoming Aware of One's Own Strength

In order to support our clients in recognizing and becoming aware of their inner strength, it is helpful to ask them, as to what enabled them to survive the traumatic event and cope with its consequences. Or, on the basis of the more concrete question suggested by Richard Tedeschi and Bret Moore (2016, p. 73), in which they recommend to stimulate post-traumatic growth: *"How have you managed to cope with what happened so far? And where is your strength most clearly shown that has helped you get through this difficult time?"*

R. Lackner, *Stabilization in Trauma Treatment*,
https://doi.org/10.1007/978-3-662-67480-2_24

24.2 Exploring and Integrating Moments of Inner Strength

Another possibility is to encourage our clients to find situations in their daily lives in which they feel strong and powerful. Frequently these are related to physical activity, success, or the setting of boundaries or assertion towards others.

Examples from practice

Vanessa, 32, feels inner strength during a mountain tour and Stefan, 29, when he does his workout. Peter, 54, experiences an inner power when playing a sonata by Rachmaninoff, and Saskia, 19, when she focuses her attention on her body, perceives it and feels grounded and centered. ◄

By our clients enabling themselves to experience such moments as often as possible, integrating them into their daily lives and being aware of them, they repeatedly experience their inner strength, which thus consolidates and deepens.

24.3 Recalling and Activating Moments of Inner Strength

Moreover, we can invite our clients to recall a moment when they felt strong and let it take effect on them and encourage them to consciously perceive their inner strength. While doing so they cn explore where in their body they first notice it or where they feel it most strongly. If an inner image, word, gesture or movement comes to mind, these can later help them to recall their inner power, activate it and re-experience it.

24.4 Imagining a Power Animal

The idea of a power animal, which is derived from different shamanic traditions, is a wonderful support for many people to get in touch with their inner power and to feel strong inside. We can suggest our clients think about which animal could give them power and strengthen them, or which powerful animal they would like to be themselves. Many, for example, think of an eagle, a tiger, a lion or a bear. Sometimes it is also another animal; however, it is crucial that our clients feel strengthened by their animal. When imagining their power animal, we can support them with the following or similar questions to develop a vivid inner picture that can be experienced by all their senses:

- *"If you see your tiger/bear … in yor mind's eye, what does it look like?"*
- *"What color is it?—How big is it?"*
- *"If you were to touch it, how would it feel?"*

- *"How does its fur feel? Is it more soft or rough ... warmer or cooler?"*
- *"If your tiger were to say something (to you), what would he say (to you)?"*
- *"If everything were possible, what would you like to do with it?"*

As with all inner images or movies, when accompanying our clients it is important to ensure that they can create a consistently positive image. To check this, we should ask them how their animal affects them. If unpleasant impressions occur, such as a threatening growl or a frightening look, it is important to assure our clients that in their imagination they can create everything exactly as they want to, so that their inner image is completely positive and pleasant for them. If they have developed a consistently positive image, it is useful to invite our clients to imagine that their power animal is with them and ask them: *"If you imagine that your tiger is with you, where is it? Is it next to you or in front of or behind you?"*

We can then further encourage them to explore how it is for them to be close to or in the presence of their animal. In general, many experience this as strengthening, reinforcing and invigorating. Finally, another possibility is to recommend they imagine being the animal themselves and explore how they feel while doing so. As usual, it is helpful to ask them about their physical sensations. By perceiving them, perhaps only vaguely and without being able to name them exactly, they usually feel their inner strength even more clearly and intensely. Additionally, we can encourage our clients to track down whether an impulse arises in them to carry out a gesture or movement or to take up a certain posture that reflects the feeling of their inner strength. These can later help them to activate and feel the inner strength again.

Example from practice

In his mind´s eye Leopold[1], 76, sees an older lion who is no longer very aggressive, but still very strong. Leopold imagines that his lion is lying on the ground next to him. He feels safe and protected in his presence. He sees him as a companion, to whom he feels connected and who evokes a calm inner strength in him. Leopold feels a powerful warmth in his stomach. He straightens up, lifts his head and looks straight ahead with clarity and confidence. ◄

24.5 Perceiving and Deepening Inner Strength through Movement

We can become aware of and deepen our inner strength through any form of movement in which we use and feel our physical strength. For instance, with simple strength exercises such as squats, sit-ups, push-ups, or when we press our hands against each other or press our back against a wall while in a sitting position. We can also feel our inner and outer strenght by standing 1 to 2 steps away from a

[1] We have already met Leopold in chap. 14.1 and in chap. 22.4.

wall with our hands on it, leaning forward, bending our arms and then pushing ourselves to standing upright with straight arms (like a push-up). Lifting weights in particular is a good way to feel our physical and so our inner strength.

Our clients could try out these or similar exercises with us or on their own to find out which one(s) give(s) them a feeling of physical and inner strength.

Other possibilities are simple endurance exercises, such as skipping rope, jumping jacks or running on the spot. Some special exercises, such as the following from yoga or Tauna, are also helpful to support our clients in becoming aware of and deepening their inner strength.

The Seated Forward Bend

The seated forward bend is a yoga exercise or asana in which we can experience a feeling of inner strength (Nathschläger 2016). We sit with our legs stretched out on the floor. With the inhalation we lift our arms over our head, stretch them and straighten our upper body and stretch it. With the exhalation we bend our straight upper body forward from the hips as far as possible. Head and back form a straight line. Then we lower our arms onto our legs and, depending on the flexibility, our hands rest on our upper or lower legs or feet. During the entire exercise our back and legs remain stretched and our feet are flexed up so that the toes point upwards. We stay in this position, keeping our shoulders and arms as relaxed as possible. Then we change to the opposite position: We put our hands behind our buttocks on the floor, our wrist pointing towards our back, our fingertips pointing away from us; then we lift our pelvis and let our head gently fall back, so that our body forms an "inclined plane" (Nathschläger 2016, pp. 97–98).

Caution: Pregnant women and people with slipped discs, sciatica, hernia inguinalis or inflammations or recent operations in the abdominal area should not do this exercise.

The Warrior

Another yoga exercise, that reinforces inner strength, is the warrior (Nathschläger 2016). We stand with our legs apart and turn our right foot 90° outwards, the left one slightly inwards. Now we stretch our arms horizontally to both sides. Our hands pull outwards, so that our arms are slightly tense and form an axis with our shoulders. Then we turn our head to the right and look over our right hand. With the exhalation we bend our right knee until it is above the right ankle joint. Our upper body remains upright. Our arms continue to pull slightly outwards. We stay in this position for a while, breathing in and out evenly. After a while we repeat this position in the other direction: We now turn our left foot outwards and our right one slightly inwards, then we turn our head to the left and look over our left hand. With the exhalation we bend our left knee. We remain in this position for a while, breathing in and out slowly.

Tauna-Body Exercise

A body exercise from Tauna, the yoga of the Andes from the Inca tradition (Delval 2014) can be very helpful, too. We stand with our feet hip-width apart with loose,

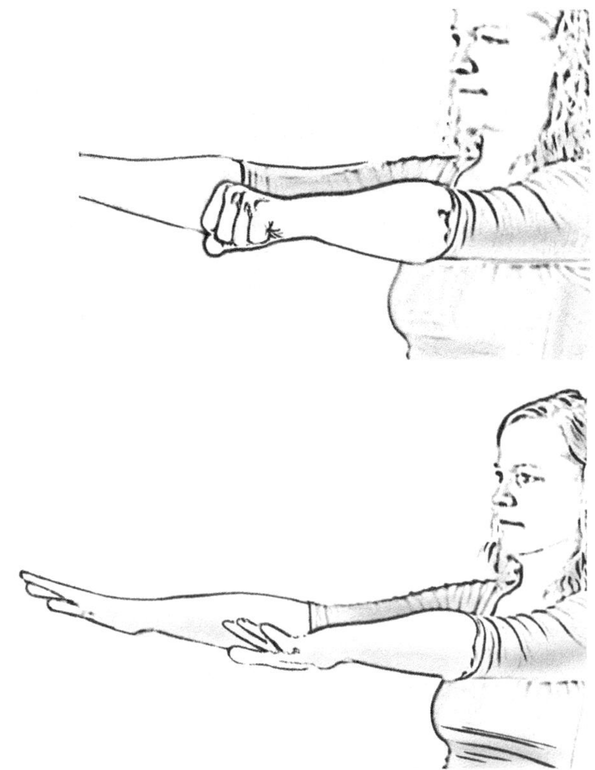

Fig. 24.1 Tauna—with arms stretched out we make fists with our hands and then sharply spread our fingers

not completely straightened legs. Our feet face forward. We stretch our arms out in front of us to shoulder level. Now we make fists with our hands and then sharply and powerfully spread and stretch our fingers while we breathe out powerfully (fig. 24.1).

We repeat this sequence of movements several times, each time forcefully breathing out and forcefully spreading our fingers. We keep this movement while we gradually move our stretched arms sideways, so that they form an axis with our shoulders. We spread our fingers energetically out of the fists a few more times. Then putting our hands up with our fingertips pointing upwards. Our hands move outwards, as though pushing something away, so that we feel tension in our arms (fig. 24.2).

Using our palms we can now clearly set a boundary around us. This exercise is well suited to making us aware of our boundaries. It can help us to distance ourselves internally from people, situations or topics that burden us. It is supportive to imagine keeping everything burdensome away from us with our upright hands.

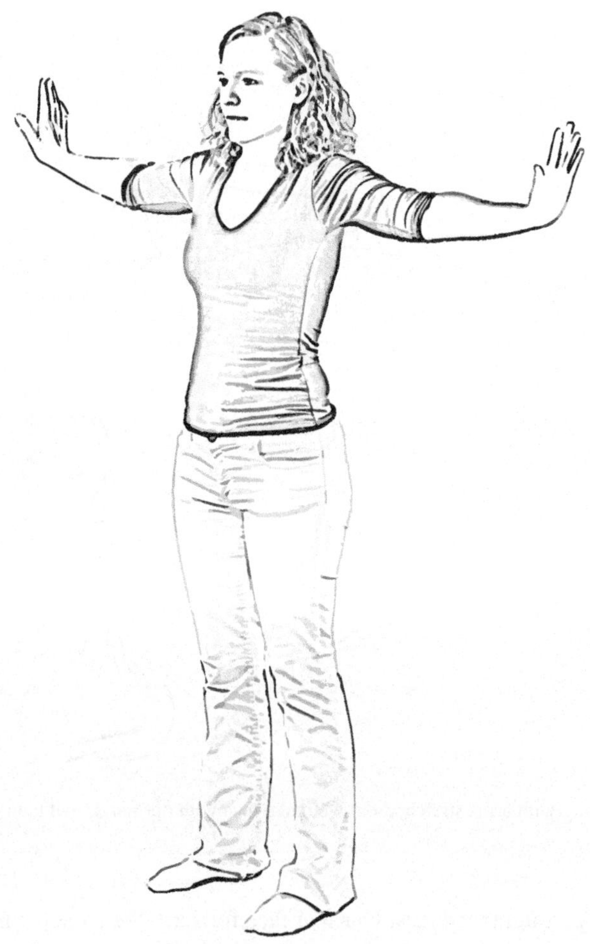

Fig. 24.2 Tauna—our stretched arms form an axis with our shoulders, our fingertips point upwards

References

Delval M (2014) Tauna — Yoga der Anden. Persönliche Mitteilung. www.melaniedelval.at (Tauna—Yoga of the Ands) Personal communication. 25 October 2014

Nathschläger AP (2016) Yoga fürs Leben. Die fünf Schätze des Yoga für den Alltag. YogaVision, Dechantskirchen

Tedeschi RG, Moore BA (2016) The posttraumatic growth workbook. Coming through trauma wiser, stronger, and more resilient. A step-by-step guide to help you. New Harbinger Publications, Oakland

Calming the Nervous System—Calming Down and Relaxing

25

Contents

By acting on our nervous system and so on our entire organism in a regulating and calming way, we contribute significantly to our psychological stability.

25.1 Perceiving Pleasant and Neutral Impressions

Many people experience perceiving impressions that they find pleasant or neutral as calming (Levine 1998); these are resources that we can use to regulate our organism and stabilize ourselves. Accordingly, it is often helpful and supportive to invite our clients to, for instance, let their gaze wander and linger on those impressions that have a positive or neutral effect on them.

R. Lackner, *Stabilization in Trauma Treatment*,
https://doi.org/10.1007/978-3-662-67480-2_25

Example from practice

For Barbara, 67, the view from the window to the sky and the opposite houses is calming and stabilizing. She has therefore made it a habit to look out of the window or observe her environment whenever she feels fear, panic, restlessness or tension. This immediately calms her body and her inner self. ◄

Listening and paying attention to pleasant or neutral sounds has a stabilizing effect, too. As do pleasant smells, for example, from spices or essential oils, or touching different objects that feel good.

We can also calm down if we find areas in our body that we register as pleasant or neutral, and focus on them and let them act on us. However, it should be noted that it can be difficult or threatening for many traumatized people to direct their attention to their body and feel it. If this is the case, then it is particularly advisable at the beginning of our joint work to draw on external stimuli as resources. If it is possible for our clients to work with body awareness, then exploring neutral sensations is very helpful (Levine 1998). If we encourage our clients to find out whether they perceive a point or area in their body that feels neutral, then this is usually very relieving for them. As a rule, this suggestion does not evoke any expectation and thus no pressure to have to feel something specific. By discerning a neutral sensation—for Constanze it was the tip of her nose (see chap. 4.3)—we can reduce even a strong activation and calm ourselves.

25.2 Conscious Breathing

We can also calm down with the help of our breath. Breathing exercises act directly on our nervous system; above all, slow and deep breathing and long exhalation stimulate the ventral vagus and consequently calm our organism (Porges 2018).

As already discussed in chap. 9.4, however, many people find breathing exercises unpleasant or even threatening; perceiving and observing our breath leads us directly into our body and our inner self. Therefore, breathing exercises can be a trigger especially for traumatized people and can evoke threatening feelings, physical sensations and/or inner pictures or flashbacks. For that reason, they should be used with particular caution. If our clients become restless or feel uncomfortable, constricted or threatened, it is necessary to interrupt and discontinue the exercise. Then other regulating interventions that convey safety and have a calming effect are necessary, such as external resources that our clients perceive as neutral or pleasant, like the view from the window, looking at a picture or listening to the ticking of a clock.

Some of our clients only find individual or a specific breathing exercise pleasant, such as observing the movement of their abdomen during inhalation and exhalation or connecting slow inhalation and exhalation with a certain image.

Unless it is difficult for our clients for health reasons, it is advisable to recommend that they breathe in and out through the nose in all breathing exercises.

This increases the nitric oxide release in our body, which reduces anxiety states (Newberg and Waldman 2012).

Example from practice

Due to some accidents, operations and hospital stays in his childhood, Clemens, 51, suffers from an extremely high level of arousal with strong restlessness, nervousness, irritability, sleep disturbances and panic attacks. At the beginning of our joint work, slow breathing and especially long exhalation are the only possibilities for Clemens to calm down. ◀

We can suggest various breathing exercises to our clients:

Slow deep breathing: When we breathe slowly, we automatically breathe deeper; this not only calms our organism, but also tormenting thoughts.

Caution: Very deep breathing, in which we breathe very deeply into our abdominal area, activates the limbic system and can trigger various emotional reactions (Newberg and Waldman 2012). Hence, traumatized people should avoid repeatedly breathing in very deeply.

Long exhalation: We exhale twice as long as we inhale; for example, we count to 2 when inhaling and to 4 when exhaling.

Variations of alternate nostril breathing from yoga (Nathschläger 2016): Unlike normal breathing, we always keep one nostril closed when doing alternate breathing. To do alternate breathing, we open our right hand, fold our middle and index fingers into our palm, and keep the other fingers stretched. Then we put our thumb on our right nostril and the tip of our ring finger on our left.

Alternate breathing with one nostril: We close our right nostril with our right thumb and breathe slowly in and twice as long out through the left nostril. We repeat this several times. Then we close our left nostril with the tip of our right ring finger, release our thumb from our right nostril and breathe slowly in and twice as long out through this nostril.

Simple alternate breathing without or with holding the breath: We close our right nostril with our right thumb and exhale slowly through the left nostril. Then we inhale slowly through this nostril, close it with our right ring finger, open our right nostril and exhale for a long time through this nostril. Now we inhale through our right nostril, close it with our thumb, open our left nostril and exhale through it. We repeat this alternating inhalation and exhalation several times. If it is agreeable for our clients, they can hold their breath between inhalation and exhalation.

Caution: Holding the breath can trigger anxiety, feelings of constriction and panic attacks. Children and pregnant women as well as all those who do not feel healthy should not hold their breath (Nathschläger 2016).

Observing the breath: for example, by placing one hand on our abdomen and/or one on our chest and noticing how they rise slightly when inhaling and sink a bit when exhaling.

Caution: Observing inhalation and exhalation can trigger anxiety, restlessness, constriction or flashbacks in some people. If this is the case, we should immediately stop and discontinue it and ask our clients, e.g., to orient themselves on the outside or feel the ground under their feet.

Breathing can be wonderfully combined with an inner image as we discussed in chap. 9.4. For instance, we can suggest our clients imagine a summer corn field through which the wind gently passes. On the inhalation, the wind gently sways the corn in one direction, on the exhalation in the other. All by itself. The image of a beach, with waves flowing on to the shore on inhalation and receding back out to sea with exhalation—or vice versa—is also very pleasant for many. By changing the speed of the waves in their imagination, our clients can experience that they can influence their breath through their inner image. The slower they let the waves come to the beach and recede back into the sea, the slower the rhythm of their inhalation and exhalation will be. Our clients can also imagine that the waves flow slowly but a little further inland to reach the beach. This can deepen their breathing and they can become even calmer. Many appreciate the image of a flower, like a lotus flower that opens on inhalation and closes on exhalation (Zhi-Chang 2002); or vice versa, depending on what is more appropriate for our clients.

Caution: For people who have experienced floods or a tsunami or who have almost drowned, imagining a beach and waves should not be used.

Of course, any other image that comes to our clients' minds or seems appropriate to us can be helpful, too.

25.3 The Relaxation Response

The Relaxation Response, a method developed by US cardiologist Herbert Benson (2020), is a proven tool that helps us relax. Herbert Benson researched the effect of meditation on our body back in the 1960s. He calls the physical changes that occur during meditation, such as reduced breathing and heart rate, relaxation response (BHI 2020). To evoke this, Herbert Benson developed his own method inspired by traditional Indian meditation techniques, but free of spiritual aspects: the Relaxation Response or Benson Meditation. We find a comfortable sitting position and gradually relax our entire body. Now we breathe slowly and consciously through the nose in and out. After each exhalation we silently say a word that has a pleasant effect on us; for example, peace, rest, wide expanse or blue. If thoughts arise during the exercise, we try to let them pass and direct our attention back to the breath and to our word. Herbert Benson (2020) recommends doing the exercise for 10–20 minutes and then staying in the sitting position for a few more minutes. However, for traumatized people it is advisable to only do this exercise for only a few minutes at the beginning or only as long as they find it pleasant.

Caution: We should not do the exercises within 2 hours after eating, as the digestive process is likely to inhibit the triggering of the relaxation response (Benson 2020).

25.4 Moving Mindfully

When we are edgy, driven or restless, it is often very difficult or even impossible for us to do exercises such as the Relaxation Response or to observe our breath; many times such interventions even intensify our restlessness and increase our level of arousal. Then we need exercises by which we can reduce or use this. So, for our clients when feeling restless, nervous or driven we should recommend exercises that reduce tension (see chap. 26) or require movement which they can notice and observe. Slow movements usually have a calming effect, as they stimulate the ventral vagus (Dana and Grant 2019).

One of these exercises is the walking meditation. Here we focus our attention on the sequence of walking, slowing it down and consciously perceiving it (Kiehas 2019). At the beginning we feel our feet and the ground under them while standing. We take a few breaths in and out. We can close our eyes or leave them open and focus our gaze a short distance in front of us on the ground. Now we take slow and deliberate steps one after the other. We consciously become aware of the movement. If we want, we can connect our breath with our walking; e.g., taking three steps while inhaling and six steps while exhaling. If thoughts arise, we consciously direct our attention back to the movement sequence of walking and to our feet and their contact with the ground. At the end while standing we become aware of our body and notice our contact with the ground.

In addition, we can calm down with any other form of ***mindful, consciously perceived movement***, like Thai Chi, Qi Gong, Yoga or dancing, simple gymnastic exercises or sport such as running or swimming. By connecting the movement with our breath, we can deepen its effect.

There is an ***exercise from the Christian tradition that is connected with the heart prayer*** which can also have a calming effect (Steinmetz 2018). We stand with our feet hip-width apart, our legs relaxed and not fully straight. Our hands are one on top of each other on our heart. With the inhalation we lift our heels from the ground (if we can stand safely) and raise our hands from our heart up over our face and head until our arms are stretched. As we exhale, we lower our heels and bring our arms down each side in semi circles, bringing our hands together in front of our abdomen and back up to our heart (Steinmetz 2018). We repeat this sequence at a comfortable pace several times.

25.5 Sea-sawing, Swinging and Rocking

We have already learned in chap. 23 that "one of the simplest ways to calm down and regulate ourselves" are swinging movements (Porges 2018, p. 158). They stimulate the vagus nerve and so the parasympathetic nervous system and consequently have a balancing effect on our body. Whether on a rocking chair, a Hollywood swing, a sitting or gymnastics ball or a simple swing, when we swing we can quickly calm our organism and become calm inside.

25.6 Singing and Toning, Humming and Whistling

We have also already spoken about the calming effect of singing, toning, humming and whistling. By automatically exhaling longer, the vagus nerve is stimulated and we can calm down (Porges 2018).

25.7 Yawning and Gargling

For the two American neuroscientists Andrew Newberg and Mark Waldman (2012), conscious yawning is one of the best tools to relax. If we imitate yawning 6 to 7 times, by inhaling with an open mouth and then exhaling for a long time, we trigger a natural yawn. On the 10th or 11th yawn, a deep relaxation with simultaneous alertness sets in (teary eyes or a running nose are natural side effects).

Furthermore, gargling stimulates the vagus nerve and thus the parasympathetic nervous system and so has a calming effect (Fasolo 2020)

25.8 Cold, Cold Water and Ice

The vagus nerve can even be stimulated by cold and so calm our organism down: e.g., by wetting the face with cold water for some time, placing a cold, damp cloth or cool pack on the neck, taking a cold shower, drinking cold water or letting ice cubes melt in the mouth (among others Fasolo 2020). As our body gets used to the cold, the activity of the sympathetic nervous system decreases and that of the parasympathetic increases.

Through repeatedly, regularly experiencing cold or through acclimatization to cold, for instance, through regular cold showers, there is an adaptation of our autonomic nervous system; the activity of the parasympathetic nervous system is increased and we are generally more relaxed (Mäkinen et al. 2008).

25.9 Naming Unpleasant Feelings and States

By naming our unpleasant feelings, we gain some distance from them and can become calmer. This has to do with the fact that naming a feeling dampens the activation of the limbic system associated with it; hence, by naming feelings they can be "tamed" ("name it to tame it") (Siegel 2012, p. 183). We can therefore use the language centers of the left hemisphere to "calm down the strongly firing right emotional areas" (Siegel 2012, p. 183).

Naming and simultaneously stimulating acupuncture points

According to Fred Gallo's Energy Psychology (2002), we can combine naming our feelings with the stimulation of four specific acupuncture points to support its calming effect: for this we slightly tap or massage the point between the eyebrows (third eye), between the nose and upper lip, in the depression between the lower lip and chin, and the point on the sternum above the thymus gland, about three fingers below the collarbone (fig. 25.1).

While we stimulate the four points in turn, we name the feeling or state, e.g., "this restlessness"; while doing so, we breathe slowly in and out. If we repeat this sequence several times, we gain distance from the respective feeling or state; strong feelings and circulating thoughts usually lose their sharpness and intensity.

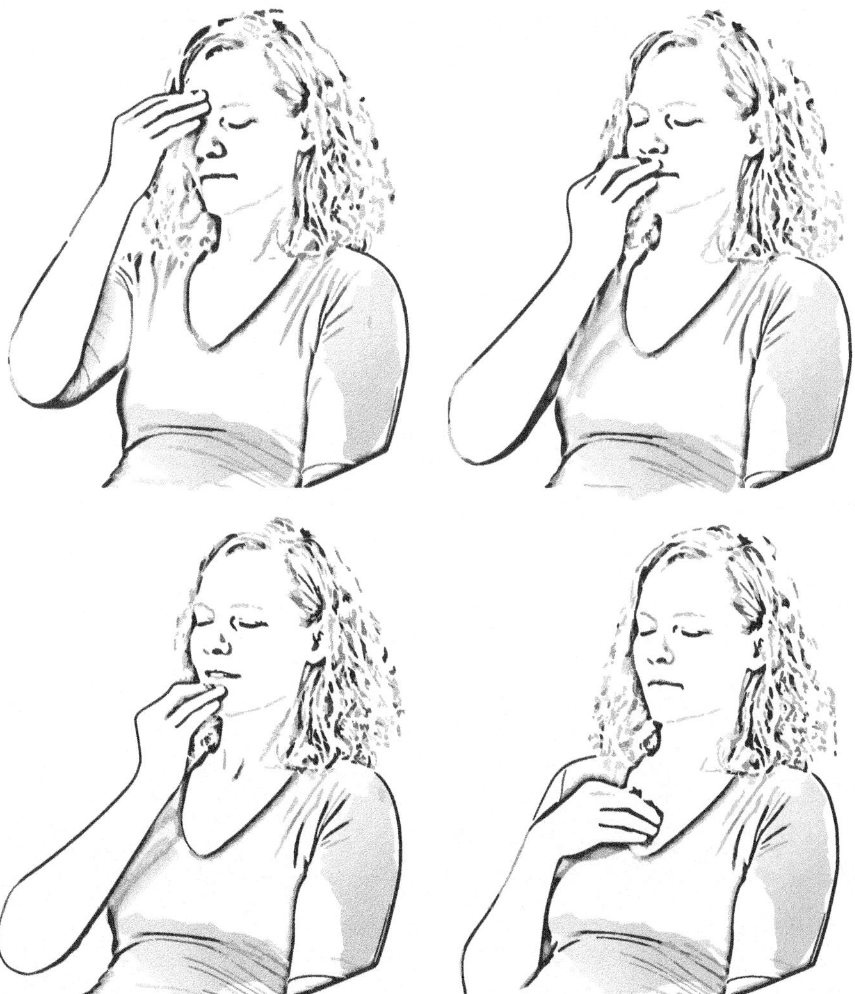

Fig. 25.1 Stimulating four acupuncture points—while breathing slowly in and out and naming the respective state or feeling

25.10 Self-contact by Touch

A wonderful way to calm ourselves can be by touch.

The so-called ***Butterfly Hug***, in which we wrap our arms around ourselves and hold our shoulders or upper arms with our hands, is a fine simple way to become calm. Additionally, we can stroke our shoulders and upper arms with our hands or gently press them (Fasolo 2020).

Healing stream: We place one hand on our abdomen between the end of the sternum and the navel and the other on our sternum (fig. 25.2). Stimulating these two areas leads to calming of our nervous system and lets us relax.

We can also place both hands on our chest, below the clavicle (fig. 25.3). This reduces restlessness, panic states and shock reactions (Eufis 2009).

Both variants can assist our clients to fall asleep. According to the teachings of Jin Shin Jyutsu, an ancient Japanese healing method, and healing stream (ibid.), the areas on which we place our hands correspond to the so-called energy gates of

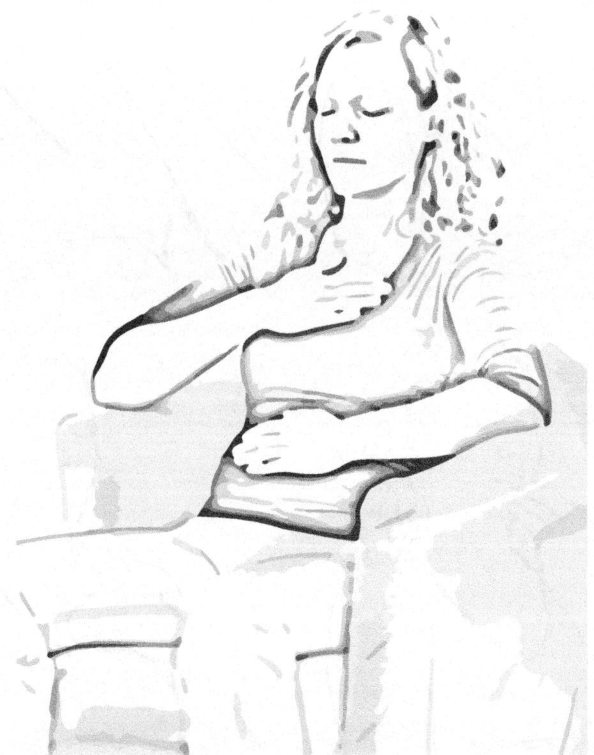

Fig. 25.2 Healing stream—calm down, relax

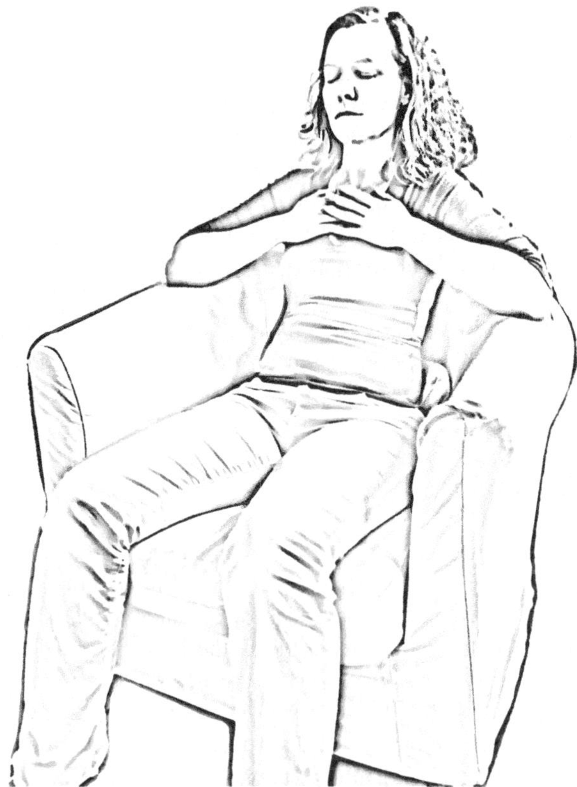

Fig. 25.3 Healing stream—calming down; relieve restlessness, anxiety, panic attacks and shock reactions

our body. By placing our hands, we activate these and so stimulate our self-regulation. It is ideal to hold these positions for ten to twenty minutes each.

25.11 Inner Images

Inner images can be a wonderful way to calm down. On one side, the already mentioned inner images, such as a field of wheat through which the wind gently passes, or a beach where the waves wash up and recede back into the sea. Or the idea of sitting on a swing and swinging back and forth and flying through the air. They can be used alone as well as in connection with our inhalation and exhalation. On the other side, we can invite our clients to imagine a situation in which they are completely at peace, calm or balanced. Or we can suggest they imagine what it would be like to be completely relaxed.

Example from practice

Ida, 62, imagines lying in a hammock in a garden in summer. She enjoys the warmth, the chirping of the birds and the gentle swaying of the hammock. She looks through the leaves of the trees into the vastness of the sky. No one demands or expects anything from her; she can just be at peace on her own. Ida feels relieved, free and light. During her imagining this, she senses a warmth in her stomach and a pleasant heaviness in her legs. Ida practices this imagery every day. It helps her to become calmer, to come into her center and to refuel. ◄

For some, the idea of a pleasant light is relaxing as is a soothing color that envelops them, flows through their body from top to bottom and gradually lets them calm down.

25.12 Meditation

Finally, meditation can be a way to become calm inside. However, as mentioned in chap. 9, meditation can be a double-edged sword for traumatized people; they can trigger threatening content, feelings, physical states or flashbacks. Therefore, short meditation times are just as advisable at the beginning as forms of meditation in which they focus their attention on a movement or on specific inner images. Furthermore, our clients should observe very carefully how they feel during meditation and break it off as soon as they feel uncomfortable or threatening content appears. Regardless of this, meditation is not as easy to implement as is frequently conveyed in self-help books. Especially at the beginning, it is very difficult for most people to keep their attention in the here and now. As a rule, we need some time and practice to learn to be present in the moment and in this way experience the positive effect of meditation. It is easier to implement those forms in which it is less effort to maintain our attention; such as the already discussed walking meditation or other forms of mindful movements. We can also encourage our clients to take a break from time to time in everyday life and perceive what they just see, smell, hear, feel or taste. Moreover, we can suggest they carry out everyday activities consciously and deliberately, as if they were meditations in everyday life; that way they can come completely into the present moment (Thich Nhat Hanh 2005). In addition, our clients can use this to train their "dual attention" (Rothschild 2002), which in turn makes it easier for them to deal with stressful feelings, thoughts and states; by observing and perceiving them, they can gain distance from them.

25.13 Hook-up

Another helpful exercise can be the Hook-up according to Fred Gallo (2002). While sitting we cross our left leg over the right one at ankle level. We stretch our arms out in front of our body, with the back of our hands touching each

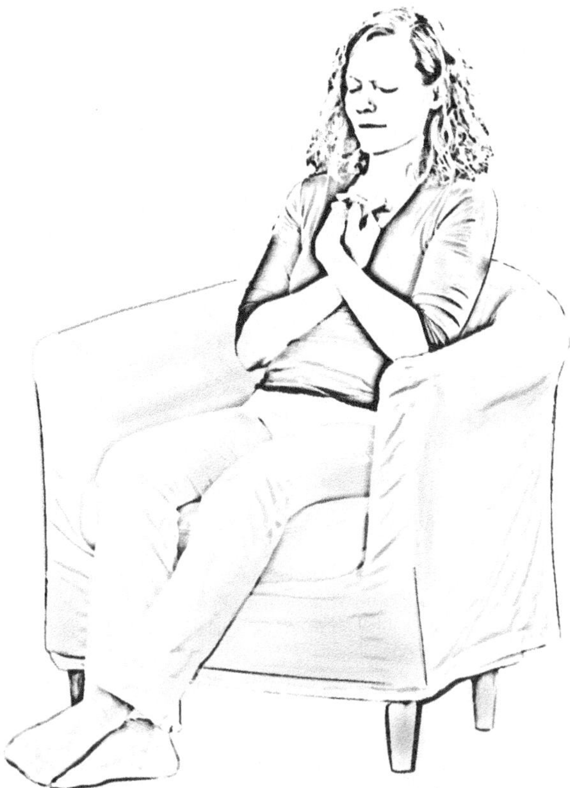

Fig. 25.4 Hook-up according to Fred Gallo—calmimg down and finding the center

other. Then we place the right wrist over the left one; now our palms touch each other. We interlace the fingers of both hands and turn them down from the elbows towards our chest, so that the outer edges of our hands touch our chest at the level of the thymus gland, about three fingers below the collarbone (fig. 25.4).

While we inhale slowly, we press our tongue against the roof of our mouth, and when we exhale we release it again. We do this for a few minutes while maintaining the position. According to Fred Gallo (2002), this exercise leads to an energetic balance of our body and allows us to calm down and find our center.

Caution: Like all breathing and meditative exercises, this can activate unpleasant or threatening content.

References

Benson H (2020) Steps to elicit the relaxation response. http://www.relaxationresponse.org/steps/. Accessed 20 July 2020

BHI (2020) Benson-Henry Institute for mind body medicine. https://bensonhenryinstitute.org/mission-history/. Accessed 20 July 2020

Dana D, Grant D (2019) Das Polyvagal-PlayLab. Hilfe für Therapeuten, die ihre Klienten im Sinne der Polyvagal-Theorie behandeln wollen. In: Porges SW, Dana D (Hrsg) Klinische Anwendungen der Polyvagal-Theorie. Ein neues Verständnis des Autonomen Nervensystems und seiner Anwendung in der therapeutischen Praxis. G. P. Probst, Lichtenau/Westfalen, pp 207–230 (The Polyvagal PlayLab: Helping Therapists Bring Polyvagal Theory to Their Clients. In: Porges SW, Dana D (Eds) Clinical Applications of The Polyvagal Theory. The Emergence of Polyvagal-Informed Therapies. 2018, W.W. Norton, New York, pp 185–206)

Eufis (Europäisches Forum für Impuls-Strömen) (2009) Basiskurs. Eufis, Linz, AT

Fasolo A (2020) 6 psychologist-approved hacks for calming your nervous system, and mind. https://www.bodyandsoul.com.au/mind-body/wellbeing/6-psychologistapproved-hacks-for-calming-your-nervous-system-and-mind/news-story/4d9d9e977c369ef471684f3508b3401c. Accessed 20 July 2020

Gallo FP (2002) Advanced energy psychology I. Trainings manual Level I. VAK, Kirchzarten, DE

Kiehas C (2019) Bewegte Meditation. Magazin für Yoga, Gesundheit und Spiritualität, 25

Levine PA (1998) Trauma-Heilung. Das Erwachen des Tigers. Unsere Fähigkeit, traumatische Erfahrungen zu transformieren. Synthesis, Essen (Waking the Tiger: Healing Trauma. The Innate Capacitiy to Transform Overwhelming Experiences. 1997, North Atlantic Books, Berkeley)

Zhi-Chang Li (2002) Setz dich hin und tue nichts. Das Buch der Entspannung. Wilhelm Heyne, München

Mäkinen TM, Mäntysaari M, Pääkkönen T, Jokelainen J, Palinkas LA, Hassi J, Leppäluoto J, Tahvanainen K, Rintamäki H (2008) Autonomic nervous function during whole-body cold exposure before and after cold acclimation. Aviat Space Environ Med 79(9):875–882. https://doi.org/10.3357/ASEM.2235.2008

Nathschläger AP (2016) Yoga fürs Leben. Die fünf Schätze des Yoga für den Alltag. YogaVision, Dechantskirchen, AT

Newberg A, Waldman MR (2012) Der Fingerabdruck Gottes. Wie religiöse und spirituelle Erfahrungen unser Gehirn verändern. Goldmann, München (How Good Changes Your Brain. 2009, Ballantine Books, New York)

Porges SW (2018) Die Polyvagal-Theorie und die Suche nach Sicherheit. Traumabehandlung, soziales Engagement und Bindung. G. P. Probst, Lichtenau/Westfalen

Rothschild B (2002) Der Körper erinnert sich. Die Psychophysiologie des Traumas und der Traumabehandlung. Synthesis, Essen (The Body Remembers. The Psychophysiology of Trauma and Treatment. 2000, W.W. Norton, New York) Own translation

Siegel DJ (2012) Mindsight. Die neue Wissenschaft der persönlichen Transformation. Goldmann, München (Mindsight. The New Science of Personal Transformation. 2010, Bantam Books, New York) Own translation

Steinmetz K-H (2018) Herzensgebet. Continuing Lessons. Scola Cordis. Vienna, AT

Thich Nhat Hanh (2005) Achtsam leben—wie geht das denn? Theseus, Berlin

Reducing and Discharging Restlessness and Inner Tension

26

Contents

Many of our clients suffer from restlessness, nervousness and tension. Some can become calm through one or another exercise that we discussed in chap. 25. Others, however, find little or no help from these; sometimes they even become more tense and restless. Then they need interventions with which they can specifically reduce their tension. Regardless of this, it is generally supportive for our clients and contributes to their stability if we consider and explore together how they can reduce tension.

26.1 Exploring and Discovering Vents

In general, I ask my clients at one of our first appointments how they deal with restlessness, nervousness and tension, and whether they have vents to reduce them. Many have no way to channel their tension and suppress it. Or they try to dampen it by, for example, smoking, food, alcohol or drugs. And some hurt themselves. Therefore, it is important to find ways together with our clients as to how they can relieve their restlessness and tension, both continuously and in acute situations. It is useful if they have different vents; on the one hand, as not every valve is equally effective or consistent, and on the other hand, as not every one is applicable at all times.

R. Lackner, *Stabilization in Trauma Treatment*,
https://doi.org/10.1007/978-3-662-67480-2_26

Example from practice

Claudia, 29, suffers from a number of post-traumatic symptoms due to a serious traffic accident as a teenager. She feels driven and restless and is often nervous and tense. It is hard for her to pay attention and concentrate, and she has great difficulty falling and staying asleep. When I asked her what she does with her restlessness, Claudia answered helplessly: "Actually nothing." I suggest that we consider together how she can reduce her tension and whether anything has ever helped her when she was restless. Claudia says that she used to run a lot before her accident. And when she was restless, she often did squats, danced or sang. Since her accident, she has completely given this up. We discuss whether she can take up one or the other again and also incorporate more movement into her daily life. Claudia decides to go running twice a week and do a quarter of an hour of exercise every day; this is feasible for her in terms of time. She also resolves to sing again and, if she is very restless, to do squats, skip rope or shake her arms and legs. ◀

26.2 Reducing Tension and Restlessness through Movement

Any form of movement is helpful in reducing tension, restlessness and nervousness. It does not have to be time-consuming activities; often a few minutes are sufficent to free oneself from restlessness or reduce it. For Claudia, for example, a few minutes of skipping rope or 30 squats are often enough to feel less tense and restless. It is very helpful for our clients if we jointly consider which exercises they can use when they are particularly restless and agitated. We should also encourage them to take some time for movement every day to relieve tension continuously and to plan regular longer units of movement, especially endurance activities, such as brisk walking, running, cycling or dancing.

To specifically reduce tension, I frequently recommend one or the other of the following exercises to my clients. They can be applied easily in acute situations. When trying them out, I suggest they do them slowly, dosed and controlled at first. This reduces the risk that they will be overstimulated by the respective exercise and consequently overwhelmed by threatening feelings, sensations or inner images. If they like one or the other exercise and it does them good, I encourage them to experiment with it playfully and, for instance, to do it more intensely or quickly. In doing so, they can explore with what intensity they have to carry out the exercise in order to reduce tension and feel safe and good at the same time.

Strength exercises

In the following exercises, we build up tension, notice it and then let it go again: For example, we press both palms against each other or squeeze a small gymnastic ball between our hands. We can push away one hand with the other, either by pressing one palm against the other or by pressing it against the inner wrist of the other hand. Or we stretch a Theraband and span it. We can also sit leaning against a wall with bent legs and press our back against it or do push-ups against a wall.

Hopping, jumping

Hopping and jumping, like jumping jacks, hopping or jumping with both legs or from one to the other, with a skipping rope or on a stepper or trampoline.

Shaking the body

We shake our arms or our entire body. We stand firmly on both feet so that we have a secure stance. Standing firmly we can also shake our legs. While shaking our arms, legs or body, we can imagine shaking off everything we want to get rid of: tension, restlessness, nervousness as well as feelings like sadness or rage.

Tiger Exercise[1]

We stand firmly on the ground with legs hip-width apart, our feet facing forward and our legs relaxed. We lift our arms and flex them at about a right angle so that our hands are at shoulder level and form claws with them, ready to attack. We bundle our strength and tense our body, as if we were preparing for a fight. We can also imagine being a tiger that wants to sharpen its claws on a tree trunk (fig. 26.1).

Now we breathe in a little deeper and then exhale vigorously while we relax down into a squat or crouch. We repeat this sequence of movements several times.

26.3 Progressive Muscle Relaxation

One of the best known exercises for reducing tension is Progressive Muscle Relaxation according to Edmund Jacobson, which is based on alternating tension and relaxation of individual muscle groups (Simhofer 2016). We tense our hand or upper arm, for example, and hold the tension for 7–10 s while we sense it; then we release the tension again and perceive the relaxation. (Detailed instructions can be found in numerous books and on the Internet.)

26.4 Creative and Playful Activities and More

Finally, we can relieve tension and restlessness through creative and playful activities or other activities that involve movement or using our body; for instance, when we

[1] I first got to know this exercise in the 1990s. Despite careful research, I could not find out where and from whom I learned it.

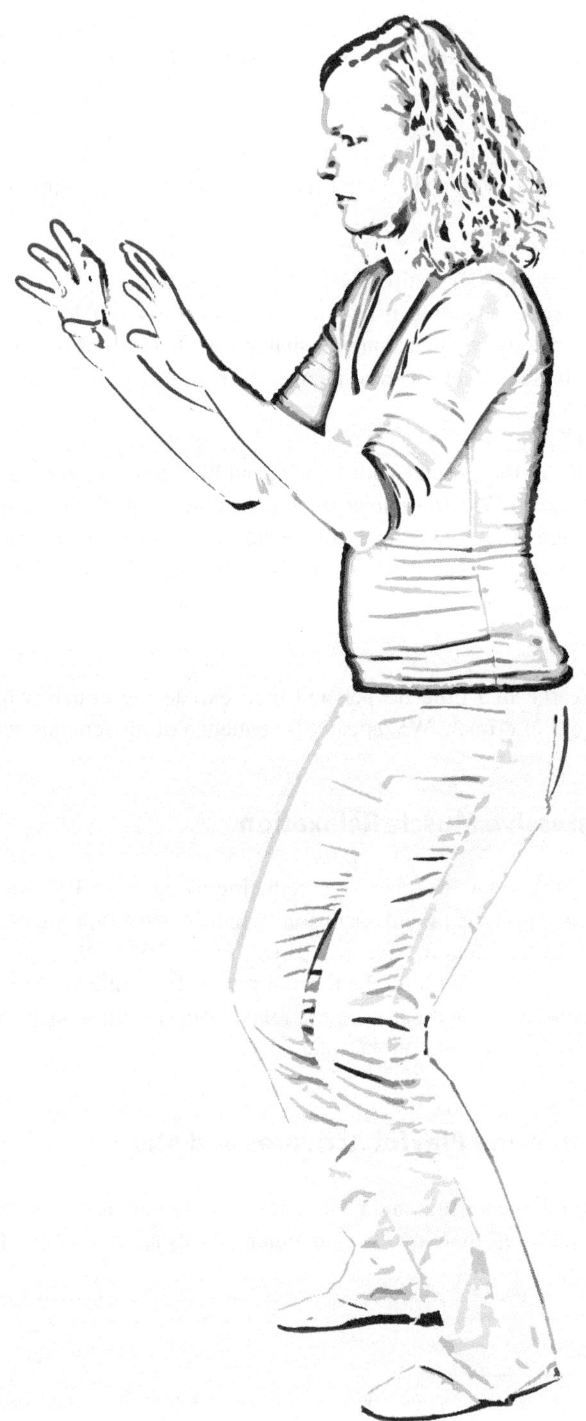

Fig. 26.1 Tiger—we flex our arms, hold our hands at shoulder height and form claws with them, like a tiger that wants to sharpen its claws on a tree trunk

- sing, play music or drum on a table or other object in a certain rhythm
- paint or work with clay
- knit or crochet
- play table tennis or table football
- do handicrafts or work in the garden

Examples from practice

Werner, 54, can reduce his tension by playing the drums, Michaela, 29, by singing and Ingrid, 46, when she plays the piano. Leonie, 24, discovers that she can relieve her restlessness and tension not only by hula-hooping, but also by knitting and baking. ◀

References

Simhofer D (2016) Progressive Muskelentspannung nach Jacobson. (Progressive Muscle Relaxation by Jacobson). www.minimed.at. Accessed 27 May 2020

27 Finding the Way Out of Dissociation

Contents

For our clients, it is already a relief and a first step towards change when we inform them that dissociations are a normal consequence of traumatic experiences. In the moment of the event, they protect us from its force and afterwards from the intensity of the memory and the associated feelings and physical sensations. For example, emotional numbness can be a protection against the unfathomable emotional pain, uncontrollable rage or unbearable guilt, enabling us to cope with and master our everyday life. But these protective and survival mechanisms have their price; they separate us from our inner self, other people and our environment and give us the feeling of not really being alive.

R. Lackner, *Stabilization in Trauma Treatment*,
https://doi.org/10.1007/978-3-662-67480-2_27

27.1 Exploring the Triggers and Signs

Dissociations decrease in intensity and frequency when we gradually integrate the "cut-off elements of the trauma into the ongoing narrative" of our lives, so that our "brain can recognize that '*that* was then and *this* is now'" (van der Kolk 2016, p. 218). To make this possible, it is important, among other things, to explore the triggers of dissociation. Accordingly, we should investigate with our clients in which situations they dissociate and what precedes it. It can be helpful if they keep a log or diary for a while, in which they record the form of dissociation (e.g. drifting away, feeling numbness), the time and place of its occurrence and the respective preceding situations and circumstances. Based on these records and observations, the triggers that cause dissociative states can usually be recognized. This makes them more understandable and controllable for our clients and they no longer feel so at the mercy of them. Moreover, it is supportive to explore how these present or what their first signs are. This enables our clients to take counter measures as soon as possible with one intervention or another and so cushion, interrupt or dissolve the dissociation. Together we can consider which exercises our clients can use to better cope with emerging dissociations. It is sensible to discuss whether anything has helped them end dissociative states before. As with the reduction of tension, it is important that our clients have several possibilities from which to choose or to which they can resort; after all, not every intervention is applicable and effective at all times. Often even several are needed to get out of a dissociative state.

If our clients suffer from persistent dissociative states, we should proceed in small, continuous steps. Depending on the form of dissociation, different approaches are useful. For instance, with constant emotional numbness, they can gradually regain access to their feelings with the aid of a positive memory. It is helpful recalling the situation at the time and their feelings and body posture or movements. In doing so, it is important to proceed in a dosed or titrated manner so that our clients are not over-activated. We can support this by encouraging them to alternately pendulate between their memory and their attention in the present moment and to observe their body and feelings.

If our clients have no access to their body, feel estranged or separated from it and can hardly or not feel it at all, they can regain contact with it over time with body exercises. To begin with, small movements, such as stretching and extending a hand or forming and making a fist, are suitable, or simple strength exercises such as slowly performing squats or lifting weights. It is beneficial if our clients carry out the movement slowly and attentively and observe it and become aware of what they feel in their body (Rothschild 2012).

27.2 Orienting in the Here and Now

One of the most effective instruments to intercept and interrupt dissociations is our orientation in the here and now.

When we notice that our clients are beginning to dissociate or are dissociated, we should ask them to direct their attention outward and consciously perceive what they can see, hear and/or feel and sense. By having a drink (of cold water), smelling a strong smell (like peppermint oil) or tasting a strong taste (e.g. a spicy candy), they can orient to the present and here and now. We should recommend this to our clients for their everyday life and suggest they consciously pay attention to what they can perceive with their senses as soon as they notice that they are beginning to dissociate or are dissociated.

Yvonne Dolan's 5-4-3-2-1 Technique

Yvonne Dolan (1991, cited in Bambach 2006) has adapted Betty Erickson's technique of self-hypnosis or trance induction specifically for sexually traumatized people. With Betty Erickson's method, which is known both as the 3-2-1 and as the 5-4-3-2-1 technique, we name three things we can see, hear and feel, then two and finally one thing (in the 5-4-3-2-1 technique five to one). Then we first imagine one thing we can see, hear and feel, then two and finally three things. Yvonne Dolan omits this imaginative part and limits her 5-4-3-2-1 method to the perception of real sensory impressions. Like Betty Erickson she recommends her clients focus their gaze on a certain point while naming things they can see in their field of vision. However, especially in cases of dissociation, it is advisable to ask our clients to look around the room and consciously direct their attention outward. We invite them to

- name five things they can see, hear and feel,
- then four, they can see, hear and feel,
- then three,
- two and finally
- one thing they can see, hear and feel.

We can do this exercise together by alternately naming the things with our clients. If they are beginning to dissociate or are dissociated, we can support them in taking up the exercise and orienting themselves outward through our participation. Even if they cannot participate due to their dissociative state, we still stimulate them to direct their perception outward. Furthermore, by doing so, we signal that we remain in contact with them.

The 5-4-3-2-1 technique can also be applied in reverse order as the 1-2-3-4-5 method (Püschel, cited in Schubbe 2006).

Example from practice

Stefanie, 36, uses one of the two methods as soon as she notices that she is drifting away, feeling estranged or cut off from the world or when everything seems unreal to her. This helps her to gradually come back to the present and into her body and to feel clearer again. ◄

27.3 Moving

Any form of movement can help to break dissociations. Asking our clients to focus their attention on their body while moving and feeling the movement and the tension of their muscles, is usually supportive. Here are some examples:

- simple movements and body exercises, like stretching out a hand and feeling it extent, making a fist, tensing and feeling the tension, pressing hands against each other, doing squats, push-ups or sit-ups, lifting weights
- walking, hopping, jumping, running, dancing
- shaking out arms and legs, shaking the body
- stamping firmly, tapping arms and legs
- stretching and extending
- making faces
- changing body position or posture: straightening up, standing up, lifting or turning the head, turning the upper body to the right and left

Example from practice

Triggered by the death of his grandfather, who sexually abused him as a child, Bernd, 34, repeatedly falls into a dissociative state; especially when he is confronted with events or situations that remind him of the abuse or his grandfather. He then has a feeling of drifting away and not being here anymore, can no longer feel his body and feels like he is beside himself. In these moments, Bernd finds it most helpful when he moves; he circles his shoulders and arms, extends and stretches himself, moves his head back and forth and consciously takes in the impressions around him. It also helps him to stamp or jump and to shake his arms and legs vigorously or to tap them. This usually enables Bernd to come back to the here and now and to feel himself and his body. ◄

27.4 Balancing and Skill Exercises

Balance and skill or dexterity exercises such as juggling, standing on one leg, balancing on a balance board or balance ball, skipping rope, hula-hoop, dribbling a ball or throwing and catching it holds our attention and brings us into the here and now.

27.5 Grounding Oneself

Grounding exercises support us in centering ourselves and are another way to break dissociative states: for instance, feeling the ground under the feet, the seat under the buttocks or the backrest in the back, feeling the contact with the ground while standing or squatting and feeling one's own weight or the gravity of the body. While doing so it can be supportive to stamp or step firmly or jump.

27.6 Singing and Whistling, Toning and Humming

Singing uplifting powerful songs, whistling, humming or toning a certain vowel or mantra, like Om, can also be helpful. Peter Levine (2011) recommends, for example, to "tone a long voo … ", to hold it until the end of the exhalation and feel the vibrations in the stomach that enhance the "sensations in the internal organs" (p. 165). The image of a foghorn, "which signals the captain in fog that the mainland is near and thus guides ship and crew *safely home*" can be a support (ibid.). Through the connection of sound and vibration, our clients can orient in the here and now and come into contact with "inner safety and trust" (ibid., p. 166).

27.7 Making Music, Clapping and Body Percussion

Playing an instrument, tapping on a table, a vessel or another object in a certain rhythm, snapping our fingers or clapping our hands helps us to be in the moment. We can also suggest our clients use their body as an instrument, as we know from Body Percussion (e.g. Keith Terry 2008). By alternating tapping their belly, buttocks, chest and upper thighs or clapping their hands, they can create a rhythm that supports them to be in the here and now and at the same time to feel their body and its boundaries.

27.8 Activating Energy Pathways and Acupuncture Points

The opening exercise for Qi Gong, tapping the meridians, is an activating, invigorating and at the same time centering exercise that can be helpful in dissociative states. There are numerous variations; one possibility is to gently tap with the right hand from the clavicle along the inside of the left arm to the hand several times, then from the back of the hand along the outside of the left arm to the shoulder. We repeat the same procedure with the left hand and the right arm. Then we tap from our lower back over our buttocks and hips, down the legs to the feet and then up the inside of the legs, over the groins to our belly. We repeat the entire sequence several times. Then with our fingertips we can gently tap several times from our forehead up over our head and finally stroke down to our neck.

The gentle tapping of the acupuncture points mentioned in chap. 25.9 (see fig. 25.1; Gallo 2002) can be supportive, too; we tap or massage the point between the eyebrows, between the nose and upper lip, the point between the lower lip and chin and that on the sternum about three fingers below the clavicle. While tapping the individual points, we breathe in and out slowly. Additionally, we can name the state; like "this drifting away" or "this being beside myself". We repeat the procedure several times.

27.9 Cold Water and Ice

Washing the face with cold water, letting cold water flow over our forearms, placing a cool pack on the forehead or neck, taking a cold shower, drinking cold water or letting ice cubes melt in the mouth are further possibilities to come into the here and now (e.g. Fasolo 2020).

27.10 Puzzles and Games with Numbers and Words

We can distract ourselves with puzzles as well as with number and word games and so find our way out of dissociative states:

- solving sudokus
- playing with numbers or calculations, e.g., counting backwards in 4s from 100
- playing with words such as "categories", in which we find and write down a city, a country, a river etc. for each letter of the alphabet, or forming word chains, in which the last letter of one word is the first of the next

27.11 Helpful Tools

Weights or heavy objects such as heavy stones or balls that we hold in our hands can help to ground us and so intercept or end dissociations, as well as cherry pit pillows or weighted or heavy blankets that our clients can put on their shoulders, thighs or feet (Wiedenmann 2020).

A rubber band that our clients can put around a wrist can be a useful tool, too; when starting to dissociate or in a dissociated state, they can pull on the rubber and then let it ping back, creating a light stimulus that helps them to return to the present moment.

27.12 The Emergency Kit

For many of our clients, their very own personalized emergency kit is a particularly important tool. Together we can think about what it should contain in order to be helpful in dissociations, but also in panic states or flashbacks.

Example from practice

Frieda's emergency kit contains very spicy peppermint candies and a few wasabi nuts, a massage ball with knobbles that she can press into her palm or roll over her arms, legs or face, and a jagged stone that she presses into her palm in the event of stronger dissociations. Frieda also has a rubber band that she can wear on her wrist; when she pulls on it and then lets it ping back, it can help her to come back to the here and now. Her emergency kit includes a lemon oil that Frieda associates with summer and sunshine and that does her good, and a peppermint oil that helps her to intercept lighter dissociations with its sharpness. Furthermore, Frieda´s emergency kit has a list of things that she can do to get out of a dissociative state: stomping her feet firmly, tapping and shaking her arms and legs, drinking cold water, washing her face with cold water and singing. Finally, Frieda's emergency kit includes a list of names and telephone numbers of people and institutions that she can call. ◄

27.13 Caution in Acute Moments

In acute dissociative states, in which our clients are hardly or not at all accessible, we should consider some points.

The most important thing is to convey our clients a feeling of safety even in these moments. Therefore, we should refrain from anything that could compromise or reduce their feeling safe. So we should always say what we are going to do. It is important to reassure our clients with a calm, clear and steady voice that they are safe here and now. Often it is sufficent if we calmly but firmly ask them to direct their attention outward and to feel the ground under their feet, to listen to sounds, or to straighten up and stretch. If they hold something in their hands or do a movement, even a very small one, such as lightly stroking one finger over another, it is useful to pick up on this and tell them our observation, for example: *"I notice that you are lightly stroking your right thumb over your right index finger."* We can also supplement this observation with a conjecture, such as: *"I have the impression that this calms you down."* Taking up the movement and performing it in the same rhythm can be a way to get in touch with our clients. This can convey a feeling of safety and make it easier for them to turn outward again. We can also encourage them to change the movement and, for instance, to extend it a little.

Different tools such as a damp cool cloth, a cool pack, a nub ball, a heavy blanket or a cherry stone pillow can be helpful, too.

Describing the current situation and naming the place, time, our function and the reason for our conversation or being together is another way to support them to come back to the here and now (Sachsse 2011).

At the beginning of our joint work we should discuss with our clients whether they suffer from dissociations and in what form and to what extent these occur. We should also clarify how we should proceed if they dissociate in our sessions and what we must not do under any circumstances.

Example from practice

Ruth, 42, suffers from frequent, sometimes severe dissociations. These occur mainly in threatening situations, when she is under pressure or when many impressions act on her. As soon as Ruth notices that she feels overwhelmed or threatened, she withdraws and tries to reduce external stimuli as much as possible; in this way she can calm down and the dissociations subside and gradually dissolve. If Ruth has no opportunity to withdraw, it can happen that she dissociates so strongly that she is no longer accessible. Then it is best for her if others let her be as much as possible and just be there; the condition then subsides after a few minutes by itself. ◀

While some, like Ruth, need peace in a severe dissociative state, others benefit from a distinct stimulus, such as a loud clap to get out of it. However, if they are dissociated, and we have agreed this beforehand, we should tell them when we are going to clap loudly.

References

Bambach S (2006) 5-4-3-2-1-Methode. In: Schubbe O (Hrsg) Traumatherapie mit EMDR. Ein Handbuch für die Ausbildung. Vandenhoeck & Ruprecht, Göttingen, pp 248–253

Dolan Y (1991) Zit. in: Bambach S (2006) 5-4-3-2-1-Methode. In: Schubbe O (Hrsg) Traumatherapie mit EMDR. Ein Handbuch für die Ausbildung. Vandenhoeck & Ruprecht, Göttingen, pp 248–253

Fasolo A (2020) 6 psychologist-approved hacks for calming your nervous system, and mind. https://www.bodyandsoul.com.au/mind-body/wellbeing/6-psychologistapproved-hacks-for-calming-your-nervous-system-and-mind/news-story/4d9d9e977c369ef471684f3508b3401c. Accessed 20 July 2020

Gallo FP (2002) Advanced energy psychology I. Trainings manual level I. VAK, Kirchstetten, DE

van der Kolk B (2016) Verkörperter Schrecken. Traumaspuren in Gehirn, Geist und Körper und wie man sie heilen kann. G. P. Probst, Lichtenau/Westfalen, p 218 (The Body Keeps the Score. Mind, brain and body in the transformation of trauma. 2015, Penguin Books, London, p 217) Quoted from original English version (p 217)

Levine PA (2011) Sprache ohne Worte. Wie unser Körper Trauma verarbeitet und uns in die innere Balance zurückführt. Kösel, München (In an Unspoken Voice. How the Body Releases Trauma and Restores Goodness. 2010, North Atlantic Books, Berkeley) Own translation

Püschel I. zit in: Schubbe O (2006) 1-2-3-4-5-Methode. In: Schubbe O (ed) Traumatherapie mit EMDR. Ein Handbuch für die Ausbildung. Vandenhoeck & Ruprecht, Göttingen

Rothschild B (2012) The body remembers. Volume 2. Revolutionizing trauma treatment. W.W. Norton, New York

Sachsse U (2011) Stabilisierung. In: Sachsse U (Hg) Traumazentrierte Psychotherapie. Theorie, Klinik und Praxis. Schattauer, Stuttgart, pp 198–259

Schubbe O (Hrsg) (2006) Traumatherapie mit EMDR. Ein Handbuch für die Ausbildung. Vandenhoeck & Ruprecht, Göttingen

Terry K (2008) Body Percussion Body Music DVD. https://www.youtube.com/watch?v=FOaJTH1jOto. Accessed 10 October 2020

Wiedenmann I (2020) Somatic Experiencing®. Training, Intermediate I, February/March 2020, Seitenstetten, AT

Feeling the Body (Again) 28

Contents

To sense one's own body and feel emobodied is an essential aspect of psychological stability. Therefore, it is important to support our clients in regaining access to their body. Besides a number of mindful body exercises "awareness-promoting questions" are helpful (Odgen et al. 2010, p. 269), which we have already got to know in chap. 9.2. By using them, we encourage our clients to explore and observe their physical sensations and reactions.

28.1 Exploring Body Sensations

While accompanying our clients we should always include questions about physical sensations, such as:

- *"How is it when you talk about it?"*
- *"What do you notice in your body?"*
- *"Where in your body do you sense this feeling the most or strongest?"*
- *"And as you think about it, what happens in your body?"*
- *"When you tell me about it, what do you feel in your body?"*

R. Lackner, *Stabilization in Trauma Treatment*,
https://doi.org/10.1007/978-3-662-67480-2_28

By asking these questions, we support our clients in focusing their attention on their body and becoming aware of it. Many find this particularly difficult at the beginning. It is important to recognize this and to appreciate it as a protective mechanism. Furthermore, it is helpful to ask about different qualities of sensations, such as: *"Does it feel pleasant or unpleasant ... or more strange or neutral?"* If they answer, for example, with "pleasant", we could then ask: *"And what tells you that it feels pleasant?"* and possibly add: *"Does it make you feel calmer, does something in you relax?"* As so often, it is crucial here, too, to proceed dosed or titrated so that our clients do not feel overwhelmed or get over-activated.

Exploring body sensations enables them to gradually get in touch with their body and to acquire the ability to become the observer. By striving to answer the questions, our clients perceive their sensations from a certain distance and experience *having* a sensation, but not *being* the sensation (Odgen et al. 2010). This is decisive for their stabilization and their entire course of recovery and supports them, among others, in dealing with states of anxiety and flashbacks.

28.2 Moving Mindfully

Any form of mindful movement that we observe attentively offers us the opportunity to connect with our body.

Slow movements

For instance, by slowly stretching and extending our hand, then closing it into a fist and opening it again, or by stretching and extending our arms, our back or our entire body.

In addition, we can access our body through exercises from trauma-sensitive yoga (Emerson 2016): while sitting by slowly moving our upper body to the right and left or leaning forward and backward, or by slowly turning our head to the right and left. We observe the movements attentively, explore which areas of our body we can feel, and experiment with the movement by slowing it down or widening it.

In a further exercise, we place our fingertips on our shoulders and move our bent arms forward and backward, so that our elbows point alternately forward and backward. Another exercise could be the seated twist pose. We sit on the floor with our legs stretched out, we raise one knee and place our foot next to the outstretched leg, either on the inside or the outside. Then we support ourselves with one hand by positioning it behind our buttocks and turn our upper body to the same side. We explore what we can sense in our body when we turn in one direction and then in the other, and when we support ourselves on one hand and then the other.

Caution: The seated twist is contraindicated in case of back or spinal injury or pain.

Strength exercises
Simple strength exercises that they carry out slowly and mindfully can also assist our clients to find access to their body again. For example, by pressing their palms together, lifting and lowering a dumbbell, doing squats, or repeatedly pushing themselves up slowly to the ball of their feet.

28.3 Touching, Pressing, Tapping and Massaging

We can also suggest our clients touch individual body parts, like their hands or arms, or lightly press, tap or massage them (Levine 2008). Or they rub their hands together firmly and notice what they feel; maybe they sense a pulsation, tingling or warmth. Or they roll a knobbly ball over their arms, face or legs and feel the sensations. Our clients could direct the shower jet onto individual body parts while showering and explore how the pressure or pulsation of the water jet feels on their skin (Levine 2011). Or walk barefoot over a meadow, on pebbles or a carpet and notice what they can feel. Many other materials and objects can be used—like feathers, cherry stone pillows or stones—to sense their body, and perceive and explore sensations.

28.4 Grounding Oneself

Another option to get in touch with our body is by grounding exercises: for instance, to feel the contact with the ground while standing, sitting or squatting, to perceive the seat or the backrest in the back while sitting and explore how it feels. We can ground ourselves by touching, holding and pressing an object. We can support our clients with these exercises by using the folllowing or similar questions:

- *"How does the ground feel; is it more warm or cool ... is it smooth or rough ... soft or hard?"*
- *"How does the glass feel that you are holding in your hand? Is it heavy or light ... warm or cool, or neither?"*
- *"When you feel the seat under your buttocks, what do you notice in your body?"*
- *"And while you become aware of the ground under your feet, what happens in your body?"*

28.5 Conscious Breathing

We put one hand on our belly and/or one on our chest. When inhaling we notice that it rises a bit and when exhaling, that it sinks a little.

We hold our hands in front of our face and blow into our palms when we exhale. What do we notice?

28.6 Singing, Toning and Humming

By toning and singing we can get into contact with our body through the resulting vibration in our head, neck and chest area. At the same time, the vagus nerve is stimulated, so that toning, humming and singing have a calming effect (Levine 2018; Porges 2017). Consequently, for many people they are a gentle way to get in touch with their body.

References

Emerson D (2016) Healing trauma through yoga. An online-e-course. Trauma Center at the Justice Resource Institute, Boston

Levine PA (2008) Vom Trauma befreien. Wie sie seelische und körperliche Blockaden lösen. Kösel, München (Healing Trauma. A Pioneering Program for Restoring the Wisdom of Your Body. 2005, Sounds True, Boulder)

Levine PA (2011) Sprache ohne Worte. Wie unser Körper Trauma verarbeitet und uns in die innere Balance zurückführt. Kösel, München (In an Unspoken Voice. How the Body Releases Trauma and Restores Goodness. 2010, North Atlantic Books, Berkeley)

Levine PA (2018) Polyvagal-Theorie und Trauma. In: Porges SW, Dana D (Hrsg) Klinische Anwendungen der Polyvagal-Theorie. Ein neues Verständnis des Autonomen Nervensystems und seiner Anwendung in der therapeutischen Praxis. G. P. Probst, Lichten/Westfalen, pp 19–42 (Polyvagal Theory and Trauma. In: Porges SW, Dana D (Eds) Clinical Applications of The Polyvagal Theory. The Emergence of Polyvagal-Informed Therapies. 2018, W.W. Norton, New York, pp 3-26)

Odgen P, Minton K, Pain C (2010) Trauma und Körper. Ein sensumotorisch orientierter psychotherapeutischer Ansatz. Junfermann, Paderborn (Trauma and the Body. A Sensorimotor Approach to Psychotherapy. 2006, W.W. Norton, New York) Own translation

Porges SW (2017) Die Polyvagal-Theorie und die Suche nach Sicherheit. Traumabehandlung, soziales Engagement und Bindung. G. P. Probst, Lichtenau/Westfalen

29 Stopping Flashbacks and Getting out of them

Contents

Just by letting our clients know that flashbacks are a very common and typical consequence of traumatic experiences, can give them great relief.

29.1 Exploring the Triggers

In order for our clients not to feel so at the mercy of their flashbacks and to be able to deal with them better, it is important to get to the source of their triggers. As with dissociations, we should explore together which situations, circumstances, impressions and stimuli trigger their flashbacks. Here, a diary or protocol can be

R. Lackner, *Stabilization in Trauma Treatment*,
https://doi.org/10.1007/978-3-662-67480-2_29

helpful, in which our clients record both the situations in which they occur and their contents. Based on these records, the triggers can usually be identified. This makes the flashbacks more understandable and controllable for our clients and allows them to avoid the triggering moments, situations and circumstances if possible. Regardless of this, it makes sense to discuss whether there has been anything so far that has helped them to cope with their flashbacks. They can then consciously use this in the future. However, usually further and different strategies are necessary. Together with our clients, we can consider which can be implemented. Many of the interventions and exercises that we have discussed regarding dissociative states are also suitable for intercepting and interrupting flashbacks. So that you don't have to go back searching, alongside others, you will find them listed and briefly explained below, sometimes slightly modified or supplemented.

29.2 STOPP

Sometimes just the thought of or saying the word "stop" or the idea of a stop sign can interrupt a flashback. Connecting the word "stop" with a few specific intervention steps, can make it even more effective.

The British psychotherapist Carol Vivyan (2009) developed the following proven STOP technique from an exercise by Joseph Ciarrochi and Ann Bailey; she uses the word STOPP as an acronym composed of the initial letters of the individual steps of this intervention:

- **S** stands for "stop and step back"—we pause
- **T** stands for "take a breath"—we breathe slowly in and out
- **O** stands for "observe"—we take an observing stance and become aware of the thoughts that are going through our mind, what we sense in our body and what we are feeling right now
- **P** stands for "pull back: put in some perspective"—we change our perspective; thoughts can be helpful, such as: "Here and now I am safe."—"It's over. Now I'm an adult and can defend myself."—"That was then. I survived it. Now I can decide for myself about my life." The thought "Flashbacks are a flare-up of the past. But I am not the flashback." can also help us to change our perspective.
- **P** stands for "practise what works"—we apply what has already proven to be effective; for instance, we shake our body, call a friend, do sit-ups, sing our favorite song or watch our favorite movie

29.3 Distracting Oneself

Often it helps to simply distract oneself; by for example

- watching a movie, reading a comic, playing a computer game, solving a sudoku
- cleaning out, tidying up, cleaning
- singing, drumming, playing the piano
- painting, craftwork, sewing, gardening or
- phoning or chatting

29.4 Orienting in the Here and Now

A key element in dealing with flashbacks is orienting to the outside as well as in the here and now. Therefore, we should recommend to our clients that, as soon as they are overwhelmed by a flashback, they should direct their attention outward and consciously observe with their senses.

The 5-4-3-2-1 and the 1-2-3-4-5 Technique
The 5-4-3-2-1 technique mentioned in chap. 27.2 by Yvonne Dolan (1991, cited in Bambach 2006) and its reversed variant, the 1-2-3-4-5 method by Ines Püschel (Schubbe 2006), can be supportive. With the 5-4-3-2-1 technique, our clients name

- 5 things they see, hear and feel, then
- 4 things they see, hear and feel, then
- 3 things they see, hear and feel, then
- 2 things they see, hear and feel, and finally
- one thing they see, hear and feel.

With the 1-2-3-4-5 method, this is done in reverse order.

Dual Awareness
We perceive our inner experience and external stimuli at the same time; i.e., we experience a flashback with all the feelings and bodily sensations and at the same time we notice our environment and know that we are in the present. The following, slightly modified protocol by Babette Rothschild (2002, pp. 192–193) can be helpful:

- I feel … (e.g. fear) and
- in my body I sense … (e.g. tension and pressure),
- because I remember … (event, without details).
- At the same time I look around and realize that I am in … (current place) and
- it is … (current year),
- I see … (some things, e.g. a yellow lamp, a red sofa) and
- hear … (e.g. the ticking of the clock),
- therefore I know that … (the event) is over.

Example from Practice

When Boris, 39, is overwhelmed by flashbacks, he tries to describe what is happening inside him. In between he names things in the outside. Sometimes that is enough, sometimes not, then he may still has to use other strategies. Depending on what comes to his mind, Boris then either plays a computer game, does his work-out, takes a cold shower, listens to his favorite music or eats a piece of ginger, which he always carries with him. ◄

29.5 Moving

Any form of movement can be a help to stop a flashback; especially when we focus our attention on the movement and our body and perceive this:

- simple strength exercises such as squats, push-ups or sit-ups, push-ups against a wall or exercises with dumbbells
- hopping, jumping, running, dancing
- shaking the whole body, shaking arms or legs, tapping arms and legs
- extending and stretching
- pulling faces
- changing body position or posture: leaving the room or place, straightening up, standing up, lifting the head and looking in a different direction

29.6 Balancing and Skill Exercises

Balance and skill or dexterity exercises such as juggling, balancing an object on one hand, balancing on a balance board or balance or sitting ball, skipping rope, throwing and catching a ball, hula-hoop require our attention and bring us into the here and now and support us to stop flashbacks.

29.7 Grounding Oneself

We can be in the moment and center ourselves and thus interrupt flashbacks with the aid of grounding exercises; for instance, by perceiving the ground under our feet, the seat under our buttocks or the backrest in our back. Or while standing feeling the contact of our feet on the ground and the gravity of our body. It can be helpful to stamp firmly, walk through the room with firm steps or jump. We can also stand with our feet apart, go into a light squat and shift our weight from one leg to the other. While doing so, it is beneficial to have our attention in our body noticing how our muscles tense and relax.

Example from practice

As soon as Rosa, 66, is overwhelmed by a flashback, she moves; she walks around, stamps firmly, perceives the ground under her feet and feels her weight. She circles her shoulders, stretches, extends and shakes her arms vigorously. While doing so, she makes herself aware that she is in the present and that the experienced belongs to the past. ◄

29.8 Making Music, Clapping and Body Percussion

Playing an instrument, drumming on a table or other object, finger snapping, clapping hands or stamping with the feet in a specific beat or rhythm holds our attention and can support us to get out of flashbacks. Besides, we can " tap" our belly, bottom, chest or upper thighs with our hands in a certain rhythm and feel our body (Body Percussion; e.g. Keith Terry 2008).

29.9 Singing and Whistling, Toning and Humming

Singing, whistling or humming calming or very powerful songs, or toning a specific vowel, a mantra, like Om, or the voo-sound (Levine 2018) are further possibilities. Longer, more complicated mantras hold our attention even more and can therefore be even more effective. Regardless of this, they usually have a centering effect and, depending on their meaning, another supportive impact.

29.10 Conscious Breathing

Sometimes it helps breathing in slowly and exhaling twice as long. This can calm our organism. For instance, by counting to 2 when inhaling and to 4 when exhaling, we focus our attention on counting and can so gain distance from the flashbacks. Furthermore, we can exhale or blow out strongly and imagine that we exhale, puff or hiss the flashbacks from us.

29.11 Cold Water and Ice

Cooling our face with a damp, cold cloth, wetting our face with cold water for a while, letting cold water flow over our forearms or head, holding a cool pack to the forehead or placing it in the neck, taking a cold shower, drinking cold water or letting ice cubes melt in the mouth calms our organism and brings us into the here and now (e.g. Fasolo 2020).

29.12 Games with Numbers and Words

Playing with numbers or words holds our attention and concentration and distracts us at the same time, so that we can gain distance to flashbacks:

- finding words from a specific category (e.g. sport) with a certain initial letter or forming word chains, like from two-part words, where the second part of the first word forms the first part of the next word (e.g. leaf tree—tree house)
- number or arithmetic games, like counting back from 100-0 in numbers divisible by 4 (100, 96, 92, …)

29.13 The Emergency Kit

In addition, the already mentioned emergency kit is very helpful for many of our clients in the case of flashbacks (see chap. 27.12).

29.14 Inner Images

Inner images can be a wonderful way to distance oneself from flashbacks.

Vault, container and co.
In German speaking countries imagining a safe is one of the standard images of trauma treatment (Reddemann 2001; Sachsse 2011). We invite our clients to imagine a safe into which they can put everything that burdens them. With the aid of the following or similar questions, we can support them in creating a consistently positive inner image:

- *"What does your safe look like?"—"What material is it made of?"—"What color is it?"*
- *"How big is it?"*
- *"How can it be locked?"—"Is that enough or does it need additional security?"*
- *"Where is your safe?"*

Once our clients have created an inner image of their safe, we invite them to put everything that burdens them in it. They can record, what burdens them: Memories, for example, as photos in an album or as a movie on a DVD, feelings in the form of a drawing or a symbol, thoughts or inner voices could be recorded on an MP3 player or stick. When they have put everything burdensome in the safe, we ask our clients to recheck whether everything that burdens them at the moment is now in the safe. If this is the case, they close it and check if it still needs more security. Sometimes, for instance, it still needs another lock or a chain that locks the safe even more securely. They can then keep the key in a safe place. It is important that we assure our clients that we will gradually deal with the contents step by step whenever they are ready to do so.

The safe should enable our clients to distance themselves from burdensome content and to decide for themselves when to deal with it. In addition, with the help of the safe they can discover that they can influence their thoughts and inner images. This in turn strengthens them in their self-determination and autonomy. As an alternative to the safe, we can suggest our clients imagine a container, a box or another lockable vessel. In principle, it is sensible to suggest several ideas and so stimulate their imagination and inner images enabling them to create an image corresponding to their innermost being as freely as possible.

Caution: The image of a safe or other container is helpful and effective for some, but not for all people. Some find it too cumbersome, or too difficult for them to imagine recording the burdensome content on a memory stick, DVD etc. Often they only experience this imagining as a relief for a short time; rarely do the contents remain locked in the safe for a long period of time. Hence, it is important to inform our clients that the safe often only offers short-term or temporary relief and that the memories and thoughts can reappear. Otherwise our clients believe that they are not able to imagine the safe well enough and therefore the contents will not remain locked up for a longer period of time.

Our practice, other real places and Hermione's bag

In my experience, far more effective and supportive than the image of a safe or container, is to recommend our clients imagine leaving behind all the emerging burdensome thoughts, memories, inner images and flashbacks in our practice room. I like to invite my clients to think about where they would put it all; e.g., in my chest of drawers, in a corner behind a plant or under the sofa. I emphasize that there is enough space for everything, just like in Hermione's bag (Rowling 2011). Harry Potter's friend Hermione has a wonderful bag in which a multitude of things fit, even Ron's father's car. This idea is supportive, relieving and also amusing for everyone; it takes away some of the heaviness and the concern of taking up space for oneself. I supplement this suggestion with my assurance that everything is well kept here and that we can always come back to it. For our clients it is also important to assure them that we will take care that the contents do not fall into oblivion or get repressed; whenever they are ready, we can pick them up again and deal with them. In addition, I suggest to them that I will ask them from time to time whether it is still good to store this burden or whether it is time to look at some of the content carefully. With this assurance we calm the inner parts of our clients, who are worried about forgetting, repressing or avoiding the experienced. It is a relief for them, not having to take care of keeping the experienced from being repressed or forgotten. My clients always gladly accept this suggestion and go back to it in between our sessions. The thought of depositing the burden in my practice room is generally not only easy for them, it also relieves them quickly and is thus rapidly effective.

For many the idea of a real place where they can keep something is easy to implement. A real place in the outside world where we can deposit the burdensome or threatening thoughts mentally creates a clear, very real spatial and thus also mental and emotional distance. In contrast, an imagined safe or other containers in which we keep all traumatic and burdensome issues remain in our mind and often make it difficult for us to establish and maintain a distance from the contents.

Draft of air, cleansing light and vacuum cleaner
It is also useful to suggest alternative images to our clients with which they can gain distance from flashbacks. For example, by imagining a draft of air or a strong wind that blows the flashbacks out of their head. Or a cleansing color or cleansing light that frees their head from the flashbacks. We can also encourage our clients to imagine spraying the flashback with a cleaning agent until it disappears (Williams and Poijula 2012), or wipe it away with a windshield wiper, just as we clean the windshield of our car from mosquitoes and spots. For some, the idea of the flashbacks being sucked up by a vacuum cleaner, is helpful, or flying away like balloons, becoming smaller until they finally disappear on the horizon.

29.15 Differentiating and Gaining Distance

Most of the time it is beneficial for our clients if they become aware that the flashback is an echo of their past and the event of that time has long gone. Special anchors on the outside that are connected to their current life can be supportive and give them safety and security, like a photo of their last birthday party, their last salary slip or just a current wall calendar.

An essential support is also the differentiation between the flashback or the traumatic event of that time and the present life or today (Dolan 1991, cited in Williams and Poijula 2012). By asking what is different today since then, our clients can realize the differences; for instance, that they were children then and could not defend themselves or run away, but are now adults and can decide whether to expose themselves to a situation or rather leave it.

Furthermore, a pictorial or symbolic representation of the differences between then and now can be supportive, especially if our clients connect it with a movement. One possibility is to mark the past and the present on the floor with a pillow or piece of paper; by consciously changing from the place of the past to the place of the present, they physically move into the present. With the help of a timeline, which we record or depict on the floor with a string, and on which we mark the flashback and the associated experience of that time and the contrast with today, our clients can move from the past to the present, look back on the past and so gain distance from it and the flashback.

29.16 Changing Flashbacks

Another possibility is to encourage our clients to change the flashback in their imagination so that it has a positive outcome (Bannink 2014). With these or similar questions we can support them in imagining a positive inner image that, so to speak, overwrites the original situation:

- *"What would you have needed then?"—"What would have been good for you?"*
- *"What would you have liked to do then?"*
- *"Who or what should have stood by you?"—"What would he or she have had to do?"*

Some of our clients imagine that they would have run away from the situation then or freed themselves. Or that someone would have helped, protected or freed and saved them. Some also imagine that the adults they are today would have stood by and stepped in for the children they were then, standing in front of them protectively and, for example, confronted the disparaging parents.

References

Bambach S (2006) 5-4-3-2-1-Methode. In: Schubbe O (Hrsg) Traumatherapie mit EMDR. Ein Handbuch für die Ausbildung. Vandenhoeck & Ruprecht, Göttingen, pp 248–253

Bannink F (2014) Post traumatic success. Positive psychology & solution-focused strategies to help clients survive & thrive. W.W. Norton, New York

Dolan Y (1991) zit. in: Bambach S (2006) 5-4-3-2-1-Methode. In: Schubbe O (eds) Traumatherapie mit EMDR. Ein Handbuch für die Ausbildung. Vandenhoeck & Ruprecht, Göttingen, pp 248–253

Fasolo A (2020) 6 psychologist-approved hacks for calming your nervous system, and mind. https://www.bodyandsoul.com.au/mind-body/wellbeing/6-psychologistapproved-hacks-for-calming-your-nervous-system-and-mind/news-story/4d9d9e977c369ef471684f3508b3401c. Accessed 20 July 2020

Levine PA (2018) Polyvagal-Theorie. In: Porges SW, Dana D (Hrgs) Klinische Anwendungen der Polyvagal-Theorie. Ein neues Verständnis des Autonomen Nervensystems und seiner Anwendung in der therapeutischen Praxis. G. P. Probst, Lichtenau/Westfalen, pp 19–42 (Polyvagal Theory and Trauma. In: Porges SW, Dana D (Eds) Clinical Applications of The Polyvagal Theory. The Emergence of Polyvagal-Informed Therapies. 2018, W.W. Norton, New York, pp 3–26)

Püschel I. zit in: Schubbe O (2006) 1-2-3-4-5-Methode. In: Schubbe O (eds) Traumatherapie mit EMDR. Ein Handbuch für die Ausbildung. Vandenhoeck & Ruprecht, Göttingen, pp 254–255

Reddemann L (2001) Imagination als heilsame Kraft. Zur Behandlung von Traumafolgen mit ressourcenorientierten Verfahren. Klett-Cotta, Stuttgart (Who You Were Before Trauma: The Healing Power of Imagination for Trauma Survivors. 2020, The Experiment, New York)

Rothschild B (2002) Der Körper erinnert sich. Die Psychophysiologie des Traumas und der Traumabehandlung. Synthesis, Essen (The Body Remembers. The Psychophysiology of Trauma and Treatment. 2000, W.W. Norton, New York)

Rowling JK (2011) Harry Potter und die Heiligtümer des Todes. Carlsen, Hamburg (Harry Potter and the Deathly Hallows. 2013, Bloomsbury, London)

Sachsse U (2011) Stabilisierung. In: Sachsse U (Hg) Traumazentrierte Psychotherapie. Theorie, Klinik und Praxis. Schattauer, Stuttgart, pp 198–259

Schubbe O (Hrsg) (2006) Traumatherapie mit EMDR. Ein Handbuch für die Ausbildung. Vandenhoeck & Ruprecht, Göttingen

Terry K (2008) Body Percussion Body Music DVD. https://www.youtube.com/watch?v=FOaJTH1jOto. Acessed 10 Oct 2020

Vivyan C (2009) https://www.get.gg/docs/STOPP.pdf. Accessed 10 Sept 2020

Williams MB, Poijula S (2012) PTB-Arbeitsbuch. Wirksame Techniken zur Überwindung von Symptomen traumatischer Belastung. G. P. Probst, Lichtenau/Westfalen (The PTSD Workbook. Simple, Effective Techniques for Overcoming Traumatic Stress Symptoms. 2002, New Harbinger Publications, Oakland)

Stopping and Leaving Thoughts Behind

30

Contents

Intrusive, threatening thoughts, memories and images usually contribute to or intensify the destabilization of our clients. Therefore, it is important to support our clients in finding ways to counteract them, to stop them and to leave them behind.

Commonly we try to suppress, ward off or fight against disturbing thoughts that intrude into our consciousness. Advice such as "Just don't think about it!" or "Just forget it!" confirms and reinforces it in us. However, trying to ward off our thoughts, does not mean they simply disappear or evaporate. On the contrary, they become stronger, more intense and more persistent. We have already discussed in chap. 12 that our thoughts intrude into our conscious mind even more by our attempts to suppress or fight them (Wegner et al. 1987). Therefore, it is not about driving away or fighting against disturbing, threatening and tormenting thoughts, memories and images, but rather about either dealing with them in a constructive way, looking at them from an observing, non-judgmental perspective or consciously directing our attention away from them and towards something else (Wegner 2003).

R. Lackner, *Stabilization in Trauma Treatment*,
https://doi.org/10.1007/978-3-662-67480-2_30

30.1 Being Aware of Thoughts and Observing them

One possibility is to notice our emerging thoughts without judging them. By doing that we can gain distance from them. It can be helpful to say to ourselves: "Ah, there's that thought again", "I know this thought" or "It's just a thought that comes and goes". It can also be useful to ground ourselves, to breathe in and out slowly and to orient ourselves in the here and now and on the outside.

30.2 Inner Images

Imaginings are another possibility to distance oneself from disturbing thoughts, inner images and memories. By, for example, letting them rise up in a hot air balloon and fly away, we no longer focus our attention on them, but on the balloon and its journey through the sky.

Letting thoughts pass by
For some of our clients, this image is already enough or a similar one, such as letting their thoughts pass by like clouds in the sky or like small paper ships floating by in a stream. Sometimes it can be relieving, to imagine that the thoughts can be "turned down" like the volume of a radio, that they murmur quietly in the background or, for example, are murmured by a tiny being. For some people to imagine a breath of air or a strong wind that sweeps through their head and takes away all the disturbing thoughts is supportive. Or imagining a cleansing color or a clarifying light that frees their head. These are just a few ideas that we can suggest to our clients. Many take up one or the other idea, others develop their own images based on our suggestions that are helpful for them.

Safe and container—real places and locations
As with flashbacks, it can be relieving to imagine putting disturbing, intrusive thoughts into a safe, container, box or other vessel and locking them in. Letting the box or container lift off in a spaceship or speed away in a sports car, usually makes these inner images even more effective. Imagining a movement or moving away holds our attention even more and thus distracts us all the more. Moreover, we gain still greater distance from our disturbing thoughts.

A real place where our clients can imagine putting their thoughts can be supportive, too, especially as this enables them to bring them outwards.

Example from practice

Marlene, 38, witnessed as a little girl how her grandfather collapsed next to her and died shortly afterwards. Since then she has had great fear of losing people she loves. She frequently suffers from the intrusive thoughts and images that something could happen to her family. ◄

I: "How about if you could just put these thoughts somewhere?"
Marlene: "That would be great."
I: "If everything is possible, and in our imagination everything is possible, where could that be?"
M: "Hm ... at the big old beech in our garden. It has a small hollow right next to the trunk, where the roots come out, that would be a good place."
I: "Ah, and when the thoughts are in the small hollow, how is that?"
M: "Good ... that's good. Then they are further away, not so much in me, somehow outside ..."
I: "Ah, then they are not so much in you. And how is it when the thoughts are outside?"
M: "Good ... then I feel somehow freer ... and lighter." (takes a deep breath)
I: "Fine, then take that in consciously. ... and while you do that, where in your body do you notice that you feel freer and lighter?"
M: "Hm ... there" (touches her chest) "... there it feels lighter."
I: "Ah, then take that in consciously too, that your chest feels lighter. ... and you know, in your imagination you can always put your burdensome thoughts and fears into the small hollow at the old beechtree, then they are further away and you feel freer and lighter."

30.3 Reinforcing Phrases and Affirmations

Inner images can be combined and supplemented with a certain sentence or affirmation, which often makes them all the more effective. Sometimes sentences can be helpful on their own through repeatedly saying or thinking them, for instance: "Thoughts come and go", "Thoughts are like soap bubbles that fly away" or "I am much more than my thoughts".

30.4 Worry Appointments

Another help can be so-called Worry Appointments (Borkovec et al. 1983). It may seem paradoxical to our clients when we recommend taking half an hour a day to specifically deal with their tormenting thoughts. However, studies show that regular Worry Appointments lead to a reduction of intrusive thoughts. A time limit of half an hour a day or two fifteen-minute appointments is advisable. Dealing with the intrusive thoughts in a controlled way, lowers the risk that they will pop up at other times (Wegner, cit. in Winerman 2011). Furthermore, the thoughts frequently lose their intensity or threat as soon as we deal with them. If tormenting thoughts appear between the set times, the knowledge of the Worry Appointments can help us to postpone the thoughts. It can be supportive to briefly note the thoughts down, and then deal with them at the appointed time.

30.5 Writing and Releasing

Journaling can be relieving, too (Borkovec et al. 1983); similarly to Worry Appointments, we deliberately deal with our burdensome, intrusive thoughts here. By writing them down, we can organize them, bring them out and distance ourselves from them. Consequently, writing can be a relief valve that also reduces the occurrence of burdensome thoughts at other times (edb.). A special "trauma diary" can be like a "filing tray" for all burdensome memories and thoughts associated with the traumatic experience (Fischer 2019, p. 65). Writing should also be limited to half an hour a day.

30.6 Focused Distraction

One of the most effective ways to reduce burdensome thoughts is the so-called Focused Distraction or targeted distraction (Sadia et al. 2009; Wegner et al. 1987). Usually, we distract ourselves from our burdensome thoughts with all kinds of other thoughts or activities. However, it is crucial that we choose a single specific positive thought to which we turn deliberately making it easier for us to distract ourselves (Wegner, quoted in Winerman 2011).

30.7 Conscious Breathing

Besides, connecting an inner image with consciously breathing in and out can be beneficial; for example, by imagining sitting on a swing and on breathing in swinging back and on breathing out swinging forward with our feet flying up to the sky, or vice versa, whichever is more appropriate for us.

30.8 Thoughts and Younger Inner Parts

It is often our younger inner parts that cannot get away from certain thoughts, memories and inner images and feel taken over or threatened by them.

Example from practice

As soon as Paula, 52, experiences something nice, has professional successes or is simply happy, she has great fear that her mother will die. Paula then feels guilty, empty and powerless and withdraws from everyone. ◄

By dealing with these thoughts and feelings and their origins, and by asking simple questions, such as *"Who says that?"* or *"If you say or feel that, do you feel as old as you are now, or do you feel younger or smaller?"*, we can help our clients to view their thoughts more in a differentiated way and to unravel them. It frequently turns out that these thoughts and feelings are linked to younger parts. And that there are also adult parts or the present adult self that thinks and feels differently. This differentiation of thoughts and feelings and their assignment to a younger, generally wounded part enables our clients to better deal with the contents of these thoughts. As soon as Paula thinks and feels that she is guilty, which unfortunately happens very often, she makes herself aware that it is the little Paula who believes this. With that these feelings and thoughts lose their overwhelming power and the thoughts of the adult Paula, which are also always there and show themselves, can gain space; they can exist alongside those of the little Paula without being suppressed and extinguished by them. This allows Paula little by little to stay more in her adult self and be more stable or become stable again more quickly. Over time, the original thoughts lose some of their significance and effect.

30.9 Thoughts and Former Attributions

Many times, the oppressive thoughts that arise are based on experiences in which we were denigrated, discriminated against, exposed, judged or ignored. These usually burrow deep into us and shape our attitude towards ourselves, life or other people, and can manifest themselves in tormenting thoughts.

Example from practice

Paula was repeatedly denigrated, insulted and exposed by her parents. They made Paula responsible for their own misfortune countless times. From an early age she heard that she was to blame for everything and good for nothing. Accordingly, Paula often and quickly suffers from feelings of guilt, self-accusations and a sense of worthlessness. ◀

Examining these sentences and thoughts and asking questions about where they came from and who said them, as well as questioning whether they ever had validity, are important steps of differentiation and assignment. Through this process, Paula was able to gradually learn to give these thoughts less importance; they never had validity, since as a small child Paula was neither responsible for her parents´ life nor their misfortune and things were demanded of her at that time that a child can never be held responsible for. So differenting the oppressive thoughts and inner images can help our clients to look retrospectively at the given circumstances anew, to evaluate them, and as a result to correct their view of themselves and to reorder their inner self. As so often, it is supportive to ask our clients what they notice in their body when they look at themselves anew. In general, this is a strengthening, calming and stabilizing body sensation. Taking this in consciously and letting it act on oneself, possibly with a movement or body posture that arises, an inner image or symbol, a sentence or word, reinforces and promotes the stabilizing effect. However, as sometimes feelings of guilt or negative self-attributions intrude during this it is helpful to invite our clients to perceive both. If both are allowed to be—the new, strengthening experience and the old, burdensome feelings and thoughts—this usually gives our clients relief and supports their process of transformation from the former to a new self-image and self-experience.

30.10 Thoughts and the Search for Explanations

Immediately after a traumatic experience, sometimes even in the moment it occurs, we try to orient ourselves and find out how it happened; we look for explanations and answers. If we do not find them, this can lead to repeated, insurmountable thoughts about the causes, course and consequences of the event. The tormenting uncertainty goes hand in hand with the feeling of helplessness in the face of the experience and often triggers feelings of guilt. Hence, it is important for traumatized people to get information and thus clarity about the event and its causes and to find answers. Understanding how, for instance, an accident happened, why their parents were violent or a parent committed suicide is crucial to calm tormenting thoughts, the repeated preoccupation with the experience as well as feelings of guilt and self-accusations. Accordingly, it is important that we encourage our clients to obtain further information and make our experience and knowledge available to them. Especially if they experienced physical, sexual and/or psychological violence and/or neglect during their childhood and/or adolescence; then it is vital to convey to them that the responsibility always lies with the perpetrators and never with the affected children. It is often very helpful and relieving for our clients to get more information about the dynamics of and reasons for violence. Through our clarification and information we can contribute to them finding answers and clarity, thus experiencing relief from their feelings of guilt and allowing their tormenting thoughts to subside.

References

Borkovec TD, Wilkinson L, Folensbee R, Lerman C (1983) Stimulus control applications to the treatment of worry. Behav Res Ther 21(3):247–251

Fischer G (2019) Neue Wege aus dem Trauma. Erste Hilfe bei schweren seelischen Belastungen. Patmos, Ostfildern

Sadia N, Riemann BC, Wegner DM (2009) Managing unwanted intrusive thoughts in obsessive compulsive disorder: relative effectiveness of suppression, focused-distraction, and acceptance. Behav Res Ther 47(6):494–503

Wegner DM (2003) Thought suppression and mental control. In: Encyclopedia of cognitive science. Macmillan, London, pp 395–397

Wegner DM, Schneider DJ, Carter SR 3rd, White TL (1987) Paradoxical effects of thought suppression. J Pers Soc Psychol 53(1):5–13

Winerman L (2011) Suppressing the "white bears". Meditation, mindfulness, and other tools can help us avoid unwanted thoughts, says social psychologist Daniel Wegner. Monit Psychol 42(9):44. https://www.apa.org/monitor/2011/10/unwanted-thoughts. Accessed 31 October 2020

31 Reducing and Overcoming Fear and Anxiety

Contents

Knowing different exercises and tools to influence, reduce and so cope with their fears contributes significantly to our clients´ stability.

Some of the exercises we have already got to know are also suitable for alleviating fear. I will only briefly mention them here and supplement them with others.

31.1 Breathing—A Key to Reducing Fear and Anxiety

For some of our clients, conscious breathing has a fear-reducing effect:

- slow inhalation and exhalation
- exhaling twice as long as inhaling

R. Lackner, *Stabilization in Trauma Treatment*,
https://doi.org/10.1007/978-3-662-67480-2_31

- observing inhalation and exhalation by placing one hand on their stomach and/or one on their chest and noticing how their body rises a bit when inhaling and falls a little when exhaling; sentences such as "I breathe in—I breathe out" or "My stomach rises—my stomach falls" can make it easier for them to keep their attention on their breath.
- breathing in connection with an inner image, such as waves that are washed up on a beach with inhalation and retreat back into the sea on exhalation (or vice versa)

In so far as it is possible healthwise for our clients to do so, we should recommend they breathe through their nose; this supports the calming effect, as it leads to an increased release of nitric oxide (Newberg and Waldman 2012).

Caution: As already mentioned several times, some people find breathing exercises unpleasant, frightening or even threatening; consequently, they are not suitable for them, so we should discard them.

31.2 Swinging, Rocking and See-sawing

Swinging and rocking movements have a calming effect on our organism (Porges 2018) and can therefore soothe our fears and anxieties.

31.3 Singing and Whistling, Humming and Toning

Singing, whistling, humming and toning individual vowels or mantras have a calming and anxiety-reducing effect. They can be easily combined with swinging and rocking and in this way reinforce these effects.

31.4 Loosening and Releasing the Tongue

By letting our tongue relax, our mouth and our jaw relax, too, then our face and finally our entire body follow; this reduces our fear (Berger 2020). Maybe our mouth opens automatically; if not, we can do this consciously and so increase the effect. To further this, we can let our gaze rest on something that lets us feel safe and supported, or sway back and forth.

31.5 Grounding Oneself

Grounding exercises support us in centering and being in the present moment and so can alleviate anxiety or fear. For instance, we consciously notice the ground under our feet, feel our gravity and weight while standing, hold something tightly with our hands or squeeze it. While doing it, we direct our attention to our body and become aware of it.

Caution: Some people find grounding exercises unpleasant or even threatening, as they focus their attention on their body and feel their fear even more intensively or the perception of their body triggers fear in them. It is helpful for them to orient themselves on the outside and in the here and now.

31.6 Orienting in the Here and Now

We direct our attention outward and consciously perceive with our senses. As mentioned in chap. 27.2 the 5-4-3-2-1 technique by Yvonne Dolan (cited in Bambach 2006) or the 1-2-3-4-5 technique by Ines Püschel (cited in Schubbe 2006) can support us.

31.7 Movement and Sport

Any form of movement and sport has a positive effect on fear and anxiety states. As studies have shown, both individual units and regular training reduce anxiety and panic disorders; moderate training 3 to 4 times a week is most effective (Knapen and Vancampfort 2014).

Caution: Too intensive training units can increase existing fears.

31.8 Perceiving the Fear and Anxiety

If our clients are fearful, it is useful to ask them to notice and observe it. That on its own can resolve the fear a bit. Then we can invite them to explore where they sense the fear most easily or strongest.

I: "Where in your body do you feel the fear most easily or strongest?"
Albin: "In the stomach, it contracts."
I: "Then observe it a little bit. … and while you do that, does it change or stay the same?"
A: "Yes, the stomach is less contracted now."
I: "Ah, it is less contracted now. And as you notice that and observe it further, what happens then?"
A: "It relaxes even more." (takes a deep breath)
I: "How is that now?"
A: "Good, now I'm much more relaxed."
I: "Fine, then consciously notice it and enjoy it."

While our clients talk about their fear, it is sensible to ask them what they feel in their body: *"And while you are talking about the fear, what is happening in your body?"*

By simply perceiving and observing, fears and other burdensome feelings usually subside a bit. Sometimes this simple exercise is enough for our clients' fear to calm down; so it can be an effective self-help intervention, too. But often it is necessary to take another intervention step.

Perceiving fear and pendulating to a resource

While our clients are noticing their body sensations associated with their fear, it is useful to invite them to explore where it feels good or neutral in their body (Levine 1998). If it is difficult for our clients to find a pleasant or neutral sensation, we can support them by pointing out: *"Sometimes it is only a small spot, for instance, an ear or the tip of the nose, that feels good or neutral."* By pendulating between the body sensations associated with fear and a body resource—a pleasant or neutral sensation—the fear and unpleasant body sensations gradually diminish. A similar effect is achieved by picking up a resource in the outside, such as looking out the window and looking at the sky; or another resource, such as a few slow, deeper breaths or the thought of something nice. This way, our clients "may consciously experience (feeling internally) for the first time, that feelings, no matter how terrible they seem, can and do change" (Levine 2011, p. 108).

I: "Where in your body do you feel the fear most or strongest?"
Albin: "In my stomach, it's tightening."
I: "Then observe that for a while. … and while you do that, does it change or stay the same?"
A: "My stomach is even more tightened now."
I: "And when you tune into your body, where does it feel pleasant or neutral right now?"
A: "Hm … in the hands, they are calm."
I: "And as you stay with your attention on your hands and feel that they are calm. … how is that?"
A: "That makes me calmer."
I: "Ah, then consciously take that in and stay with it for a while. … and when you tune into your stomach again, how does it feel now?"
A: "A bit better."

Exploring and perceiving a neutral or pleasant body sensation, a resource from outside or an alternative one can be utilized by our clients on their own for self-regulation when they experience fear or anxiety.

31.9 Fear, Anxiety and Inner Parts

Many times our fear is linked to one of our younger inner parts. Therefore, when dealing with fears, it is helpful to explore with our clients whether it is one of their younger inner parts that is feeling fearful. The following question can be a support in this regard: *"When you notice this fear or think about it, do you feel as old as you are now or do you feel younger?"* We can also first encourage our clients to explore what body sensations they experience in connection with the fear and then ask if they feel younger or smaller. If it is a younger part that is related to the fear, it makes sense to determine what this would need, what could calm him or alleviate his fear. We can then accompany our clients on an imaginative level in making up for what is necessary (Arntz and Weertman 1999).

I: "When you notice the fear, how old do you feel, as old as you are now or younger?"
Norbert: " Younger … maybe 8 or 9."
I: "So still a little boy?"
N: "Yes, right."
I: "What should we call the little boy, just Norbert or little Norbert?"
N: "Norbi. That was my nickname."
I: "Norbi. So I may call the little Norbert Norbi?"
N: "Yes, that´s okay."
I: "Fine. What would be good for Norbi, what would he need?"
N: "He would just need someone who is there and tells him that everything is alright … and holds him … just takes him in his arms and hugs him."
I: "Who could do that?"
N: "Hm … I don't really know. … best of all my grandfather. I always liked to be with him. He always told me so many stories and showed me so much."
I: "Is it possible for you to imagine that your grandfather is there and tells the little Norbi that everything is alright and takes him in his arms and holds him?"
N: "Yes … that's possible. He is sitting in his old red armchair and I sit next to him and cuddle up to him. It's a bit tight, but it's nice."
I: "Nice. And how is it right now when you sit next to your grandfather?"
N: "Good. … everything is fine there, nothing can happen. I'm just safe there."
I: "And as you experience that everything is fine and you are just safe, where in your body do you feel that?"
N: "Everywhere. That makes me calmer." (takes a deep breath) "… and I can also breathe better now." (takes a deep breath in and out)
I: "Fine. Then take it in consciously and let it work on you."

The imaginative making up for what was not possible or for needs that were not or insufficiently satisfied has a far-reaching, corrective and thus healing effect. By doing this as a daily or repeated exercise, our clients not only experience positive moments and thus have the experience of being able to influence their well-being. They can also gradually nourish and satisfy unfulfilled needs, such as that for safety and security; in this way the painful experiences are counteracted by the positive or corrective ones. These experiences can be significantly supported and reinforced by consciously being aware of their bodily sensations.

31.10 Imagining Fear and Anxiety-Free Moments

Recalling and imagining a moment in which our clients were free of fear or anxiety, or allowing a vision of what it would be like if they were fear-free, can be very helpful. Both the taking up of an already experienced moment and the anticipation of a desired state, assist our clients in overcoming their fears and anxieties. We can invite them to imagine themselves on an inner screen, as if they were free of fear or had only little fear. For some people, it is easier and more appropriate to start with the idea of not having to leave all fear behind immediately, but to keep a little of it. This usually has a relieving and calming effect; all the more so if the fear is associated with feelings of guilt and these increase when imagining being fear-free. We can support our clients in imagining the most life-like vivid image possible by asking them questions, such as what they look like, what they are wearing and how they are moving.

Example from practice

Naida, 41, who fled from Iran as a young woman, imagines herself walking freely and buoyantly through the streets. When asked "If you see yourself in your inner eye, how do you feel then?", she describes herself as powerful and carefree. She feels a lightness in her upper body and a tingling in her legs. ◄

By imagining this daily, Naida can experience fear-free moments again and again; additionally, it contributes to her feeling less frightened over time. It is beneficial for her to think of this image in everyday life, especially when walking, and to remember her upbeat movements.

31.11 Imagining Protection and Safety

When they feel frightened, imagining something that surrounds them protectively or makes them feel safe and protected can be supportive and relieving for our clients (see chaps. 23.3 and 23.4).

31.12 Activating Acupuncture Points and Healing Streams

Furthermore, the activation of four acupoints described in chap. 25.9 can help our clients to reduce their fears and anxiety (Gallo 2002). While lightly tapping or massaging between the eyebrows (third eye), between the nose and upper lip, between the lower lip and chin, and at the level of the thymus gland on the sternum (about three fingers width below the clavicle), we breathe in and out slowly and name the fear "this fear" or "this anxiety" (fig. 25.1).

Similarly, it can be helpful to place our hands above our breasts at the level of the 2nd to 5th rib and maintain this position for about 20 minutes. According to the teachings of Jin Shin Jyutsu and healing stream, this has a calming and anxiety-reducing effect (Eufis 2009). This position can also be helpful when falling asleep (fig. 25.3).

31.13 Prayers

For people who are religious or have a spiritual approach, prayers can be supportive, too. These can be easily combined with inner images.

Example from practice

For Marlies, 32, belief in a higher power is very important. In a car accident she barely escaped with her life. Since then, Marlies suffers from great fear. When exploring and trying out different possibilities that could assist her in everyday life to deal with or reduce her fears, I take up Marlies' belief in a higher power, which she has already mentioned several times. Marlies immediately confirms it could be helpful for her to entrust her fear to the higher power and to give herself up to it affirmatively. From then on, Marlies repeatedly imagines that she is held by the higher power and puts her fear in its hands. She says a prayer and makes a request, both having a calming and comforting effect on Marlies. ◄

References

Arntz A, Weertman A (1999) Treatment of childhood memories: theory and practice. Behav Res Ther 37:715–740

Bambach S (2006) 5-4-3-2-1 Methode. In: Schubbe O (Hg) Traumatherapie mit EMDR. Ein Handbuch für die Ausbildung. Vandenhoeck & Ruprecht, Göttingen, pp 248–253

Berger D (2020) Simple movements to ease your anxiety. https://www.youtube.com/watch?v=fKv1qgOYkDk. Accessed 15 September 2020

Dolan Y (1991) zit. in: Bambach S (2006) 5-4-3-2-1-Methode. In: Schubbe O (Hg) Traumatherapie mit EMDR. Ein Handbuch für die Ausbildung. Vandenhoeck & Ruprecht, Göttingen, pp 248–253

Eufis (2009) Impulsströmen, Basiskurs. Europäisches Forum für Impuls-Strömen, Linz, AT

Gallo FP (2002) Advanced Energy Psychology I, Trainingsmanual Level I. VAK, Kirchzarten, DE

Knapen J, Vancampfort D (2014) Evidence for exercise treatment of depression and anxiety. Int J Psychol Rehabil 17(2):75–87

Levine PA (1998) Trauma-Heilung. Das Erwachen des Tigers. Unsere Fähigkeit, traumatische Erfahrungen zu transformieren. Synthesis, Essen (Healing Trauma. A Pioneering Program for Restoring the Wisdom of Your Body. 2005, Sounds True, Boulder)

Levine PA (2011) Sprache ohne Worte. Wie unser Körper Trauma verarbeitet und uns in die innere Balance zurückführt. Kösel, München (In an Unspoken Voice. How the Body Releases Trauma and Restores Goodness. 2010, North Atlantic Books, Berkeley) Own translation

Newberg A, Waldman MR (2012) Der Fingerabdruck Gottes. Wie religiöse und spirituelle Erfahrungen unser Gehirn verändern. Goldmann, München (How Good Changes Your Brain. 2009, Ballantine Books, New York)

Porges SW (2018) Die Polyvagal-Theorie und die Suche nach Sicherheit. Traumabehandlung, soziales Engagement und Bindung. G. P. Probst, Lichtenau/Westfalen

Püschel I zit in: Schubbe O (2006) 1-2-3-4-5-Methode. In: Schubbe O (Hg) Traumatherapie mit EMDR. Ein Handbuch für die Ausbildung. Vandenhoeck & Ruprecht, Göttingen

Schubbe O (Hg) (2006) Traumatherapie mit EMDR. Ein Handbuch für die Ausbildung. Vandenhoeck & Ruprecht, Göttingen

32 Stopping and Dissolving Panic Attacks

Contents

Many of the interventions and exercises from chaps. 27 and 29 can be a help in panic attacks, too. Those that in my experience are particularly effective and helpful I have listed and briefly summarized below.

32.1 Exploring the Triggers

By exploring with our clients in which situations they are overwhelmed by panic attacks, these become more understandable and predictable for them. Recording the individual attacks and the respective circumstances can be helpful. Recognizing the triggers enables our clients to possibly avoid such situations or to shape them according to their needs; for example, by paying attention to sitting

R. Lackner, *Stabilization in Trauma Treatment*, https://doi.org/10.1007/978-3-662-67480-2_32

in a certain seat in a meeting. Furthermore, our clients can prepare for the respective situation and, with the aid of one or the other strategy or exercise, counteract a possible panic attack or recall a few tools they can draw on if necessary. Among others, strategies that have previously helped can be useful here. Therefore, it is important to discuss with our clients how they have dealt with panic attacks so far. As with dissociations and flashbacks, a repertoire of different interventions is generally required for panic attacks.

32.2 Cold Water and Ice

Drinking cold water, letting ice cubes melt in the mouth, wetting the face with cold water for a while, letting cold water flow over our arms, holding a cold wet cloth or a cool pack to the forehead or neck, taking a cold shower activate the parasympathetic nervous system and therefore have a calming effect on our organism and can help us to intercept panic attacks (e.g. Fasolo 2020).

32.3 Grounding Oneself

Grounding exercises support us to come into the here and now and so to cushion panic attacks. For example, by consciously feeling the ground under our feet, standing firmly or stamping, or feeling the seat under our buttocks and thus perceiving the body and its weight. Or by taking something in our hand, holding or squeezing it, focusing our attention on the object and noticing how it feels.

32.4 Moving and Changing Body Posture

- extending and stretching
- shaking arms and legs, shaking the body
- air boxing
- changing body posture: straightening, standing up
- changing the direction of view
- leaving the place or room

32.5 Orienting in the Here and Now

Consciously directing attention outward and into the here and now and perceiving with our senses is another way to interrupt panic attacks. The 5-4-3-2-1 method by Yvonne Dolan (cit. in Bambach 2006) and its reverse variant, the 1-2-3-4-5 method by Ines Püschel (cit. in Schubbe 2006), mentioned in chap. 27.2 can be supportive.

32.6 Inhaling Slowly—Exhaling for a Long Time

Slow inhalation and exhalation as well as long exhalation have a calming effect on our organism (Porges 2018); for instance, we can count to 2 when inhaling and to 4 when exhaling. In this case, sentences like "I breathe in—I breathe out" or "slowly inhaling—slowly exhaling" can be helpful. Connecting the breath with an inner image such as the image of a corn field swaying gently in the wind can provide additional support.

Caution: For some people, observing their breath intensifies their fear and panic, because they perceive their breath, heartbeat and body more intensely.

32.7 Singing and Whistling, Humming and Toning

Singing, whistling, humming and toning also calm our organism (Porges 2018). In addition, they hold our attention and assist us to distract ourselves from panic and fear and the associated inner images and thoughts.

32.8 Activating Acupuncture Points

Activating the four acupuncture points of Energy Psychology according to Fred Gallo (2002) can be supportive in panic attacks, too (see chap. 25.9); massaging or lightly tapping the point between the eyebrows (third eye), between the nose and upper lip, between the lower lip and chin, and the point above the thymus gland (on the sternum about three fingers below the collarbone). In this case, we breathe slowly in and out and name the state aloud or silently; e.g., "this panic" or "this fear".

32.9 Counteracting Thoughts

Sometimes even just the thought is helpful that we are safe here and now and that the panic attack is a mere echo of a previous experience that has nothing to do with the current situation.

32.10 Inner Images that Give Us a Feeling of Safety

Furtmermore, inner images that give us a feeling of safety and support can also contribute to the panic attack subsiding. For example, the idea of having someone with us who protects or calms us. Or the idea of something that surrounds us and protects us, such as a protective light, a protective shell or a protective force.

Examples from practice

Ingeborg, 72, imagines her deceased husband at her side, and Gunther, 49, Saint Michael who protects him. And for Lena, 23, the idea of a safety net that catches her, helps. ◄

32.11 An Anchor on the Outside

Objects or impressions on the outside that give us safety and support can be a kind of safety anchor for us, helping us to cushion or stop a panic attack, like a photo of a beloved person, a talisman or mascot, or a symbol.

32.12 STOPP

Another way to intercept and end panic attacks is the "STOPP" technique by Carol Vivyan (2009) previously mentioned in chap. 29.2:

- **S** "Stop and step back"—we pause
- **T** "Take a breath"—we breathe slowly in and out
- **O** "Observe"—we observe what we perceive, the thoughts that go through our mind and what we feel
- **P** "Pull back: put in some perspective"—we change our perspective; the following thoughts can be helpful: "Here and now I am safe"—"This is a panic attack, it will pass"—"I know this: the panic comes and it will go away again."
- **P** "Practise what works"—we apply what has already proven to be successful; we drink cold water, ground ourselves, breathe slowly in and out, walk up and down, tone Om

32.13 The Emergency Kit

The emergency kit mentioned in chap. 27.12 can be a special help.

References

Bambach S (2006) 5-4-3-2-1-Methode. In: Schubbe O (Hg) Traumatherapie mit EMDR. Ein Handbuch für die Ausbildung. Vandenhoeck & Ruprecht, Göttingen, pp 248–253

Dolan Y zit. in: Bambach S (2006) 5-4-3-2-1-Methode. In: Schubbe O (Hg) Traumatherapie mit EMDR. Ein Handbuch für die Ausbildung. Vandenhoeck & Ruprecht, Göttingen, pp 248–253

Fasolo A (2020) 6 psychologist-approved hacks for calming your nervous system, and mind. https://www.bodyandsoul.com.au/mind-body/wellbeing/6-psychologistapproved-hacks-for-calming-your-nervous-system-and-mind/news-story/4d9d9e977c369ef471684f3508b3401c. Accessed 20 July 2020

Gallo FP (2002) Advanced energy psychology I, trainingsmanual level I. VAK, Kirchzarten, DE

Porges SW (2018) Die Polyvagal-Theorie und die Suche nach Sicherheit. Traumabehandlung, soziales Engagement und Bindung. G. P. Probst, Lichtenau/Westfalen

Püschel I zit in: Schubbe O (2006) 1-2-3-4-5-Methode. In: Schubbe O (Hg) Traumatherapie mit EMDR. Ein Handbuch für die Ausbildung. Vandenhoeck & Ruprecht, Göttingen

Schubbe O (Hg) (2006) Traumatherapie mit EMDR. Ein Handbuch für die Ausbildung. Vandenhoeck & Ruprecht, Göttingen

Vivyan C (2009) https://www.get.gg/docs/STOPP.pdf. Accessed 10 September 2020

Loosening and Releasing Immobility

33

Contents

Our clients frequently feel frozen, paralyzed or immobilized. Even just knowing that the immobilization is a natural, instinctive survival reaction of our body, which protects us, when fighting and fleeing are not possible and/or we are in shock, can offer them relief. Likewise informing them that freezing is a common reaction to a trigger, when we were frozen in the moment of the traumatic event. This allows our clients to better comprehend their reaction of paralysis and to better understand themselves.

33.1 Perceiving and Releasing Immbolity

In order to release themselves from the state of freezing, it is necessary to support our clients in becoming aware of "their own physiological paralysis and closure" (Levine 2011, p. 141). By inviting them to notice and observe the immobility, it can gradually be released. In doing so, it is helpful to ask our clients, for example:

R. Lackner, *Stabilization in Trauma Treatment*,
https://doi.org/10.1007/978-3-662-67480-2_33

"And as you notice the freezing, what happens then?" By consciously perceiving and feeling the immobility, our sympathetic nervous system is activated; this can be seen by, for instance, small, gentle movements. If we notice a movement, even if it is a very small one, in our clients, we should make them aware of it and encourage them to explore it. If this is not the case, we can also stimulate our clients: *"And while you observe feeling paralysed, maybe an impulse arises to move."* Or we initiate a movement directly by asking: *"If your body could move a little, where would it want to move?"* (Zanotta 2018, p. 131). Similarly, we can also ask: *"If your body could move, how would it want to move?"* If our clients describe a movement without carrying it out, it is useful to invite them: *"Would you like to try to allow this movement and to do it slowly and attentively?"* With our request to carry out the movements slowly and mindfully, we dose or titrate the process. Our clients then experience their movements consciously and with control. This usually has a very relieving and healing effect.

By consciously experiencing the immobility, the sympathetic nervous system is activated and with it our defense and flight mechanisms, which had been blocked by being frozen. Therefore, during allowing movements, feelings of indignation and rage, powerlessness, or of sorrow and pain often appear, which were the original reactions to the traumatic event hidden underneath the paralysis. By encouraging our clients to perceive and allow these feelings and to pendulate from these feelings to a resource and back again, we can titrate the process guiding them gently through it.

Example from practice

Clara, 39, fell into an unbearable immobility state due to the death of her stepfather, who had sexually abused her for years as a girl. She feels paralyzed and frozen. While she observes this state, I ask her if she perhaps feels an impulse to move. She begins to move her hands very slowly and then her arms; first in small and increasingly in expansive movements, as if she wanted to defend and protect herself. While Clara allows these movements and carries them out consciously, intense feelings of pain and sorrow emerge in her. By pendulating repeatedly from these to an external resource, namely the view from the window and the feeling of the carpet under her feet, Clara can allow and express the pain and sorrow; as a result, little by little they resolve and gradually the rage at her stepfather and what he did to her appears. Clara can allow this feeling, which is accompanied by strong defensive movements of her arms. Again, we slow down the process by my repeatedly asking Clara to repeat her movements in a controlled manner and direct her attention to her resources in between. Increasingly, her current life and her life partner come in as strengthening resources. In this way the rage which Clara expresses by controlled powerful punches into the air and onto the sofa armrest, gradually dissipates. Finally, Clara looks relaxed and present; she feels relieved, strengthened and liberated. ◄

33.2 Imagining the Opposite of Immobility

The process of resolving immobilization can also be initiated by Peter Levine's question (o. J.) about the opposite of freezing. This can be shaking the body, or stretching, screaming or running. Sometimes it is also hitting out or pushing away. Or the image of breaking out, freeing oneself or flying away. Again, it is useful to invite our clients to allow these movements and to carry them out in a controlled manner in their imagination or even in reality. By encouraging them to sense inside and to perceive emerging feelings and body sensations, we support this process. By pendulating to a resource, we can dose and shape it gently.

33.3 Imagining not Being Frozen

Another possibility is to ask our clients how it would be for them not to feel frozen. In this way we encourage them to imagine a corresponding inner image and to sense the feelings and body sensations evoked by it. Alternatively, we can invite our clients to recall a situation in which they were not frozen and to imagine it and let it take effect on them. It is also useful to motivate them to notice movement impulses and to consciously allow and carry them out in a controlled way.

33.4 Reassuring Safety in the Here and Now

Assuring that they are safe and secure in the here and now and that the danger is over can contribute to our clients' frozen state subsiding.

Example from practice

Sabine, 51, is in a highly activated state due to a multitude of early chronic traumatizations; her body reacts quickly to various triggers by freezing. Assuring that she is safe and secure here and now calms Sabine relatively quickly and leads to her frozen state decreasing and gradually resolving. ◄

33.5 Imagining Safety and Security

Imagining that they are in a place where they feel completely safe and secure, or having someone with them who gives them safety and security, can also be supportive.

33.6 Grounding Oneself

Grounding exercises, such as consciously being aware of the ground under their feet or the seat surface under their buttocks can give our clients a feeling of support and safety and thus contribute to their immobility subsiding.

Example from practice

Otto, 49, freezes when certain topics are discussed, for instance, when he talks about his hot-tempered boss or a dominant colleague. It helps him to ground himself by feeling the ground under his feet. This gives him safety and calms him down and leads to his freezing subsiding again. ◄

33.7 Conscious Breathing

By observing how their chest and belly rise and falls slightly when breathing, our clients can still feel the movement in their body despite their immobility and thus get in touch with their vitality. By consciously observing the movement during inhalation and exhalation, their breathing usually calms down and deepens, and the movement of their chest widens a bit and becomes more perceptible. Furthermore, through conscious breathing, our clients can calm down and experience a feeling of safety. This can contribute to their freezing decreasing.

Caution: Breathing exercises can trigger restlessness, tension or constriction and fear and thus increase the state of immobility.

33.8 Singing and Whistling, Humming and Toning

In addition, our clients´ immobility can be resolved by singing, whistling, humming or toning; e.g. with the voo-sound suggested by Peter Levine (2011) which we have already encountered. This sets our face, throat and neck area as well as our upper body into slight pulsation which we can perceive as vibrations. These can slightly activate us and bring us into contact with our vitality. Furthermore, it can bring about a feeling of safety and inner stability, which let us calm down and counteracts our immobility.

Example from practice

Yussi, 46, has got into the habit of toning the sounds O or U, sometimes also Om or voo, as soon as he notices that he becomes rigid and is frozen. This usually helps him to find his way out of this state. ◄

33.9 Perceiving External Stimuli and Impressions

Consciously perceiving and observing pleasant or neutral external stimuli, like a neutral sound or a pleasant, safety-imbuing smell, can also be a support.

33.10 Activating Acupuncture Points

If possible, despite their rigidity, lightly tapping or massaging the acupuncture point above the thymus gland (about 3 fingers width below the collarbone) can be beneficial for our clients. Activating the four acupuncture points described in chap. 25.9 (between the eyebrows, between the nose and upper lip, between the lower lip and chin and above the thymus gland; fig. 25.1) can be of help (Gallo 2002). In doing so, our clients can repeatedly name the immobility aloud or silently—"this paralysis" or "this being frozen"—and inhale and exhale slowly in between.

References

Gallo FP (2002) Advanced energy psychology I. Training manual level I. VAK, Kirchstetten, DE

Levine PA (2011) Sprache ohne Worte. Wie unser Körper Trauma verarbeitet und uns in die innere Balance zurückführt. Kösel, München (In an Unspoken Voice. How the Body Releases Trauma and Restores Goodness. 2010, North Atlantic Books, Berkeley) Own translation

Levine PA (o. J.) Ron–Flying Dutchman: renegotiation of developmental trauma. SE™-Demo. Somatic Experiencing Demo Media Library Rental, Boulder

Zanotta S (2018) Wieder ganz werden. Traumaheilung mit Ego-State-Therapie und Körperwissen. Carl Auer, Heidelberg (Somatic Ego State Therapy™ for Trauma Healing: Whole again. 2024, Routledge, New York) Own translation

34 Alleviating Depression, Powerlessness and Hopelessness

Contents

To alleviate and transform feelings of sadness, powerlessness and hopelessness as well as depressive mood, the following interventions can be helpful as well as all those discussed in chaps. 22, 23 and 24.

34.1 Allowing and Acknowledging

As with all burdensome feelings, the first step in alleviating sadness, inner emptiness, powerlessness and hopelessness is to allow and acknowledge them; only then can they be transformed and resolved. By recognizing and appreciating these feelings as appropriate reactions to their traumatic experiences, we support our clients in accepting them and developing compassion for themselves. This is by no means self-pity, which is weakening, but rather an attitude towards oneself that

R. Lackner, *Stabilization in Trauma Treatment*,
https://doi.org/10.1007/978-3-662-67480-2_34

is characterized by respect and appreciation of the experience and the associated pain, thus strengthening and supporting their self-esteem and self-care.

34.2 Being Mindful

Regularly used mindful exercises can have a positive effect on depression (e.g. Hofmann et al. 2010). Therefore, it makes sense to suggest one or the other appropriate exercise to our clients, such as consciously observing their breath, doing mindful activities or movements such as Qi Gong, or consciously perceiving with the senses.

Caution: As discussed in chap. 9, for some of our clients mindfulness exercises are unpleasant or threatening and sometimes they can worsen existing depression.

34.3 Exploring Body Sensations

When our clients become aware of and explore their depressive mood, powerlessness, inner heaviness and helplessness, they frequently feel a heaviness or pressure in their body; their legs, for instance, feel leaden or their shoulders feel heavy. When we ask them what they feel in the rest of their body or where it feels different, they usually discover areas that they perceive as neutral or even pleasant.

Example from practice

Alexander, 54, suffers from major depression. He feels paralyzed, helpless and powerless. While he perceives this, he notices that his legs and arms feel very heavy. On my question how the rest of his body feels, Alexander notices that his stomach and back are neutral. He is amazed to find out that he has always felt completely and exclusively heavy and leaden. Recognizing that this is not the case, but that apart from the heaviness he also senses a neutral feeling, gives him relief and lets him feel lighter. ◄

By discovering neutral or pleasant body sensations, our clients often experience, like Alexander, that they are not exclusively or continuously burdened, heavy or depressed, but also have pleasant, vital, healthy and strengthening parts in themselves.

34.4 Following the Body's Movement Impulses

While our clients are feeling their depressive mood, heaviness and powerlessness and the associated body sensations, it is healing to ask them: *"And as you are noticing this, what would your body most like to do?"* Frequently then the impulse arises to run, "to leave the body" or to scream. Alexander, for instance, would most like to run off his powerlessness and helplessness. By inviting our clients to imagine that they are carrying out these impulses to move, they no longer feel powerless or helpless. Alexander increasingly feels liberated when he imagines running and shedding the powerlessness. On my suggestion, he makes running movements with his feet while imagining (Levine 1998); this reinforces his feeling of liberation and ability to act.

34.5 Imagining Consolation

We can suggest to our clients to consider: *"If everything is possible, and in our imagination everything is possible, what would be good for you?"* Often the need for rest, comfort, security and safety or lightness arises. By then asking, for example, *"What does it take for you to feel safe/secure?"* or *"Who or what could give you comfort/security/safety?"*, we encourage our clients to imagine a positive inner image that allows them to refuel, catch up on what was missed and renourish themselves. This can be very liberating and freeing for them and an important step towards relieving their sadness, depression or inner emptiness. As usual, it is useful to recommend our clients keep this imagery up as a daily exercise for a while and in doing so to consciously be aware of their feelings and body sensations. A gesture, sentence, word or symbol associated with the image can serve as an anchor and make it easier for them to recall and re-experience the corresponding feelings.

34.6 Considering Positive Aspects

Especially with dejection, sadness, depressive mood or inner emptiness, it is advisable to support our clients in focusing on what is successful and pleasant in their lives. This is by no means about denying or diminishing their pain or suffering; rather, it is about supporting them to broaden their view and open up to something positive again. Even through seemingly small aspects or moments, they can gain a somewhat more positive view of themselves and their lives. It can be as helpful to explore resources, such as collecting and writing down beautiful encounters, special experiences and successes or doing the "three blessings". In this exercise we write down three things that have gone well every day, which has been proven to reduce depression (Seligman 2012).

34.7 Reviving Moments of Vitality

Our clients can also get in touch with positive feelings and re-experience them by picking up, recalling and reliving moments in which they felt lively, happy or confident. By noticing the body sensation associated with the feeling, this can be experienced more intensely. A suitable movement or body posture can additionally strengthen it and later serve as an anchor to reactivate it.

During this imagining our clients sometimes experience nostalgia or sadness that they have lost or have not had these feelings for a long time. By allowing them, they can gradually decrease and dissolve. We can support our clients by making them aware that they feel joy or lightness here and now again. These feelings have not evaporated, dissipated or been lost, but can still be experienced by them and revived and strengthened once again, for example, by means of the imagination.

Example from practice

Sania, 23, lost her parents in a traffic accident at an early age. She feels a lot of sadness, pain, inner emptiness and lostness. Sania remembers how as a little girl she ran joyfully through her grandmother's garden, played with the cats and lay in the grass. In reliving this memory, initially Sania only slightly feels the joy, carefree and liveliness she experienced then. After a while these feelings increase substantially. At the same time, sadness and pain come up for her that this beautiful time is over and her grandmother and parents are no longer alive. By being able to allow both the sadness and pain as well as the joy and happiness, the sadness and pain can gradually decrease. Increasingly, she perceives a strength and vitality in her body. She now looks more relaxed, present and centered. By reliving this memory in her imagination daily for a while Sania can reconnect to her former aliveness and revive and strengthen it. This is an important step for Sania that also helps her to process the loss of her parents. ◀

34.8 Imagining Feeling Alive

In addition, inviting our clients to imagine what it would be like if they were joyful, satisfied or happy can be a support to stimulate or revive these feelings. Like on an inner screen, they can then imagine what they look like, how they move and what they are wearing when they are joyful, satisfied or happy. With that it is supportive to encourage them to notice the feelings and associated body sensations that arise. Sometimes our clients have doubts or objections, for example, that this is just a fantasy and not real; we can sensitively refute these: *"I can very well understand that you have these doubts. But you are experiencing these feelings here and now and can feel them in your body, and that is quite real."*

34.9 Changing Body Posture

Another possibility is suggesting to our clients to adopt a body posture that contradicts the depressive mood, sadness or powerlessness. We discussed in chap. 5 that "a certain posture not only enables the 'appropriate' emotion, but also makes the 'inappropriate' emotion impossible" (Pasquarelli and Bull 1951, quoted in Storch 2006, p. 48). So we can encourage our clients to straighten up, lift their head, extend and stretch, or experiment with other movements. If they sense inside while doing so, they can become aware that their mood and feelings change.

34.10 Allowing Visions of the Future

The vision of a goal, a state or an objective that our clients want to achieve or develop can be helpful, too, in counteracting, soothing or cushioning and mitigating their dejection, sadness or depression. It can be helpful to write down the vision and visualize it daily (see also chaps. 18.4 and 18.5).

34.11 Sport and Movement

Movement and sport have been proven to alleviate depression (Rosenbaum et al. 2015). Accordingly, we should encourage our clients to do some form of movement or sport that they like or enjoy; starting with short sessions of about 10 minutes that they can easily integrate into their daily life (Craft and Perna 2004).

34.12 Tonglen

For some people, a variation of the technique of Tonglen practiced in Tibetan Buddhism is helpful. In this extended form of compassion meditation, we imagine inhaling the burden and suffering of a person as a dark energy, taking it into our "heart center" and sending it out as "white energy" with the exhale and letting it flow back to him (Olvedi 2008, p. 252).

In a modified form, we can imagine inhaling our pain, our sadness and depression into our heart, taking it into our heart center, transforming it into light, and letting it flow out of us with the exhale.

Caution: For some people, this exercise is unpleasant or threatening; they have the feeling of taking in their pain even more and thus intensifying or solidifying it.

References

Craft LL, Perna FM (2004) The benefits of exercise for the clinically depressed. Primary Care Companion J Clin Psychiatr 6(3):104–111

Hofmann SG, Sawyer AT, Witt AA, Oh D (2010) The effect of mindfulness-based therapy on anxiety and depression: a meta-analytic review. J Consult Clin Psychol 78(2):169–183

Levine PA, Frederick A (1998) Trauma-Heilung. Das Erwachen des Tigers. Unsere Fähigkeit, traumatische Erfahrungen zu transformieren. Synthesis, Essen (Waking the Tiger: Healing Trauma: The Innate Capacity to Transform Overwhelming Experiences. 1997, North Atlantic Books, Berkeley)

Olvedi U (2008) Mo. Das Orakel der Tibeter. Wegweisende Antworten auf alle Lebensfragen. O. W. Barth, Frankfurt/Main

Pasquarelli L, Bull N (1951) Experimental investigations of the body-mind continuum in affective states. J Nerv Ment Dis 113:512–521. Cited in: Storch M (2006) Wie Embodiment in der Psychologie erforscht wurde. In: Storch M, Cantieni B, Hüther G, Tschacher W Embodiment. Die Wechselwirkung von Körper und Psyche verstehen und nutzen. Hans Huber, Bern, pp 35–72

Rosenbaum S, Sherrington C, Tiedemann A (2015) Exercise augmentation compared with usual care of post-traumatic stress disorder; a randomized controlled trial. Acta Psychiatr Scand 131(5):350–359

Seligman M (2012) Flourish. Wie Menschen aufblühen. Die Positive Psychologie des gelingenden Lebens. Kösel, München (Flourish: A Visionary New Understanding of Happpiness and Well-being. 2011, Free Press, New York)

Storch M (2006) Wie Embodiment in der Psychologie erforscht wurde. In: Storch M, Cantieni B, Hüther G, Tschacher W Embodiment. Die Wechselwirkung von Körper und Psyche verstehen und nutzen. Hans Huber, Bern, pp 35–72

Dealing with Anger and Rage 35

Contents

By their unpretictability and uncontrollability, rage, anger, annoyance, irritability and aggressive reactions often destabilize our clients. Therefore, it is important to support them in finding ways to deal with their rage in a positive way or to relieve it.

A first important step is to acknowledge rage as an appropriate reaction to the injustice and suffering they have experienced. Rage is generally a form of self-protection and defense of our boundaries and integrity. In this sense, there is also the term of "sacred rage", which is justified and necessary to protect oneself, to stand up for something or someone and to go one's own way (Quartier 2018). By conveying this to our clients, they can better understand their rage, accept it as appropriate and use it or the power underlying it as a resource. We can discuss how they can, for example, express their rage constructively and appropriately in boundary violations by others and how they can use their rage, for instance, as a driving force in sports or social engagement. Finally, above all it is about exploring with our clients which vents they already have or which ones they could (also) use to reduce their anger and rage.

R. Lackner, *Stabilization in Trauma Treatment*,
https://doi.org/10.1007/978-3-662-67480-2_35

35.1 Perceiving and Observing Rage

If we manage to perceive and observe our rage, preferably without judging it, we can gain distance from it allowing it to subside. Slow, deep inhalation and long exhalation can help us with this.

35.2 Vents for Rage

As with the relief of tension, movement is also an essential and particularly helpful vent for dealing with rage and aggression. Any form of movement supports us to reduce stress hormones, to dampen the increased level of arousal and to lessen rage and anger as well as aggressive impulses. Special exercises for the cardiovascular system "activate the circuits of the frontal lobes" of our brain and release our anger or make it almost impossible to "stay angry" (Newberg and Waldman 2012, p. 283). Consequently, we should recommend our clients incorporate movement into their routine; ideally daily, with it being sensible to plan shorter daily movement units and to supplement them with, for instance, one longer one per week.

As always, it is crucial that our clients find a form of movement that suits them and that they enjoy, and experience as beneficial and relieving. It should be noted that intense training, which increases heart and breathing rate significantly, can be a trigger and is therefore usually unsuitable for traumatized people (Rothschild 2002). Strength exercises and moderate endurance training are generally more appropriate for them.

Rage and anger as well as aggressive impulses can be specifically directed and channeled by movement. This way, our clients can experience that they can influence their rage and its intensity and frequency. As a result, they experience that they are not helplessly exposed to it, which in turn strengthens and consolidates their stability.

Strength exercises

For many traumatized people, the practice of simple body exercises such as squats, sit-ups, push-ups or lifting weights is very supportive. With these they can not only reduce rage and aggression; they can feel their strength, too, and, over time, increase their muscle tone. Babette Rothschild (2002) points out that people with a higher muscle tone can better tolerate a higher level of arousal. Moreover, increasing muscle strength increases self-confidence and reduces feelings of vulnerability and helplessness. Additionally, strength exercises help us to center ourselves and to feel more embodied. As with many exercises, conscious awareness and feeling of our body or the movements is also supportive.

Short endurance exercises

To reduce anger and rage, short endurance exercises such as skipping rope, trampolining, using a stepper, jumping jacks, running on the spot or skippping (running on the spot lifting the knees) are suitable.

Shaking

Powerful shaking of our arms and legs or shaking of our entire body can be a vent for our rage, too. It is useful to carry out the movements in a controlled way and consciously be aware of them. In doing so, we can imagine shaking off our rage and anger.

Tiger Exercise

As we already discovered in chap. 26, we can reduce our rage and anger doing the Tiger Exercise. We stand with feet hip-width apart, bend our arms at about a right angle and lift them slightly so that we hold our hands at shoulder level. We bundle our strength, tense our body and form paws with our hands (see fig. 26.1). We can imagine a tigress or a tiger who wants to sharpen his claws on a tree trunk or prepare for a fight. We take a deep breath and then exhale powerfully while we relax into our knees or go down into a squat. While exhaling, we imagine puffing our rage out of us. By doing the movement mindfully and pausing repeatedly to notice what we feel, we can titrate the discharge of our rage.

Swinging movements with Smoveys®

As we swing the Smoveys back and forth, we take a deep breath and exhale strongly. While moving we imagine our rage swinging out of us. Through periodically stopping and sensing inside, our rage can "carefully and yet vigorously" be released (Zanotta 2018, p. 163).

35.3 Exploring the Triggers

In order to better cope with their rage, it is useful to explore with our clients in which situations they become angry, irritated or upset or react aggressively, and what triggers it. Often rage and anger burst out of them uncontrollably and unpredictably, so that they feel overwhelmed and helpless. If we investigate the causes together, explore and get to the bottom of them, usually clear, understandable triggers can be found. Many times these are situations in which our clients feel threatened in some way and their boundaries are violated. Or moments when they feel helpless. Once the triggers are identified and thus concrete and tangible, our clients no longer feel so at the mercy of their rage and can better understand it and their corresponding reactions and consequently themselves.

Example from practice

When playing around with his 9-year-old son Timo, Gabor, 52, often experiences moments of sudden rage and a desire to hit out. "Thank God", says Gabor, he is able to suppress it. But the rage he feels in these moments weighs heavily on him; he doesn't want to be like this. He feels helpless, ashamed and guilty. I ask Gabor when the playfulness, which he definitely likes, starts to wane and which moment it is, that makes him suddenly angry. Gabor notices that it becomes critical for him when Timo punches him in his upper body. That is very bad for him; it reminds him of how his father often punched him in his arms or back when he was angry with him. I suggest to Gabor to find a strategy for such situations, as well as to work with the feeling that arises in him in such a situation.

The strategy was relatively quickly found: Gabor intends to explain to Timo that he does not want him to punch him in his upper body. And he wants to agree on a stop signal with him. If it should happen despite the stop that Timo punches Gabor, he intends, depending on the situation, to take a few steps away or stand up, consciously breathe out and notice his breath. He will tell Timo, too. ◄

35.4 Following the Body's Movement Impulses

When our clients tell us about a situation in which they were angry, we can suggest they recall the situation and notice the rage that arises.

I: "When you remember a situation in which your father punched you, what happens inside you?"

Gabor: "… everything inside me tightens up."

I: "And when you notice and feel a bit that everything inside you tightens up, what happens then?"

G: "Everything tightens even more. ... and it makes me furious."

I: "Yes, and if you notice that it makes you furious, what would you like to do with the fury?"

G: "… punch back."

I: "Would you like to imagine punching back?"

G: "… no, I can't do that. I can´t hit someone. I don't want to do that."

I: "Yes, I understand. How about if you just imagine the movement, so that you just punch into the air?"

G: "Yes, that's a good idea."

I: "If you want, you can also carry out the movement and actually punch into the air, not just imagine it."
(Gregor punches a few times into the air, at first hesitantly, then more forcefully)

I: "How is it now when you do that?"

G: (takes a deep breath in and out) "Good. That feels good. I have to do it a few more times … even harder … "

I: "Try to do the movement very consciously and slowly, so that your body can follow it well."
(Gregor punches slowly into the air, takes a few deep breaths in and out and then ends the movement)

I: "How is it now?"

G: "Good, that was good, now it feels lighter, freer."

Catching up and carrying out the original action impulses of their body is usually very liberating for our clients; they then not only experience "what it would have felt like to fight back or run away" (van der Kolk 2016, p. 261); they also experience the liberation and relief through the completion of an unfinished action.

This can happen through doing a movement, as with Gabor, or by simply imagining it.

35.5 Allowing and Releasing Rage through Imagery

Example from practice

Franz, 44, has been suffering from severe anxiety, insecurity and self-doubt since a panic attack 3 years ago. In the course of our work, it becomes clear that Franz was denigrated, humiliated and treated without love from an early age by his father; he never received recognition or praise from him. Even today he feels insecure and tense in his presence. Gradually, Franz becomes aware of how much his father hurt, unsettled and frightened him. He gradually begins to feel rage towards his father; sometimes also towards his mother, who did not protect him from his father. At the same time, Franz does not want to allow this sudden rage and fights against it; meanwhile he has a good relationship with both of them. Both have changed a lot over the years. I assure Franz that here and now in the therapeutic context, the rage is allowed. After what he has experienced, it is understandable; when we experience injustice, boundary violations and injuries, rage is an appropriate reaction. In therapy, it is important and relieving to allow it and give it space. This is often a healing step. Franz can hardly accept these arguments. Only my assurance that it is neither about assigning blame nor condemning or badmouthing his parents makes it possible for Franz to take up my suggestion. Likewise my explanation that by allowing the rage to be released, something can change and be freed within him.

I: "As you notice the rage right now, where in your body do you sense it most or strongest?"

Franz: "In my hands, there is a tension … actually in the whole body, especially in the jaw, I often clench my teeth together."

I: "As you feel the rage in your body and just observe and perceive it … how is that?"

F: "… then it gets even stronger …"

I: "Mhm, and if everything is possible—and in our imagination everything is possible—what would you most like to do with the rage?"

F: "Hit somewhere."

I: "Ah, do you want to imagine that you hit somewhere? … is that possible?"

F: "… I would most like to give my father a punch. … but I don't do that, now he's old. … but I would tell him my opinion …"

I: "Ah, and is it possible that you imagine that you tell your father your opinion?"

F: "Yes, that's possible. … what was he thinking treating a little child—his child!—like that? How can you do that? Such an asshole." (while Franz continues speaking, he lightly hits the armrest of the sofa)

I: "Try to hit the armrest a little slower with your fist and consciously be aware of it."
(Franz hits slowly but harder on the armrest with the fist, while he breathes deeply in and out)

I: "How is that now?"

F: "That feels good …" (Franz breathes deeply in and out, and hits repeatedly slowly but strongly on the armrest) "… you hurt me so much. … you don't treat your child like that. … that is absolutely the limit …"

I: "How is it when you tell your father that?"

F: "That feels good, I've never done that before, I would never have dared." (sits up a bit)

I: "Then consciously be aware of it and also notice that you are now sitting a bit more upright."

F: "… absolutely useless. … as a father you were really useless. … I won't let you make me feel small anymore." (Franz repeatedly breathes deeply in and out; after a while he only hits the armrest from time to time, now clearly lighter, gradually he breathes slower again)

I: "How is it now?"

F: "Good … I feel somehow stronger. … and he is no longer so big … now we are on an equal footing. … I wouldn't have thought that it would be so liberating. … he is no longer threatening to me, somehow neutral. … that's good."

For Franz, the experience of being able to say everything to his father in his imagination that he had never been able to say before, as well as consciously expressing his rage by hitting the armrest in a controlled manner, is very relieving. Since then he can approach his father more freely and relaxed. ◄

Franz was able to direct and channel his rage towards his father in his imagination by telling him everything that was in his heart. However, for some people this is not possible; then it is necessary to suggest they have someone—a helper—at their side who takes over this task. We can ask the question: *"Who or what could help you to tell your father your opinion, or even take over the task of doing it?"* Many then think of a certain person or—in situations from childhood—frequently their own adult self. If this is not the case, we can stimulate our clients´ fantasy by making a few suggestions, such as: *"This could be, for example, an ancestor or a spiritual figure, an angel or a father figure or someone completely different."*

In Franz's case, the rage could be resolved well in this session and he could leave relieved; often, however, it can only be partially discharged. Then it is necessary to find a way to dampen the rage for the moment so that our clients can calm down and end the session well; images such as the following can be helpful here: *"Could it be helpful if you imagine the rage like a volcano that could now discharge a little? It has let off some steam and is now a bit calmer; and in our next session it can discharge again."*

It is also sensible to address our clients´ innermost being directly and assure them that we will take care of the rage, will not forget or push it away, and that it has a place here and can show itself: *"So that your innermost self knows that we take care of the rage here in our sessions. It can show itself here and is seen. In the time between our sessions it can rest, knowing that it has a place here."* With this or a similar intervention we speak to the inner part of our clients that is angry and assure him that he is welcome here; this usually calms him down and our clients can cope better with their rage between our sessions. Even the awareness that it is a part in them that is angry and not them in their entirety is often relieving.

35.6 Venting

Some traumatized people have the need to get rid of their rage by hitting or kicking something. To do this safely and without the risk of injury, it is useful, for example, if they hit a pillow or punching bag, beat a sofa with a knotted cloth or stamp firmly on the ground. It is essential that our clients carry out the movement attentively and in a controlled manner; being aware that the rage is an appropriate reaction and they can now let it out and free themselves from it. A mere venting without conscious awareness and control of the movement is of little use and carries the danger that the rage increases and consolidates. For the same reason and to prevent overactivation, our clients should limit their venting in time (Fischer 2019).

35.7 The Necessity of the Consciously Experienced Expression of Rage

It is decisive in which consciousness we express our rage; if we do this consciously, attentively and while perceiving our body, this has a very relieving effect, in that we experience that we can control and regulate our body and our feelings. Furthermore, we give our body the opportunity to make up for something that was not possible before. With this conscious, attentive and body-awareness approach, we can channel our rage in very different ways. Be it in our imagination, through movement or through singing and toning, making music or creative expression such as painting, writing or handicrafts. Even conscious breathing or blowing out can be a helpful outlet. For some people, however, it is less harmonious to express their rage; for them it is more appropriate to deal with it in another, more transforming way. Thus, for some it can be supportive, like in the Buddhist practice of

Tonglen, to inhale the rage into their heart, to accept it and to let it out again (see chap. 34.12). Others imagine shaking off the rage like tar pitch or that it flows out of them and drains away.

References

Fischer G (2019) Neue Wege aus dem Trauma. Erste Hilfe bei schweren seelischen Belastungen. Patmos, Ostfildern

Newberg A, Waldman MR (2012) Der Fingerabdruck Gottes. Wie religiöse und spirituelle Erfahrungen unser Gehirn verändern. Goldmann, München (How Good Changes Your Brain. 2009, Ballantine Books, New York)

Quartier T (2018) Heilige Wut. Mönch sein heißt radikal sein. Herder, Freiburg im Breisgau

Rothschild B (2002) Der Körper erinnert sich. Die Psychophysiologie des Traumas und der Traumabehandlung. Synthesis, Essen (The Body Remembers. The Psychophysiology of Trauma and Treatment. 2000, W.W. Norton, New York)

Van der Kolk B (2016) Verkörperter Schrecken. Traumaspuren in Gehirn, Geist und Körper und wie man sie heilen kann. S. 261. G. P. Probst, Lichtenau/Westfalen (The Body Keeps the Score. Mind, brain and body in the transfomation of trauma. 2015. Penguine Books, London. p. 261). Quoted from original English version (p 261)

Zanotta S (2018) Wieder ganz werden. Traumaheilung mit Ego-State-Therapie und Körperwissen. Carl-Auer, Heidelberg (Somatic Ego State Therapy™ for Trauma Healing: Whole again. 2024, Routledge, New York)

Exploring and Being Aware of Our Boundaries

36

Contents

In traumatic experiences, our boundaries are always violated, often our physical, always our mental. Therefore, discerning our boundaries is an important stabilizing and healing step.

36.1 Being aware of Our Physical Boundaries

One way to support our clients in being aware of their boundaries is to invite them to tap, feel or stroke their body and to sense its boundaries. By doing this and becoming aware of their physical boundaries, they can center themselves, be with themselves and thus develop a feeling for their boundaries.

36.2 Extending and Stretching Oneself

In addition, we can suggest to our clients to stretch and extend themselves and to explore and perceive their boundaries while doing so; initially perhaps only with small and increasingly with expansive and all-round movements. For some this can be a challenging and difficult process, in which they come up against their

R. Lackner, *Stabilization in Trauma Treatment*,
https://doi.org/10.1007/978-3-662-67480-2_36

inner boundaries. Through a careful, well-dosed or well-titrated approach, trying out and experimenting, these inner boundaries can slowly loosen and our clients can get a feeling for their outer boundary. During this process they can become aware, for instance, that they need more space around them and that they have to set their boundaries further out to feel safe and comfortable. The image of a large old tree with its expansive crown can be supportive here. By noticing the movements and body posture that arise, our clients often develop a new understanding of themselves and their boundaries.

36.3 Imagining Our Boundaries

Another possibility is to encourage our clients to explore and feel their boundaries on an imaginative level. For example, by imagining that they are surrounded by their very own space and investigating how big this has to be for them to be just right, and imagining a boundary around that. They consciously become aware of this and let it take effect on them. Many experience a feeling of centering, safety and strength. The experience of the imagined boundary can be supported by a movement; e.g., by our clients defining their boundary around them with their hands or marking it on the ground with a string. By paying attention to their body sensations and feelings, their boundary and its effect on them can become even more tangible.

36.4 Something Protective that Surrounds Us

Imagining something protective that surrounds us (see chap. 23.3), can be a help, too, in perceiving our own boundaries, protecting ourselves and setting boundaries.

Example from practice

Grete, 72, imagines being surrounded by a blue ball. This calms her; she feels centered, present and protected. Through practicing this image Grete increasingly succeeds in keeping her distance in difficult situations, setting better boundaries for others and keeping burdensome things away from her. ◄

36.5 Being Aware of Our Boundaries and Setting them

An exercise from Tauna, the yoga of the Incas (Delval 2014), which we got to know in chap. 24.5, is another way to recognize and set our boundaries. We stand with our feet facing forward hip-width apart, our legs relaxed and not fully extended. We stretch our arms straight out in front of us to shoulder level and make fists with our hands. Now we stretch and spread our fingers forcefully and breathe out strongly (fig. 24.1). We repeat this sequence of movements several times, each time exhaling strongly while stretching and spreading our fingers out forcefully. While doing this we gradually bring our arms out to our sides, so that they eventually form a line with our shoulders. We stretch and spread our fingers out from the fists a few more times and then put our hands up with our fingertips pointing up. Our hands push outwards, so that we feel a slight tension in our arms (fig. 24.2). Now we draw a boundary around us and our space with our palms. We sense inward and notice our body sensations and feelings. This exercise can be combined with the idea of keeping everything away from us that burdens us.

We can do only part of this exercise: We stand with our feet hip-width apart, our arms stretched forward horizontally at shoulder level. We raise our hands with our fingertips pointing upwards. Now we slowly bring our arms out to our sides. We draw or set a boundary around us with our palms. We sense inward and notice how we feel.

References

Delval M (2014) Tauna–Yoga of the Ands. Personal communication. 25 October 2014. www.melaniedelval.at

Releasing Guilt

37

Contents

Due to their experiences our clients frequently suffer from feelings of guilt. These often have a destabilizing effect; hence it is important to address, discuss and counteract them.

It can be helpful for our clients to obtain (additional) information about the event in order to gain more clarity about its cause and course. If they have experienced violence or neglect, it is—as has already been emphasized several times—essential that we take a partisan stance and convey to them that the responsibility for any form of violence always lies with the perpetrators and never with the survivors. With our clear stance that, for example, children and adolescents are never responsible for the happiness or misfortune of their parents, we can contribute to reducing their feelings of guilt.

37.1 Inner Dialogue with the Deceased

When people experience a traumatic event in which someone else dies, they often develop a so-called survivor´s guilt (Niederland 1964); they then feel guilty for having survived and for still being alive. This "phenomenon" was first described by the German-American psychiatrist William Niederland in survivors of the Holocaust. Survivor's guilt is an incredible burden, robbing affected people of their joy of life and vitality and questioning their right to live. Moreover, children

R. Lackner, *Stabilization in Trauma Treatment*,
https://doi.org/10.1007/978-3-662-67480-2_37

tend to generally relate the loss of a person to themselves and feel responsible and guilty for their death.

A very helpful and relieving way to meet this guilt is to invite our clients to imagine what the deceased would say to them if he or she knew or heard how guilty they feel for surviving or continuing to live.

I: "If little Bruno were here now and heard how guilty you feel that he had to die and you are alive, what would he say to you?"

Bernhard [1]: "… he would look at me with his cheerful eyes and say that I should enjoy life. … and that it was his destiny to go so early. … and that it is good for him and that he is doing well."

I: "How is it for you when Bruno tells you that?"

B: (has tears in his eyes) "… that touches me very much that he says that. … he feels so free and cheerful … for him it's good. For him it's not bad that he died so early. I feel that so clearly. … he is doing well and he wants me to do well, too."

I: "For him it's good and he wants you to do well, too."

B: "Yes, exactly." (takes a deep breath)

I: "As you let that have an effect on you, how is that?"

B: "It makes it easier, it takes away some of the heaviness" (takes a deep breath) "… and it's also like a mission to Bruno. To honor him I have to learn that I am allowed to be well … that I am well!"

I: "Yes, to honor him you have to learn that you are well. When you say that and become aware of it, how does that feel?"

B: "Good. Yes, that's good."

I: "Fine, then take that in consciously. … and while you do that, where in your body do you feel that it's good?"

B: "In my heart, it's lighter now."

I: "Fine, then also take that in consciously that your heart is lighter now."

37.2 Handing over the Guilt to a Higher Power or Entity

For many people, it can be very relieving to hand over their guilt or feelings of guilt to a higher power or entity. We can encourage our clients: *"If there were a higher power or entity to whom you could hand over your guilt, in whose hands you could lay the guilt, how would that be?"* If we know that our clients have a spiritual or religious approach, we can directly address their faith: *"You told me that your faith is very important to you; is it conceivable for you to lay your guilt in the hands of God?"* or *"How would it be if you were to place the guilt in the hands of a higher power?"* Again, we can ask about the feelings and bodily

[1] We have already met Bernhard in chap. 2.1.

sensations. Mostly, this idea is very relieving, liberating and comforting and is accompanied by the resolving of physical tension, pressure or tightness. By allowing our clients to experience these changes in their feelings and body sensations, they usually intensify. In general, it is very supportive and stabilizing for them if they repeat this image as a daily exercise for a while.

37.3 Rituals

Rituals too can be helpful for our clients to better deal with their guilt or feelings of guilt. They frequently contribute to the feelings of guilt subsiding and the heavy weight of them reducing. For example, putting the guilt in a fire can be very relieving; by burning something that symbolizes the guilt or is associated with it, or writing the guilt statement on a piece of paper and putting it in the fire.

If it is a transferred responsibility or guilt, it is often very healing to return it to the responsible persons or perpetrators on an imaginative level. The effect of imagining this can be reinforced by a corresponding movement or a symbolic action and a sentence such as "I hand you back your guilt, it is your responsibility".

References

Niederland WG (1964) Psychiatric disorders among persecution victims; a contribution to the understanding of concentration camp pathology and its after-effects. Williams & Wilkins, Baltimore

References

Overcoming Shame

38

Contents

Traumatic events are frequently accompanied by the experience of shame; particulary sexual, physical and psychological violence, as well as neglect. Shame is often intertwined with feelings of guilt and is intensified by them.

Shame is a very painful, hard to grasp feeling; when we feel ashamed, we feel worthless, unworthy, have the feeling of not having the right to be there, and feel excluded and not belonging (e.g. Brown 2020).

Shame is like a state of collapse or shutdown, triggered by the activation of the dorsal vagus branch (e.g. Levine 2019), and is expressed on a physical level, among other things, by a feeling of weakness and powerlessness. We let our head and shoulders droop, feel empty, sometimes dizzy, and can no longer think clearly or are dissociated. The world around us seems threatening and we avoid eye contact; if someone asks us to look at him or her, it is difficult or even impossible for us to do so or it intensifies our feeling of shame if we follow the request. Therefore, it is advisable to offer our clients a sitting position that makes it easier for them to avoid our gaze; Peter Levine, for example, suggests an angle of 90° between the chairs (ibid.). My seats are facing each other slightly, at an obtuse angle.

R. Lackner, *Stabilization in Trauma Treatment*,
https://doi.org/10.1007/978-3-662-67480-2_38

38.1 Shame and Clarification

Our clients often feel ashamed of their symptoms. They feel strange, odd or not right and are afraid of not being "normal" or becoming "crazy". They frequently feel misunderstood by others or are disparaged or seen as weak or weird because of their symptoms; this further intensifies their feelings of shame. By clearly conveying to our clients that their symptoms are an expression of their coping with their traumatic experience, we contribute to their feelings of shame diminishing a bit. An in-depth clarification is therefore a means of countering shame, especially when it comes to traumatization by any form of violence. Even very specific information can be enormously relieving for our clients. For instance, regarding the extreme shame- and guilt-laden and confusing fact that those affected by sexual violence can be sexually aroused during the sexual assault (Briere 1992). This is a normal and natural physical reaction and by no means an expression of their consent or even their desire (Levin and van Berlo 2004).

38.2 Shame, Connectedness and Dignity

When shame is associated with the feeling of not being lovable and separated from or not belonging to others, it is the connection to another person or the experience of being seen, heard and respected by another person and being in contact with him or her that counteracts the shame (Brown 2020). By meeting our clients with respect and partnership, they can experience being accepted. This is an important prerequisite for them to develop self-respect and dignity again.

38.3 Exploring and Experiencing the Opposite of Shame

Besides that, it is also important to "gradually" deconstruct "the psychophysiological and postural shame state" and to reconstruct "those of pride and dignity" (Levine 2019, p. 33). In order to do this it can be helpful to encourage our clients to change their body posture by inviting them, for example: *"Would you like to try out what it's like to move a bit and change your posture?"*, and then asking, *"And as you change your body posture, what happens?"* Our clients usually notice that their feeling of shame changes and gives way to another one, such as relief, sadness or even rage.

Another possibility is to suggest our clients take up a body posture that is contrary to or the opposite to shame (Levine 2017, quoted in Zanotta 2018). By doing so, they experience that they can influence their feeling of shame with a deliberate opposite posture.

In addition, we support our clients in transforming their feeling of shame with questions such as: *"What is the opposite of shame for you?"* or *"What does dignity mean to you?"* and inviting them to take up a corresponding body posture.

38.4 Re-experiencing a Situation that was Free of Shame

We can also suggest to our clients to remember a situation in which they felt proud, dignified or confident. By recalling this experience and letting it take effect on them, they can relive the pride, self-respect or dignity. As so often, this experience can be intensified by their consciously becoming aware of the body sensations they feel. Usually their body posture changes; they straighten up, lift their head or stretch themselves. A word, an inner image or a symbol that reflects this experience can further strengthen it and later serve as an anchor to reactivate it and to find their way out of a state of shame.

38.5 Grounding Oneself, Conscious Breathing and Movement

If our clients feel shame, they can counteract it by, for example, grounding and feeling the ground under their feet, moving, stretching and orienting themselves to the outside. Noticing a body part that feels neutral or pleasant can be supportive, too, as well as the idea of having someone or something with them that stands reassuringly by them.

38.6 Shame and Younger Inner Parts

Frequently, it is younger parts in us that make us feel shame. Therefore it is useful to explore with our clients whether they feel younger or smaller when they experience shame. If this is the case, we can investigate together what the younger part needs and what could be helpful for it to feel safe and accepted. Commonly it is, for instance, to be seen and to be assured that they are okay and loved. After we have discussed from whom the younger part should get attention, affection or assurance, we can invite our clients to an appropriate imagery. When they allow this imagining and notice the feelings and body sensations that arise, the feeling of shame usually subsides.

Example from practice

Lisa, 34, experiences strong feelings of shame as soon as someone criticizes her in an unfriendly or condescending way or makes an accusation. She then collapses into herself, feels guilty, ashamed and would most like to disappear or dissolve. Through exploring her feelings of shame, Lisa is able to recognize that it is the small and younger Lisa who reacts with shame; in her childhood and youth she was humiliated, condemned and insulted countless times by her parents in front of others. As punishment she often only got bread and water to eat and was locked up for hours. She imagines a kind fatherly figure giving comfort and security to the little Lisa and reassuring and encouraging her. Lisa gradually perceives peace and strength that she feels as warmth in her belly. ◄

References

Briere JN (1992) Child abuse trauma. Theory and treatment of the lasting effects. Sage, Newbury Park

Brown B (2020) Definitions. https://brenebrown.com/definitions/. Accessed 7 September 2020

Levin RJ, van Berlo W (2004) Sexual arousal and orgasm in subjects who experience forced or non-consensual sexual stimulation—a review. J Clin Forensic Med 11:82–88

Levine PA (2017) Scham und Stolz. Seminar, 12.–15.08.2017. Weggis, CH. Cited in: Zanotta S (2018) Wieder ganz werden. Traumaheilung mit Ego-State-Therapie und Körperwissen. Carl Auer, Heidelberg (Cited in: Somatic Ego State Therapy™ for Trauma Healing: Whole again. 2024, Routledge, New York)

Levine PA (2019) Polyvagal-Theorie und Trauma. In: Porges SW, Dana D (Hrg) Klinische Anwendungen der Polyvagal-Theorie. Ein neues Verständnis des Autonomen Nervensystems und seiner Anwendung in der therapeutischen Praxis. G. P. Probst, Lichtenau/Westfalen, pp 19–42 (Polyvagal Theory and Trauma. In: Porges SW, Dana D (Eds) Clinical Applications of The Polyvagal Theory. The Emergence of Polyvagal-Informed Therapies. 2018, W.W. Norton, New York, pp 3-26) Quoted from original English version (p 16)

Zanotta S (2018) Wieder ganz werden. Traumaheilung mit Ego-State-Therapie und Körperwissen. Carl Auer, Heidelberg (Somatic Ego State Therapy™ for Trauma Healing: Whole again. 2024, Routledge, New York)

Understanding and Replacing Self-Harming Behavior

39

Contents

Self-harming or self-destructive behavior is usually based on profound traumatic experiences in childhood and/or adolescence; in particular through physical, sexual and/or psychological violence and neglect.

On one side, we can understand it as an expression of fight and flight impulses that are triggered by the activated memories (Fisher 2019). Our clients flee, for example, by taking drugs or having unprotected sex with different partners. Or they fight by inflicting injuries on themselves or, e.g. by driving dangerously. On the other side, we can see the self-destructive behavior as an attempt to reduce inner tension, to free oneself from unbearable feelings such as shame or guilt, to stop intrusive thoughts or flashbacks or to feel oneself again. In this sense, it serves to "regain self-control in the storm of thoughts and feelings" (Sachsse 2011, p. 87). Furthermore, self-harming can also be a form of self-punishment or an appeal to the environment. Sometimes they also reflect the need to be special or invulnerable.

In all this, self-harming behavior is usually an expression of a wounded younger part; so often self-harm is triggered "by the distress of younger parts associated with the experience of traumatic attachment" (Fisher 2019, p. 176).

Example from practice

Christine, 49, was severely neglected, denigrated and repeatedly humiliated by her parents in her childhood. If someone treats her condescendingly or deprecatingly and confronts her in a hostile and disrespectful manner, this triggers a flood of feelings and thoughts in Christine that overwhelm her; she then fears

R. Lackner, *Stabilization in Trauma Treatment*,
https://doi.org/10.1007/978-3-662-67480-2_39

she will be destroyed and feels worthless, unloved and abandoned. This leads to great despair and pain and at the same time rage and hatred. She tries to stop or end all this, among other things, by scratching herself until she bleeds, pulling out her hair and/or stubbing out cigarettes on her body. ◄

In order for our clients to be able to deal better with their self-harming impulses and not to feel so at the mercy of them, it is important to explore the triggers and get to the source of them.

Exploring the triggers

Exploring the triggers allows our clients to recognize why and how the impulse to self-harm arises. By exploring the respective situations in more detail or investigating the response they cause in our clients and by asking whether it is their younger parts reacting, the self-harming behavior usually becomes understandable and plausible. It can be supportive if our clients keep a log or diary for a while in which they write down the respective circumstances and the type of self-harm. By doing this, the triggers or occasions for their self-harming behavior can be easily recognized. For example, it can show that it is a high inner tension, a deep inner injury or an unbearable inner emptiness that leads to our clients harming themselves. And that it is a younger inner part that is incredibly angry or sad or feels abandoned. Depending on the underlying theme, we should then recommend interventions and exercises that they can use in those moments, for instance, to calm or comfort themselves or their inner parts. We can then draw on all the interventions and exercises discussed so far: If inner tensions are the triggers, exercises and interventions from chap. 26 are recommended, for rage those from chap. 35 and for dissociative states those from chap. 27. For flashbacks those from chap. 29 and for fear or panic those from chaps. 31 or 32 are helpful. For intrusive and ruminating thoughts the interventions from chap. 30 and for feelings of guilt those from chap. 37 are suitable.

References

Fisher J (2019) Die Arbeit mit Selbstanteilen in der Traumatherapie. Junfermann, Paderborn (Healing the Fragmented Selves of Trauma Survivors. Overcoming Internal Self-Alienation. 2017, Routledge, New York) Quoted from original English version (p 141)

Sachsse U (2011) Selbstverletzendes Verhalten. In: Sachsse U (Hg) Traumazentrierte Psychotherapie. Theorie, Klinik und Praxis. Schattauer, Stuttgart, pp 80–91

Understanding and Changing Suicidal Thoughts

40

Contents

When our clients tell us about suicidal thoughts or attempts, we sometimes think that they want to die as a "whole being" (Fisher 2019, p. 173). However, suicidal thoughts and attempts usually "reflect the point of view or impulse of one part but not necessarily all" (ibid.). Often they are not an expression of the desire to die, but rather of the desire not to have to continue living as up to the present moment or of the thought and feeling of not being able to continue living like this.

That is why it is important to find out with our clients which part or parts do not want to continue living. In order to do this, the following questions can be helpful: *"If there is a part in you that does not want to continue living and if it would tell us something, what would it say?"* and *"And are there any other parts besides this one that want to live? ... Sometimes the part that wants to live is very quiet, withdrawn or holding back."* This can show, for example, that one part is very wounded and can no longer bear its pain and therefore does not want to live anymore. In addition, it can be that another part is trying to protect the wounded one from further disappointments and wounds and allows suicidal thoughts (Fisher 2019). Or it can be that one part feels incredibly exhausted and powerless and does not want to and cannot live anymore; and another part is protecting it by seeing suicide as an escape. By asking differentiated questions and exploring, we can better understand the reasons for the suicidal thoughts and attempts. These can include deep grief, unbearable pain, not being seen, deep loneliness or a feeling of hopelessness. Based on this, we can find out with our clients what the respective parts need, what would be good for them and help them. Accordingly, we should then suggest interventions and exercises that we have discussed, for example, in

R. Lackner, *Stabilization in Trauma Treatment*,
https://doi.org/10.1007/978-3-662-67480-2_40

chap. 23 Feeling safe and protected, in chap. 28 Feeling the body (again) or in chap. 31 Reducing and overcoming fear and anxiety.

In addition, we should support and strengthen those parts that want to continue living, by paying attention to what they need (Reddemann 2011). In order to empower them, suitable exercises are those that we discussed in chap. 22 Exploring, activating, strengthening and expanding resources and in chap. 24 Gaining inner strength, or those that we will discuss in chap. 41 Doing something good for oneself.

References

Fisher J (2019) Die Arbeit mit Selbstanteilen in der Traumatherapie. Junfermann, Paderborn (Healing the Fragmented Selves of Trauma Survivors. Overcoming Internal Self-Alienation. 2017, Routledge, New York) Quoted from original English version (p 138)

Reddemann L (2011) Psychodynamische Imaginative Traumatherapie PITT – Das Manual. Klett-Cotta, Stuttgart

Doing Something Good for Oneself

41

Contents

In conclusion I would like to mention a few further exercises that can be beneficial to our clients. Just as I round off the book with something positive, we should end each session with our clients with something positive; be it a centering grounding exercise, a short strengthening inner imaging or the conscious noticing and allowing oneself to be affected by a new insight or inner strength. I usually give my clients one or the other encouraging suggestion to take away; for example, to repeatedly be aware of a strengthening thought, to collect pleasant moments in everyday life or to do something good for themselves.

Making a wonderful day

Many of our clients benefit from making a very special, beautiful day on which they only do what brings them joy and well-being, on which they follow their interests and needs and let themselves be pampered (Bannink 2014). Just the fact that we recommend this and encourage them to do so touches many deeply; they feel recognized and accepted on a deep level and experience that they are worth it to do nice things for themselves. An evening or a few hours that our clients design according to their needs are just as precious, if a whole day would overwhelm them or is not possible for them in terms of time.

Being connected to earth and sky

Sitting or standing, we imagine being connected to the earth as well as to the sky. Everything that does us good flows to us from both of them. We can, e.g. allow the idea that a beam of light or similar runs along our spine, which reaches the sky

R. Lackner, *Stabilization in Trauma Treatment*,
https://doi.org/10.1007/978-3-662-67480-2_41

through our crown and as an extension of our coccyx into the earth. From the sky we receive, e.g. confidence and lightness and from the earth strength and peace.

Being connected to a star
While sitting we become aware of the contact with the ground and imagine that a beam of light or similar runs along our spine to our crown, from there to the sky and to our very personal star; this lets us receive everything that does us good, strengthens us, calms us, gives us confidence or security and connectedness (Lyon 1990).

Asking what others like and appreciate about us
For some of our clients it is very supportive and reinforcing getting positive feedback from people who are close and precious to them telling them what they appreciate and like about them. It is useful if our clients write down the feedback in their resource book so that they can always refer to it, draw on it, read it and let it take effect on them. This is particularly helpful in those moments when they are sad, depressed or desperate, or feel lost and worthless.

Swinging back and forth on the back
We lie on our back, bend our knees, pull our thighs towards us so that they touch our stomach; our knees are now close to our chest. We hug our bent knees with our arms and pull them even closer to our upper body. We try to relax our body as much as possible. Then we swing or roll alternately to the right and to the left (Lachner 2010). This usually has a calming, comforting effect.

Connected to our ancestors
Some of our clients find it very strengthening to imagine that their ancestors are standing behind them giving them strength and love, and support and empower them.

Stimulating the Vagus nerve—the Half-Salamander Exercise
With the head up, facing forward, we let our eyes wander to the right, our head remains facing forward. Then we tilt our head to the right, so that our right ear is near to our right shoulder. We continue to look to the right. We hold this position for 30-60 s. Then we straighten our head and look straight ahead. Now we let our eyes wander to the left. Then we tilt our head to the left, so that our left ear is near to our left shoulder. We hold this position for 30-60 s. Then we straighten our head again and look straight ahead. With this exercise from Stanley Rosenberg (2017) we improve our breathing; this signals to our brain that we are safe and in turn stimulates the ventral vagus branch and thus our parasympathetic nervous system.

Giving oneself emotional security
We hug ourselves by clamping our hands under our armpits or placing them on our chest. We spread our thumbs away from our palms and place them on our upper chest area just below our collarbone (fig. 41.1). We hold this position for

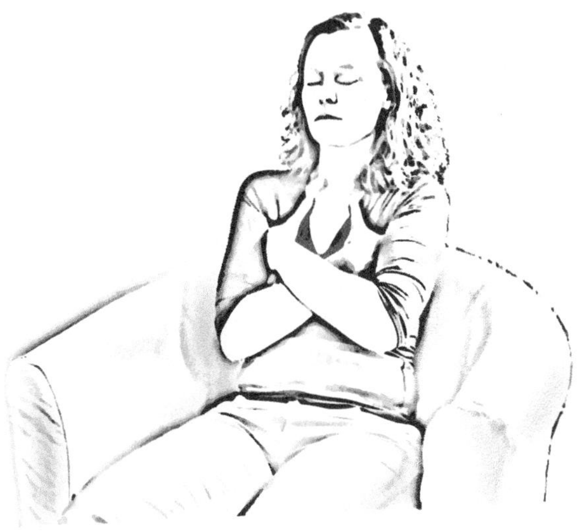

Fig. 41.1 Healing stream—giving oneself security

10-20 minutes. According to the teachings of Jin Shin Jyutsu or healing stream, it gives us security, support and comfort (Url 2019).

Gratitude

If it is appropriate for our clients, it can be very supportive for them to consciously make themselves aware of what they are grateful for every day. These can be very small things, like a flower blooming on the side of the road or an encounter with someone at a supermarket checkout, or big ones, like a success, a talent given to them, or a great love. According to Positive Psychology, gratitude is one of the most effective tools to strengthen our well-being (Seligman 2012).

Conclusion

Many more stabilizing and strengthening exercises and interventions could be added. The possibilities of stabilizing, empowering and strengthening our clients in their autonomy are unlimited. So with this book I also want to encourage you to find further possibilities, maybe in your own way that can be helpful for your clients.

All the best in doing so and in accompanying your clients.

References

Bannink F (2014) Post traumatic success. Positive psychology & solution-focused strategies to help clients survive & thrive. W.W. Norton, New York

Lachner A (2010) Yoga. Continuing class. Buddhist Center, Vienna, AT

Lyon U (1990) Yoga and meditation. Continuing class. Buddhist Center, Vienna, AT

Rosenberg S (2017) Accessing the healing power of the vagus nerve. Self-help exercises for anxiety, depression, trauma, and autism. North Atlantic Books, Berkley

Seligman M (2012) Flourish. Wie Menschen aufblühen. Die Positive Psychologie des gelingenden Lebens. Kösel, München (Flourish. A Visionary New Understanding of Happiness and Well-Being. 2011, Free Press, New York)

Url W (2019) Impulsströmen (Healing Stream). Training. Advanced 1. Europäisches Forum für Impulsströmen, Niederkreuzstetten/AT

Acknowledgements

This book owes its existence to many people.

First of all to all the people who have entrusted themselves to me, who let me participate in their story and whom I have been allowed to accompany. From them I have learned so much about trauma, traumatization and overcoming it. They inspire and enrich me and let me repeatedly recognize even more of what can be stabilizing, strengthening and healing.

To all those people from whom I was allowed to learn in the context of my training and further education, who supported and promoted me and who have had a profound impact on my professional path. Above all Richard Gelles, at whose Family Violence Research Program at the University of Rhode Island, USA, I was allowed to be a Research Fellow for one year and from whom I learned, among other things, to question and work on topics thoroughly. Eli Newberger from the Children Hospital in Boston, USA, at whose department I was a guest this year and from whom I learned so much about the dynamics and diagnostics of sexual abuse of children. Beate Wimmer-Puchinger from the Ludwig Boltzmann Institute for Women's Health Research, Vienna, Austria, who supported me as a young scientist and enabled me to carry out some projects that were close to my heart, and who was my dissertation advisor. Brigitte Lueger-Schuster from the University of Vienna, who invited me to work on a book project on children and trauma, from which the series *Wie Pippa wieder lachen lernte*[1] arose, and through which I came to Hemayat, an association for survivors of war and torture. Ulrich Sachsse, at whose Trauma Department of the LKH Göttingen, Germany, I was allowed to be a guest psychologist for 2 months and could expand my training in Guided Affected Imagery and who gave me the important advice to do a training in EMDR. Laurence Heller, with whom I completed my first module in Somatic Experiencing® and who has greatly deepened and expanded my understanding of trauma and traumatization. All the participants of the Trauma Curriculum of the Austrian Academy of Psychology where I give trainings, through whose questions and positive feedback the idea for this book came about.

[1]Published by Springer-Verlag in 2005.

R. Lackner, *Stabilization in Trauma Treatment*,
https://doi.org/10.1007/978-3-662-67480-2

Ilse Ositha Behensky, my long-term supervisor and therapist, who accompanied me in processing my own traumatic experiences and immediately heartily reinforced my idea for this book. Gabriele Maria Steiner, who always supported me with advice and encouraged me to write the book, and who repeatedly backed me up with many positive feedbacks.

Daniela Pucher, who accompanied me while writing; helped me to develop a clear concept with her questions, gave me many hints for better readability and always encouraged me anew with her positive feedback. Kerstin Barton and Renate Eichhorn from the Springer-Verlag, who liked the idea of the book right away, had confidence in me, supported me with questions and gave me enough time with a lot of patience. Sieglinde Pohle for the proofreading and Felix Loerch for the support in the last steps before printing and publication. Gerhard Vay for the graphic design and Elisabeth Bolius for the photos the drawings are based on.

My thanks go to all the people who are dear and close to me and who have supported me in the writing of this book and backed me up. My sister Katharina Lackner for her support and suggestions. And above all my son Paul, who experienced the ups and downs first hand during the writing, met them with a lot of lightness and humor and always encouraged and nudged me to complete it.

My parents, Gerda and Hans Lackner, who gave me so much on my way, which also flows into this book. And my spiritual companions. In gratitude.

The manufacturer's authorised representative in the EU is Springer Nature Customer Service Centre GmbH, Europaplatz 3, 69115 Heidelberg, Germany. If you have any concerns regarding our products, please contact ProductSafety@springernature.com

Printed and bound by CPI Group (UK) Ltd, Croydon, CR0 4YY
28/04/2026
02098519-0001